Rheumatology and Ophthalmology

Rheumatologists routinely express a desire for a better understanding of ophthalmology to enhance their care of patients whose rheumatologic diseases manifest with ophthalmic complications. Ophthalmologists feel the same, seeking to understand the systemic impacts that autoimmune diseases have for their patients. As part of the Interdisciplinary Rheumatology book series, *Interdisciplinary Rheumatology: Rheumatology and Ophthalmology* is a dialogue between expert rheumatologists and ophthalmologists that provides readers with the skills to diagnose and manage a range of inflammatory eye conditions in patients with both systemic rheumatic and ocular-limited disease. With knowledge from this book, rheumatologists and ophthalmologists will be better able to collaborate effectively in the care of these complex patients.

Dr. Laura J. Kopplin is Associate Professor of Ophthalmology at the University of Wisconsin-Madison School of Medicine and Public Health. She completed a fellowship in uveitis and ocular immunology at the Casey Eye Institute – Oregon Health & Science University and the Devers Eye Institute in Portland, Oregon. Her research interests include epidemiology and risk factors for inflammatory eye diseases, clinical trials of uveitis therapeutics, biomarkers for uveitis outcomes, and clinical management of ocular inflammatory disease. She is the subcommittee chair of the American Academy of Ophthalmology Preferred Practice Pattern – Uveitis Panel. She is also the co-host of *Headlight in the Fog: The Uveitis Podcast*.

Dr. Joanne Valeriano-Marcet is Professor of Medicine at the University of South Florida in Tampa, Florida. She completed her fellowship in rheumatology at Mount Sinai Medical Center. Her awards have included the Parker J. Palmer "Courage to Teach" Award for Program Director Excellence from the ACGME and the Outstanding GME Program Director Award from USF, and she has been named among the Best Doctors in America. She has published widely and served on the ACGME Working Group to develop Rheumatology Milestones 2.0.

Interdisciplinary Rheumatology Series

Edited by Jason Liebowitz and Philip Seo

Rheumatology and Cardiology
Edited by Vaneet K. Sandhu

Rheumatology and Nephrology
Edited by Karina D. Torralba, Duvuru Geetha, and Anisha B. Dua

Rheumatology and Pulmonology
Edited by Marcy B. Bolster and Kristin B. Highland

Rheumatology and Ophthalmology
Edited by Laura J. Kopplin and Joanne Valeriano-Marcet

To access more books in the Interdisciplinary Rheumatology Series, visit:
https://www.routledge.com/Interdisciplinary-Rheumatology/book-series/IRJL

Rheumatology and Ophthalmology

INTERDISCIPLINARY RHEUMATOLOGY

Edited by

Laura J. Kopplin, MD, PhD
Joanne Valeriano-Marcet, MD

CRC Press
Taylor & Francis Group
Boca Raton London New York

CRC Press is an imprint of the
Taylor & Francis Group, an **informa** business

First edition published 2026
by CRC Press
2385 NW Executive Center Drive, Suite 320, Boca Raton, FL 33431

and by CRC Press
4 Park Square, Milton Park, Abingdon, Oxon, OX14 4RN

CRC Press is an imprint of Taylor & Francis Group, LLC

Library of Congress Cataloging-in-Publication Data
Names: Kopplin, Laura J., editor. | Valeriano-Marcet, Joanne, editor.
Title: Interdisciplinary rheumatology. Rheumatology and ophthalmology / edited by Laura J. Kopplin and
    Joanne Valeriano-Marcet.
Other titles: Rheumatology and ophthalmology
Description: First edition. | Boca Raton, FL : CRC Press, 2025. | Includes bibliographical references and index. |
    Summary: "Ask rheumatologists what one thing that they most desire is and they will say: I wish I knew more about ophthalmology so I could care for patients whose rheumatologic diseases manifest with ophthalmic complications. Ophthalmologists feel just the same, seeking to understand the implications that autoimmune diseases have for their patients. As part of the Interdisciplinary Rheumatology book series, this book is a dialogue between rheumatologists and ophthalmologists providing a masterclass from world-renowned experts. Led by a team of international editors with in-depth knowledge and cutting-edge research on topics like vasculitis and systemic lupus erythematous, among others. Key Features: 1. Provides a clinical approach to the patient with ophthalmic manifestations of rheumatic disease. 2. Details cutting-edge research with inputs from the world's leading experts, for both ophthalmologists and rheumatologists. 3. Discusses possible future directions for research and advancement."— Provided by publisher.
Identifiers: LCCN 2024061347 (print) | LCCN 2024061348 (ebook) | ISBN 9781032592367 (hardback) |
    ISBN 9781032592312 (paperback) | ISBN 9781003453710 (ebook)
Subjects: MESH: Eye Diseases—etiology | Autoimmune Diseases—complications |
    Rheumatic Diseases—complications | Eye Diseases—immunology
Classification: LCC RC927 (print) | LCC RC927 (ebook) | NLM WW 140 | DDC 616.723—dc23/eng/20250306
LC record available at https://lccn.loc.gov/2024061347
LC ebook record available at https://lccn.loc.gov/2024061348

ISBN: 978-1-032-59236-7 (hbk)
ISBN: 978-1-032-59231-2 (pbk)
ISBN: 978-1-003-45371-0 (ebk)

DOI: 10.1201/9781003453710

Typeset in Palatino
by Apex CoVantage, LLC

To my loved ones and friends – thank you for the support and distractions that helped me finish this project with a smile. To team Uveitis – you've got flare and a permanent place in my heart. And most especially to my daughter, Amelie – you are my everything.

– Laura J. Kopplin

To my dear parents – thank you for guiding me along life's journey. To my beloved family – thank you for the joy and balance you bring to my life.

– Joanne Valeriano-Marcet

Contents

Preface

Interdisciplinary Rheumatology: Rheumatology and Ophthalmology is one book in a series examining the specific organ manifestations of a range of rheumatic diseases through the perspectives of both rheumatologists and their interdisciplinary partners.

In this book, we explore the unique aspects of the eye in autoimmune diseases. The first chapters lay the foundation for understanding the basic physiology and pathophysiology of the eye as well as the general approach to the diagnosis of ocular complications in rheumatic diseases. Subsequent chapters examine the specific ocular manifestations of a spectrum of rheumatic diseases, their management, and highlight the important interplay between the two disciplines in diagnosis and treatment. The final chapters review ocular inflammation in patients without associated rheumatologic conditions and in the pediatric population. The book provides both rheumatologists and ophthalmologists with a deeper understanding of these complex diseases and their ocular complications viewed through the lens of experts from both disciplines. We are grateful to our authors, who united across fields to share their knowledge and make this challenging topic accessible.

Laura J. Kopplin
Joanne Valeriano-Marcet

Acknowledgments

We are especially grateful for the opportunity to work with our dedicated authors and colleagues from around the world. The collaborative effort to integrate the ophthalmologic and rheumatologic perspectives into a comprehensive and cohesive text was as seamless as we hope the care of patients with these conditions should be. A special thank you to Jason Liebowitz and Philip Seo for spearheading this book series and for inviting us to be co-editors. Your mission of enhancing interdisciplinary care is a cause both of us share as a passion. A final thanks to the patients we have cared for, learned from and who inspire us to continue making advances in the evaluation and management of these complex disorders.

Contributors

Esen Akpek, MD
Wilmer Eye Institute
Johns Hopkins University School of Medicine
Baltimore, MD

Karen R. Armbrust, MD, PhD
Department of Ophthalmology and Visual
    Neurosciences
University of Minnesota
and
Department of Ophthalmology
Veterans Affairs Health Care System
Minneapolis, MN

Noor Bazerbashi, MD
Department of Medicine, Rheumatology
Morsani College of Medicine
University of South Florida
Tampa, FL

Meghan Berkenstock, MD
Wilmer Eye Institute
Johns Hopkins School of Medicine
Baltimore, MD

Sean T. Berkowitz, MD, MBA
Vanderbilt Eye Institute
Vanderbilt University Medical Center
Nashville, TN

Lorenzo E. Bosque, MD
Drexel University College of Medicine
Philadelphia, PA

Tina Brar, MD
Department of Medicine, Rheumatology
University of South Florida
Veterans Affairs Tampa Health Care System
Tampa, FL

Justine Cheng, MD
Casey Eye Institute
Department of Ophthalmology
Oregon Health and Science University
Portland, OR

Eric Crowell, MD, MPH
Mitchel & Shannon Wong Eye Institute and
    Ascension Seton Medical Center
The University of Texas Dell Medical School
Austin, TX

Rebka Ephrem, MD
Perelman School of Medicine
University of Pennsylvania
Philadelphia, PA

Anna Flts, MD
Rowan-Virtua School of Osteopathic
    Medicine
Stratford, NJ

Christina Flaxel, MD
Casey Eye Institute
Department of Ophthalmology
Oregon Health and Science University
Portland, OR

Sapna Gangaputra, MD, MPH
Vanderbilt Eye Institute
Vanderbilt University Medical Center
Nashville, TN

Shivani Garg, MD, PhD
Department of Medicine
Division of Rheumatology
University of Wisconsin
School of Medicine and Public Health
Madison, WI

Debra A. Goldstein, MD
Department of Ophthalmology
Northwestern University Feinberg
    School of Medicine
Chicago, IL

John Gonzalez, MD
Department of Ophthalmology
University of California San Francisco
San Francisco, CA

Thomas Grader-Beck, MD
Wilmer Eye Institute
Johns Hopkins University School of Medicine
Baltimore, MD

Rachel Guess, MD
Division of Rheumatology/Immunology
Department of Pediatrics
Washington University
St. Louis, MO

Rajiv Gupta, MBBS, MS
Department of Ophthalmology and
    Visual Sciences
Manipal University
Malaysia

Rula A. Hajj-Ali, MD
Department of Rheumatology
Cleveland Clinic
Cleveland, OH

Lynn M. Hassman, MD, PhD
Department of Ophthalmology
University of Colorado
Denver, CO

Lynn E. Harman, MD
Department of Ophthalmology
Morsani College of Medicine
University of South Florida
Tampa, FL

Lingling Huang, MD, PhD
Shiley Eye Institute
Department of Ophthalmology
University of California San Diego
San Diego, CA

Prarthana Jain, DO, MPH
Rheumatology, Allergy & Immunology
University of North Carolina at Chapel Hill
Chapel Hill, NC

Timothy M. Janetos, MD, MBA
Department of Ophthalmology
Northwestern University Feinberg
    School of Medicine
Chicago, IL

Beth L. Jonas, MD, FACR
Rheumatology, Allergy & Immunology
University of North Carolina at Chapel Hill
Chapel Hill, NC

Maleewan Kitcharoensakkul, MD
Division of Rheumatology/Immunology
Department of Pediatrics
Washington University
St. Louis, MO

Taylor L. Koenig, MD
Department of Rheumatology
Cleveland Clinic
Cleveland, OH

Jason Kolfenbach, MD
Division of Rheumatology
University of Colorado
Denver, CO

Kara C. LaMattina, MD
Department of Ophthalmology
Boston Medical Center
Boston, MA

Grace A. Levy-Clarke, MD
WVU Eye Institute
Department of Ophthalmology and
    Visual Sciences
West Virginia University
School of Medicine
Morgantown, WV

Norberto Mancera, MD
Florida Eye Specialists and Cataract
    Institute
Brandon, FL

Curtis E. Margo, MD
Department of Pathology and
    Cell Biology
Department of Ophthalmology
Morsani College of Medicine
University of South Florida
Tampa, FL

George Mount, MD, MHPE
Division of Rheumatology
University of Washington
School of Medicine
Seattle, WA

Veena Patel, MD
Rheumatology Department
Ascension Seton Medical Center
The University of Texas Health
Austin, TX

Cassidy Pinion, MS, CCRA
WVU Eye Institute
Department of Ophthalmology and
    Visual Sciences
West Virginia University
School of Medicine
Morgantown, WV

Amy E. Pohodich, MD
Casey Eye Institute
Department of Ophthalmology
Oregon Health and Science University
Portland, OR

Julia A. Pulliam, OD, FAAO
Department of Ophthalmology and
    Visual Sciences
Washington University School
    of Medicine
St. Louis, MO

Amit Reddy, MD
Department of Ophthalmology
University of Colorado
Denver, CO

Rennie L. Rhee, MD
Division of Rheumatology
University of Pennsylvania
Philadelphia, PA

Christopher R. Rosenberg, MD
Casey Eye Institute
Department of Ophthalmology
Oregon Health and Science University
Portland, OR

Saitiel Sandoval Gonzalez, MD
Stein Eye Institute
Department of Ophthalmology
David Geffen School of Medicine at UCLA
Los Angeles, CA

Jason Michael Springer, MD, MS
Department of Medicine
Division of Rheumatology and Immunology
Vanderbilt University Medical Center
Nashville, TN

Eric Suhler, MD, MPH
Casey Eye Institute
Department of Ophthalmology
Oregon Health and Science University
Portland, OR

Kirby Taylor MD, MS
Mitchel & Shannon Wong Eye Institute
    and Ascension Seton Medical Center
The University of Texas Dell Medical School
Austin, TX

Akshay Thomas, MD, MS
Tennessee Retina
Nashville, TN

Edmund Tsui, MD
Stein Eye Institute
Department of Ophthalmology
David Geffen School of Medicine
    at UCLA
Los Angeles, CA

Ilknur Tugal-Tutkun, MD
Eye Protection Foundation Bayrampasa
    Eye Hospital
and
Istanbul University
Istanbul Faculty of Medicine
Department of Ophthalmology
Istanbul, Turkey

Zachary S. Wallace, MD
Division of Rheumatology, Allergy, and
    Immunology
Massachusetts General Hospital and
    Harvard Medical School
Boston, MA

Kimberly M. Winges, MD
Department of Ophthalmology
Veterans Administration Portland
    Health Care System
Portland, OR

Yusuf Yazici, MD
NYU Grossman School of Medicine
New York, NY

1 General Overview of the Eye in Health and in Autoimmune Disease

Curtis E. Margo, Lynn E. Harman, and Grace A. Levy-Clarke

1.1 INTRODUCTION

The eye bears a considerable measure of injury from autoimmune disease, particularly the corneal-scleral tunic and the uveal tract. This immunological susceptibility may at first seem paradoxical, since the eye has been viewed for over 70 years as the prototypical organ of immune tolerance. Then again, the idea of immune tolerance appears at variance with the observation that sympathetic ophthalmia and phacoantigenic uveitis were two of the earliest examples of autoimmune disease. Since observational contradictions such as these are what feeds scientific curiosity, one can understand why the eye is seen as immunologically fascinating.

Various organs and tissues of the body are now known to invoke different immune responses to the same or similar stimuli, a phenomenon loosely referred to as *regional immunity*. Any phase of the immune arc (i.e., afferent, processing, or efferent) can be influenced by regional factors. The eye, however, cannot be seen as a single organ or tissue in this regard. Researchers have identified five different immunologic microenvironments within the eye: (1) conjunctiva; (2) anterior segment (i.e., anterior chamber, iris, ciliary body, and vitreous); (3) cornea and sclera; (4) retinal pigment epithelium (RPE) and choriocapillaris; (5) and choroid. In terms of differences in immune function, these anatomic territories vary from subtle to profound.

Before reviewing the anatomic and physiologic features of the eye relevant to the innate and adaptive immune systems, the historical foundations for understanding the panuveitic inflammatory disorder of sympathetic ophthalmia as an autoimmune disease is presented. The unique interaction of the systemic immune system and the eye is put on display when sympathetic ophthalmia is viewed from the perspective as an organ-limited autoimmune disease.

1.2 HISTORICAL BACKDROP FOR OCULAR AUTOIMMUNITY

The idea of autoimmunity was downplayed if not outright rejected during the early decades of the 20th century due in large part to the influence of Paul Ehrlich (1854–1915), who believed the existence of autoantibodies was incompatible with life. Much of his prestige as a biologist was tied to creating the side-chain theory of antibody production, which eventually matured into the clonal selection theory of antibody specificity. Some claim his groundbreaking perception marked the beginning of modern immunology. When Ehrlich expressed the implausibility of self-antibodies with the term *horror autotoxicus*, a disparaging label describing the dreadful outcome if autotoxins were to exist, the warning was taken seriously and the subject only tepidly debated.[1] Ehrlich's reasoning was sound, based on animal studies, the new science of blood typing, and the recently developed complement fixation assay. Experiments he performed with Julius Morganroth (1871–1924) showed that animals reacted to blood from other members of their species, developing isoantibodies, but not to their own red cells. These results reinforced in Ehrlich's mind that any type of autoantibody was incompatible with survival. His denunciation of the possibility of autoimmune disease came just a year before Paul Uhlenhuth (1870–1957) reported autoantibodies directed against the crystallin lens in 1903 and 8 years before Anton Elschnig (1863–1939) provided evidence that an intrinsic substance coming from an injured eye (a supposed intraocular molecule) could cause inflammation in the normal opposite eye.[2]

The condition Elschnig was studying was *sympathetic ophthalmia*, a clinical syndrome well known to learned eye physicians at the time. The disorder was first described in medically sophisticated detail by William Mackenzie (1791–1868) in 1840.[3] The characteristic histopathology of sympathetic ophthalmia as bilateral granulomatous uveitis was later documented in 1905 by Ernst Fuchs (1851–1930). In a series of prescient studies in 1910, Elschnig argued that injury of one eye can induce an "anaphylactic" reaction in both the traumatized eye and healthy eye, a pathway that essentially defines the general concept of an autoimmune process. These early insights into the nature of non-infectious ocular inflammation remained a curiosity until mid-century, when several landmark discoveries gave birth to another novel concept called *immune tolerance*. Investigators in the 1940s returned to the eye to study why experimental allogenic skin grafts survived so well in the ocular milieu of the anterior segment.[4] Part of the answer lay in the yet-to-be-discovered fact that much of the eye is sequestered from the systemic immune system early in embryologic development. It is as if the eye was foreign to the immune system that was created to protect it. The biologic compromise seemed understandable. The eye could exist in harmony with the apparatus of systemic immune

DOI: 10.1201/9781003453710-1

surveillance as long as its internal contents remained isolated. Under such circumstances, the eye would be more susceptible to intraocular infection, but that was the biological trade-off.

1.3 RELEVANT OCULAR ANATOMY

From a teleologic vantage point, it is easy to appreciate why the eye would develop a vigorous means of preventing infection and limiting inflammation in order to preserve vision. Even a mild infection or inflammatory reaction could result in detrimental loss of visual function. Since vision confers obvious survival advantage, the eye appears to have evolved as an immune-favored organ, although the definition of *immunologic privilege* has varied over time. The eye is anatomically delimited by its outer corneal-scleral tunic, but the conjunctiva that covers the sclera and attaches tightly to the cornea at the limbus contributes substantially to its immunologic protection.[5]

The conjunctiva is vascular and contains lymphatic channels that function in the passage of cells in the afferent and efferent immune response. The tear film that washes the epithelial surfaces of the eye contains lysozyme, an enzyme able to destroy bacterial cell walls; lactoferrin, an iron-binding protein that has bacteriostatic properties; and immunoglobulins that can serve to neutralize bacteria and viruses by forming immune complexes that augment opsonization and/or promote chemotaxis. A resident population of inflammatory cells in the conjunctiva consists of both B and T lymphocytes, scattered mast cells, and dendritic cells (both Langerhans and non-Langerhans).[6] The density of these cells varies by region, but the vast majority are found in the substantia propria, or loose connective tissue between the epithelium and sclera. Lymphoid follicles are not normally present, nor are many plasma cells, which tend to reside in accessory lacrimal glands between acinar cells. All antibody isotypes can be found in the tear film, but IgA and subclasses of IgG predominate. Effector molecules like complement and kininogen precursors also exist within the conjunctiva.

The closest regional nodes are preauricular and submandibular. Neither lymphatics nor lymph nodes are found in the orbit. The lymphoid tissue in conjunctival and lacrimal gland are referred to as conjunctival and lacrimal gland–associated lymphoid tissue (CALT), analogous to mucosa-associated lymphoid tissue (MALT) elsewhere in the body.[7] CALT appears to bestow similar immune protection and immune regulatory functions as other mucosal collections of lymphoid tissue in the gut, respiratory tract, and genitourinary system.

Conjunctiva and sclera change abruptly at the limbus in transition to cornea, where goblet cells, lymphatics, and blood vessels suddenly stop. White scleral collagen transforms rapidly to nearly transparent corneal stroma, a so-called porthole to the retina that also acts as a powerful converging lens. The unique features of the anterior segment of the eye were expanded in 1948, when Peter Medawar (1915–1987) showed how favorable the cornea and anterior chamber were in terms of accepting allogenic skin grafts. His studies shifted attention away from the optical properties of the eye to its role in modulating immune responsiveness.[8]

The obvious structural feature of the cornea – its lack of vascular and lymphatic channels – was thought to be a prime contributing factor as to why allogenic transplants were not readily rejected. But the tolerance that the cornea displayed toward transplanted tissue was far more complex. Corneal keratinocytes (epithelial cells), keratocytes (stromal fibroblasts), corneal Langerhans cells, and endothelial cells all display class 1 major histocompatibility complex (MHC) antigens. Corneal Langerhans cells contain class 2 MHC antigens, and other corneal cells can express them when induced.[9] Langerhans cells, dendritic cells, and macrophages all serve as ocular antigen-presenting cells (APCs).

The cornea central to the limbus lacks lymphatics and vascular channels, so macromolecules can enter the cornea only through diffusion. The same applies to immunoglobulins. Langerhans cells present at the limbus are not found centrally. Like the sclera, the central cornea has no APCs. The immune privilege that the cornea possesses is mediated in part by Fas ligand (CD95), under control by cytotoxic T lymphocytes, which stimulate programmed cell death of target cells (i.e., apoptosis). An understanding of the immune-friendly environment of the cornea, initially observed in the 1940s with experimental skin grafts and then later with the high success rate of corneal transplants, had to wait until the basic science of antibody-dependent delayed hypersensitivity was realized decades later.

The remaining parts of the eye differ from the cornea in terms of antigenicity and exposure to the systemic immune system. The lens consists of mostly non-nucleated cells (lens fibers) that are sequestered from the systemic immune system within weeks of conception by a continuous thick basement membrane. Albeit thin at first, this basement membrane (also known as lens capsule) thickens over time. Only an anterior monolayer of lens epithelial cells possesses MHC class 1 antigens. Of the three major crystallin proteins in lens fibers (α, β, and γ), α is the most common.[10] Despite post-natal isolation of lenticular cells from the immune system, antibodies to crystallin lens proteins can be found in the plasma of normal individuals.

The blood–ocular barrier, which is made up of zonula occludens of the pigment epithelial cells and the absence of fenestrations in the retinal blood vessels, prevents large molecules from entering the inner neurosensory layer of the eye. These anatomic features are similar in structure and function to the blood–brain barrier, which is designed to physically impede antigenic exposure to select tissues. For the eye, this includes retina and vitreous. Vessels within the uveal tract (iris, ciliary body, and choroid) are fenestrated, however. Lymphatic channels are not present in the uveal tract, and uveal tissue contains no resident lymphocytes.

Like the cornea, sclera is almost entirely collagen, a hypocellular tissue without an intrinsic vascular bed. Most nutrients that support scleral fibroblasts arrive through diffusion from neighboring vascular networks (i.e., episcleral and uveal tract).

The retina is an extension of the brain with exquisitely sensitive light-detecting photoreceptors known as *rods* and *cones*. It was generally assumed for much of the 20th century that the retina was not patrolled by the immune surveillance system. Rather, it was protected like the brain from the outside world by the blood–retinal barrier.[11] The so-called immune naivety of the retina was inferred from the behavior of the brain when it came to accepting allogenic grafts (i.e., displayed immune tolerance). Immune naivety was further inferred from the observation that the blood–brain barrier protects the central nervous system from direct injury during severe anaphylaxis. These preconceptions changed, however, when it was shown that astrocytes can react to T lymphocytes and that activated T lymphocytes can enter the CNS and mediate inflammatory reactions. The role that glial cells play in reinforcing the blood–ocular barrier in the retina has also expanded. Astrocytes can stimulate contact between vascular endothelial cells, nearly obliterating intercellular spaces and making vessels less permeable.[12] Retinal pigment epithelial (RPE) cells can be induced to express MHC class II molecules, but the absence of normal lymphocytes in this area leaves the question open to functional significance. The RPE expresses the complement regulatory protein CD46 on its basilar surface, suggesting a role in modulating complement activation arising from the choroid.

Elucidation of molecular pathways intrinsic to the eye that promote and modulate immune response and inflammation tends to lag behind revelations from morphology. The tissue proteases of the kallikrein/kinin system, for example, have been found in cells of the retina, ciliary muscle, and trabecular meshwork.[13] These particular serine proteases act on kininogens to yield bradykinins, which have modulating effects on inflammation. Their influence in particular clinical settings is being actively explored.

The optic nerve, which consists of axons of the retinal ganglion cells mixed with neuroglial support cells including oligodendrocytes, is covered by a thick fibrous membrane (meninges) made up of pia mater, arachnoid, and dura mater. The optic nerve, unlike all other cranial nerves, is not a peripheral nerve but a white tract of the brain and is thus susceptible to similar types of immune injury. It will not be discussed further in this chapter.

1.4 INNATE IMMUNE SYSTEM

The innate immune system is a native or "preprogrammed" reaction to extrinsic antigens based on highly conserved receptors within species. The major triggers to the ocular innate immune system are similar to those in other tissues and include such diverse stimuli as the molecular components of bacterial cell walls, exotoxins, and mechanical trauma. Innate immunity provides a means by which neutrophils are rapidly activated, recruited, and deployed to protect tissues. Neutrophils, in turn, activate endothelial cells that rapidly generate other innate immune provocateurs such as selectin, integrins, and immunoglobulin superfamily molecules, which direct neutrophils through small vascular channels to sites of injury. The processes, in general, are stereotypic and have less importance in the pathogenesis of autoimmune disease than acquired immunity, although a variety of cytokines have roles in both innate and acquired immunity. The eye is particularly vulnerable to the uncontrolled fury of the preprogrammed innate immune system. Purulent inflammation and the cytokine storms that develop within eyes after infection or injury can progress rapidly to phthisis bulbi.

1.5 CONCEPT OF OCULAR IMMUNE PRIVILEGE

Tasked with improving the care of burn patients, biologist Peter Medawar became interested in the problems of cutaneous transplant rejection soon after Britain entered World War II. He discovered the inability to successfully graft severely burned patients with skin from healthy donors was related to the proteins on nucleated cells, later called histocompatibility antigens. The one exception to that rule was with identical (maternal) twins. Medawar also assumed that by transplanting skin between animal twins (calves in the case of his experiments), he could distinguish maternal from fraternal twins. To his surprise, neither type of twin rejected skin transplants. Macfarlane Burnet (1899–1985), in 1949, immediately appreciated the implications of these results as showing that "immunologic self" was not intrinsically determined but instead was acquired early during embryological development.[14]

The groundbreaking corollary to the clonal selection theory that Burnet and Medawar helped to establish was known as the "clonal deletion theory," which basically states that self-reactive cell clones are deleted during ontogeny. Though widely accepted by 1960, the theory would need to be tweaked several times to better explain how and why self-reacting antibodies can emerge later in life.[15, 16]

When Rolf Zinkernagel and Peter Doherty discovered that T cells interact with antigens only in the presence of certain MHC self-proteins, it drew a sharp distinction between their function and that of B cells.[17] The interaction between T and B cells took time to decipher, particularly how the phenomenon of MHC restriction was linked to MHC polymorphism.[18, 19] The MHC, both class I and II, is expressed through human leukocyte antigens (HLAs). Class I antigens are found on most cells of the body, but class II are present on lymphocytes and dendritic cells (antigen presenting cells). Correspondingly, cytotoxic T cells recognize class I MHC antigens, while helper T cells recognize class II. Cluster of differentiation (CD) cell surface markers CD4 and CD8 are proteins found on the T cell membrane next to the T cell receptor. The genetic loci that code for HLA antigens, found on chromosome 6, are highly polymorphic. This small but non-lethal variation in genetic code of surface antigens has given scientists a natural tool to study such things as disease association within a population.

Various correlation studies in humans have shown that specific HLA class I and II alleles are associated with a number of disorders, including uveitis syndromes. Some of these associations are particularly strong. Over 90% of persons with birdshot chorioretinopathy, for instance, express HLA-A29. HLA-B27 is associated with anterior uveitis, both idiopathic and syndromic (e.g., ankylosing spondylitis). Single-nucleotide polymorphisms (SNPs) have also been correlated with specific HLA susceptibilities. A SNP of tumor necrosis factor (TNF)-α, for example, has been correlated with increased susceptibility to anterior uveitis in persons who are HLA-B27 positive.[20]

Not long after the functional differences in lymphocytes were discovered, breakthroughs in understanding the regulatory features of soluble factors released during inflammation emerged. These factors were later referred to as *cytokines* and include interleukins (ILs), chemokines, interferons, mesenchymal growth factors, and a family of peptides called tumor necrosis factor (TNF). They function by binding to specific cell surface receptors and differ from hormones by being found in concentrations one thousand times less. After attaching to surface receptors, they trigger a cascade of intracellular events mediated through transcription factors. Shortly after the start of the 21st century, nearly separate genes coding for cytokines had been identified. Knowledge of their roles in protective immunity as well as their harmful effects has accelerated. The majority of cytokines and other soluble mediators that affect the eye in uveitis are derived from the circulation and are not endogenous to the eye (Table 1.1). Perhaps the most thoroughly studied immunomodulating cytokine is IL-6. With its signaling pathway known, the development of biologics that inhibit the pathway have been able to favorably alter the course of autoimmune disease without interfering with the protective role of IL-6. Research into targeted therapies such as this was conducted on systemic disease but is now turning to ocular immune-mediated disorders.

As the study of cytokines was underway, so too was investigation into how naïve T cells interact with T cell receptors and antigens presented by dendritic cells under the influence of key interleukins and growth factors (e.g., IL-12, IL-4, TGF-β, and IL-6). Under appropriate conditions, naïve T cells could transform and proliferate into Th1, Th2, T reg cells, and Th17, which in turn produce their own host of cytokines.[21, 22] Pathways are dependent on sequential or concurrent exposure to specific cytokines (Figure 1.1). For example, naïve CD4 T cells in the presence of IL-1β, IL-6, and TGF-β produced by an antigen-presenting cell will result in Th17 cells. The first assumed pathogenic T lymphocyte was Th1, which was induced through exposure to IL-12 and IFN-γ. The next discovered was Th2, whose induction was influenced by IL-4. Studies in laboratory animals with experimental autoimmune uveitis (EAU) showed that Th2 were less injurious to the eye than Th1. In fact, Th2, under certain circumstances, displayed a suppressor function. Using mostly rodent models of EAU, investigators discovered that Th17 may be the dominant pathogenic effector cell rather than Th1. Under normal circumstances, these same inflammatory pathways that are used to

Table 1.1 Major Cell Source of Cytokines and Other Soluble Peptide Mediators Involved in Ocular Injury*

Resident Intraocular Cell Types

Cell Type	Major Cytokine or Soluble Peptide Mediator	Major Final Ocular-Specific Actions
Ocular nerves	Substance P	Alters pain appreciation; alters vascular permeability
Ocular nerves	Vasoactive intestinal protein	Suppresses T cells and macrophages; influences ocular immune privilege
Retinal pigment epithelium (RPE)	Transforming growth factor (TGF)-β	Regulator of immune privilege; suppresses T cell and macrophages; fibrous tissue proliferation and scar formation
RPE	Platelet-derived growth factors (PDGFs)	Affects fibrous proliferation, scarring, and fibrosis
RPE	Macrophage chemotactic protein (MCP)-1	Involved in recruiting and activating macrophages and T cells
Non-pigmented ciliary epithelium	TGF-β	Fibrous proliferation; scar formation; regulator of ocular immune privilege
Vascular endothelial cells	Too numerous to list	Endothelial-derived cytokines and peptides ubiquitous in innate and acquired immune responses
Fibroblasts	TGF-β	Fibrous proliferation; scar formation; regulator of ocular immune privilege

Circulating or Non-Ocular Cell Types

Cell Type	Major Cytokine or Soluble Peptide Mediator	Major Final Ocular-Specific Actions
Macrophage	Interleukin (IL)-1α; IL-6; MCP-1; tumor necrosis factor (TNF)-β; TNF-α	Macrophages affect diverse inflammatory pathways by producing numerous types of cytokines and peptides
T lymphocytes	IL-6; IL-4; TNF-β; TGF-β	Alters vascular permeability; affects neutrophil migration; multiple action on B cells; involved in immune privilege regulation
CD4 lymphocyte	IL-4; TNF-α	Induces Th2; blocks Th1
Th2 cells	IL-5; IL-10	Recruits eosinophils; blocks Th1
Natural killer (NK) cells	Interferon (IFN)-γ	Activates macrophages; stimulates neutrophil and macrophage responses
Many types of leukocytes	IFN-α	Preventative role in virus infections; inhibitor activity against neoplastic cell growth
Mast cells	Substance P; IL-4; IL-6	Alters vascular permeability; affects leukocyte migration; inducer of B cells
Platelets	PDGFs	Affects fibrous proliferation and scar formation

* Table includes major but select examples. Injury includes autoimmune but soluble inflammatory mediators also found in infection, trauma (surgical and accidental), neoplastic, and vascular.

protect against foreign antigens would appear to easily result in permanent injury to the transparent tissues of the eye if not tightly regulated. How the eye controlled immunologic injury was the next puzzle waiting to be solved.

1.6 ANTERIOR CHAMBER IMMUNE DEVIATION

By mid-century, two seemingly unique sets of ocular immunologic mysteries persisted – the success of corneal transplants and the pathogenesis of sympathetic ophthalmia. Could the key to understanding these phenomena be related? Edward Zimm (1863–1944), an Austrian ophthalmologist, performed the first human corneal transplant in 1905, but it was not until 1948 that *immunologic rejection* was described as a cause of graft failure.[9] Although immunologic tolerance to allogenic corneal tissue is not absolute, there is considerable dampening of the immune response. Delayed-type hypersensitivity was known to be the principle mechanism of graft failure by the early 1970s, but why was it muted in the cornea and anterior segment of the eye?

Expanding on the work of Medawar using an ocular tumor transplant model, Kapan and Streilein, in the late 1970s, explored the biological basis for this impaired immune reaction.[23] Following tumor

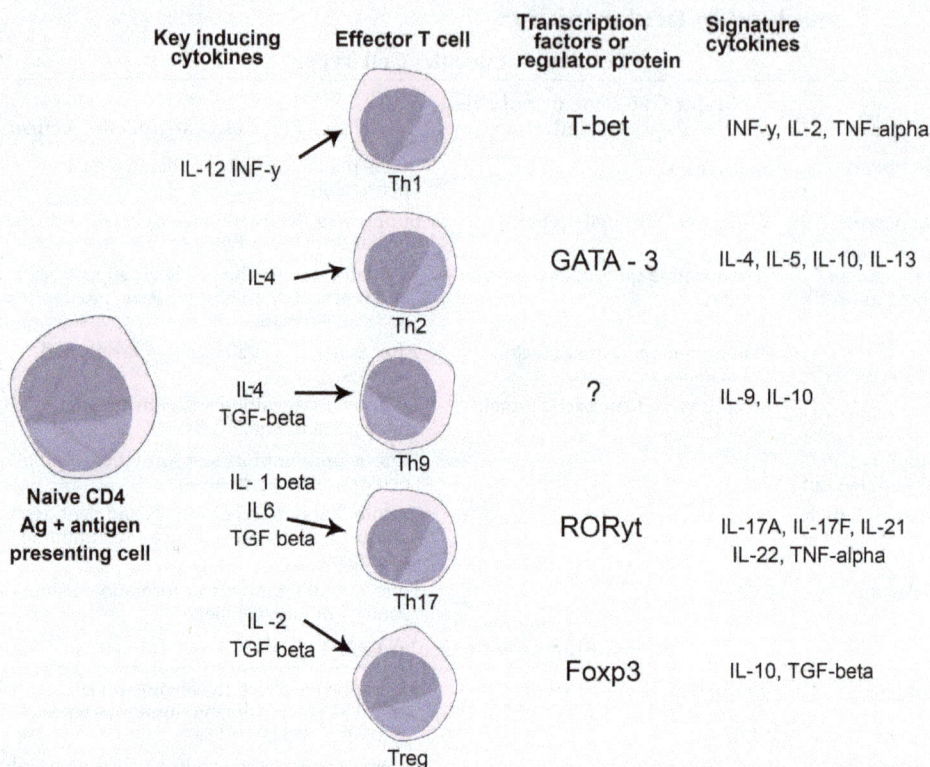

Figure 1.1 Examples of how various T helper cells (Th) are produced. Key cytokines (interleukin [IL], transforming growth factor [TGF]-β) induce naïve CD4 cells to become Th1, 2, 9, 17, and Treg. They are further acted upon by transcription factors or regulator proteins to produce characteristic patterns (signatures) of cytokines. Examples displayed in this sampling include T-bet (encoded by *T-bet gene*), GATA3 (encoded by *GATA3* gene), RORγ† (encoded by *retinoic acid receptor-related isoform γ† gene*), and Foxp3 (encoded by *forkhead box protein P3* gene).

implantation into the anterior chamber, a host of findings were observed, beginning with impaired delayed hypersensitivity.[24] Other observations included reduced or absent T cell response; the presence of primed cytotoxic T cell precursors in the spleen; splenic T cells that could suppress T cell induction; and detectable serum antibodies to tumor antigens. This combination of aberrant findings was called *anterior chamber–associated immune deviation* (ACAID).[23] Further studies showed that splenectomy prevented ACAID from developing, indicating that intracamerally injected tumor antigens are able to get into the circulation. These discoveries stressed the role that an ocular–splenic interaction played in the down-regulation to foreign antigens in the eye. Muted delayed hypersensitivity also heightened awareness that immune privilege likely increased the vulnerability of the eye to intraocular infection.

Further investigation into ACAID shed light into contributing variables. Expression of MHC class 1 and 2 was found to be low in the anterior segment of the eye.[9] Antigen presenting cells (i.e., Langerhans cells, macrophages, and dendritic cells) and other sentinel mediators of the immune response must largely be recruited from the peripheral corneal and limbus. For that to happen, cells must either traverse avascular tissue or travel through new vessels. New vessels, however, are inhibited by the release of anti-angiogenic substances.[25] Even after antigen-presenting cells reach their foreign target, they must overcome a variety of immunomodulating molecules and cytokines that block or impede their phenotypic maturation.[26] Normally, this process is referred to as priming and occurs in both host and donor antigen processing cells. Among the many implicated proteins are: Fas-ligand, a transmembrane protein belonging to the tumor necrosis family; TNF related aptosis inducing ligand (TRAIL), an apoptosis-inducing ligand; programed death ligand 1 (PD-L1), a

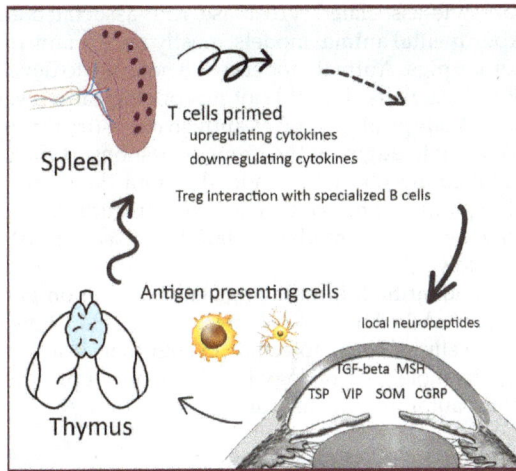

Figure 1.2 Simplified overview of anterior chamber immune modulation. Following injury, antigens are presented and proceed via trabecular meshwork and limbal lymphatics through the blood to thymus and spleen, or directly to the spleen, where costimulatory antigen-presenting cells (APC) (e.g., CD 80/86/40) are up-regulated to facilitate trafficking. In the spleen, T cells are primed by host-derived APC involving a combination of up-regulated and down-regulated cytokines. Treg (CD25) interacts with specialized B cells (e.g., Qa-1 peptide) and natural killer (NK) cells. Proliferating T cells, representing the effector arm of the arc (usually Th1 or Th17), are transported via the bloodstream to the eye. There, they encounter local neuropeptides in the aqueous like transforming growth factor (TGF)-β, melanocyte-stimulating hormone (MSH), thrombospondin (TSP), vasoactive intestinal protein (VIP), somatostatin (SOM), and calcitonin gene-related peptide (CGRP) that dampen the inflammatory response.

transmembrane protein known to inhibit adaptive immunity; α-melanocyte-stimulating hormone (MSH), a member of the melanocortin family with immune modulating properties; thrombospondin (TSP)-1, a protein involved in chemotaxis; and transforming growth factor-β, a multifunctional cytokine (Figure 1.2).[9, 27, 28] By constraining the capture of alloantigens through the release of anterior segment neuropeptides and other immunomodulatory molecules, APCs are unable to consummate T cell presentation. The development and maintenance of ocular immune privilege has thus been ascribed to a subset of regulatory T cells, or Treg.[28–30]

Treg is considered a collection of T helper cells that is able to down-regulate other T cells. Functioning essentially as a suppressor-type T cell, Treg is produced in the thymus during development and can be identified by its concurrent cell surface expression of forkhead box P3 (Foxp3), CD4, and CD25 rather than a cytokine profile.[21, 22]

1.7 SYMPATHETIC OPHTHALMIA

Sympathetic ophthalmia is a rare but quintessential example of an autoimmune disorder. Other than rare extraocular manifestations like vitiligo, it represents a primary and isolated autoimmune disease of the eye, a phenomenon attributed to its antigenic isolation since early embryogenesis. Clinically sympathetic ophthalmia is a process initiated by a penetrating ocular injury in one eye that results in bilateral granulomatous inflammation in both eyes. In an era before meaningful therapies existed, the pan-uveal inflammation resulted in bilateral blindness. In more than 90% of cases, inflammation in the second uninjured, or sympathizing, eye occurs within 12 months of the inciting event.[3] Historically, most cases occurred following accidental trauma. Now, a substantial proportion of cases follow elective intraocular surgery.[31] Trauma plays a critical role in the pathogenesis of sympathetic ophthalmia because it allows previously isolated intraocular antigens access to the systemic immune system where they are perceived as "foreign."

The role that trauma (accidental or surgical) plays in exposing intraocular antigens to the systemic immune system supported the conceptual importance of sequestered intraocular peptides and proteins in pathogenesis. The first contender for sequestered antigen was retinal S-antigen (arrestin), followed by interphotoreceptor retinoid-binding protein and later by a host of other candidates (e.g., recoverin, rhodopsin, melanocyte-associated tyrosinase, RPE-associated antigen).[32] These antigens were identified through experimental animal models, mostly mice (many of which are trans-genetic and knockout), rats, and guinea pigs. Animal models were not easy to develop because many manifest pan-ocular inflammatory reactions that did not morphologically resemble the human condition. The induction phase of EAU typically involves antigen exposure through repeated extraocular injections with Freund's adjuvant to augment the immune response. Often, a second or third agent like pertussis toxin or heat-killed mycobacteria is added to spur the reaction along. While information related to most cytokine pathways has come from rodent studies, tyrosinase-related protein 1 has been used to create an experimental model of Harada's disease in dogs (see Vogt–Koyanagi–Harada syndrome in what follows).[20, 21]

Once trigger antigens were identified, immunologists homed in on genetic predispositions for sympathetic ophthalmia (e.g., HLA-11, HLA-DR4/DRw53, HLA-DR4/DQw3, HLA-DRB1*4, etc.) and pieced together a cascade of cellular and molecular events that, if left unchecked, culminate in blinding uveitis.[32-34] Though its molecular biology is still a work in progress, sympathetic ophthalmia has become an exemplary autoimmune disorder.

1.8 CELLULAR AND MOLECULAR MEDIATORS

The pro-inflammatory cellular mediators of most types of immune-mediated uveitis are CD4+ T helper cells, primarily Th1 and Th17. Other CD4+ T helper cells play lesser roles. Experimental models indicate that Th17 serves as a key modulator and produces IL-17, -21, -22, and TNF-α. Th1 associated cytokines include IL-1α, IL-1β, TNF-α, IL-2, and interferon-γ. Interleukin-1, IL-6, and TNF-α are major pro-inflammatory cytokines in uveitis.[20-22] Although cytokine expression has been mostly studied in animal models, cytokine responses in humans and their profiles vary depending on type of uveitis. In the future, these profiles could be used to classify syndromes. Th2 cellular response is also known to occur in animal models and in humans but tends to be associated with anti-inflammatory response as seen in atopic disease. Its cytokine profile includes elevation of IL-4, IL-5, and IL-10. The Th2 response itself appears to be promoted by IL-4, IL-13, and IL-33, which can result in downstream antibody production. In all types of ocular inflammation, cytokine concentrations are higher in the eye than peripherally and will vary within compartments (e.g., aqueous, vitreous), usually correlating with the nidus or severity of inflammation. In the future, the ability to sample tissue outside the eye (e.g., tears) that reliability correlates with intraocular cytokine concentrations would eliminate the risk of harvesting intraocular samples.

1.9 PHACOANTIGENIC UVEITIS

Perhaps no clinical or uveitic entity is shrouded in as much uncertainty as phacoantigenic uveitis.[34] Animal experiments by Uhlenhuth in the early 20th century demonstrated serum antibodies directed against lens proteins, using bovine lens and rabbits as hosts. To his surprise, the rabbits also developed antibodies to lens proteins from a variety of other animals as well. In 1922, Frederick Verhoeff (1874–1968) and Albert Lemoine (1884–1957) published an article describing a form of lens-induced inflammation in 12 patients they called *endophthalmitis phacoanaphylactica*.[35] The morphologic findings of granulomatous inflammation directly at lens fibers were consistent with a hypersensitivity reaction to lens protein. Acquired immunity was further implicated through positive intradermal skin tests they performed on patients.

Most investigators think of phacoantigenic uveitis as an autoimmune condition, in large part through the process of exclusion.[34, 36] Its study has been complicated by the fact that few cases are ever diagnosed clinically, before the eye or the lens is surgically removed.

1.10 VOGT–KOYANAGI–HARADA SYNDROME

Between 1906 and 1929, Alfred Vogt, Y. Koyanagi, and E. Harada reported eight patients with varying manifestations of bilateral uveitis, vitiligo, white hair, hearing loss, and cerebrospinal fluid (CSF) pleocytosis.[37] Three years later, the condition was unified (and memorialized) as a uveo-meningeal eponym called Vogt–Koyanagi–Harada (VKH) disease. Clinicians have debated the minimal diagnostic criteria for VKH syndrome. Most accept bilateral panuveitis associated with one of four neurological or auditory findings (meningismus, tinnitus, hearing loss, or CSF pleocytosis) or one of three abnormal integumentary findings (poliosis, vitiligo, or hair loss), any of which occurs in the absence of a history of trauma.[38]

The pathogenesis of VKH appears autoimmune. The early morphologic findings of non-necrotizing granulomatous uveitis are indistinguishable from sympathetic ophthalmia (absent the penetrating wound in the inciting eye). The neurological, auditory, and integumentary findings suggested a link to the uveal tract through the association of melanin. As the search for putative melanocyte-specific peptides continued through the years, genetic predispositions were suspected due to geographic variation in incidence.[39] Substantially greater proportions of uveitis patients are affected with VKH syndrome in Japan, Brazil, and Saudi Arabia than elsewhere in the world. As strong associations with HLA-DR4 among Japanese and HLA-DR1 among Hispanics in California provided further evidence of genetic susceptibility, investigators confirmed the inflammation was cell mediated through T lymphocytes. More recent investigation has identified tyrosinase-related proteins-1 and -2 as potential target autoantigens in humans, although the search for other melanin antigens continues.[40] Much still needs to be learned about how such intracellular molecules become targets of immunological attack and what is shared in terms of intraocular and extraocular uveal self-antigens.

1.11 AN OVERVIEW OF AUTOIMMUNE DISEASE AND THE EYE

If ocular inflammation is *not* due to infection, trauma, secondary to neoplasm, or drug related, one must consider autoimmune disease and idiopathic immune-mediated inflammation. Essentially every tissue of the eye and ocular adnexa have been documented as vulnerable to autoimmune assault.[34, 41–44] Several immune-mediated inflammatory disorders of the eye are suspected as being autoimmune, but conclusive evidence remains elusive. Examples would include Susac's syndrome, birdshot chorioretinopathy, Cogan syndrome, and acute zonal occult outer retinopathy.

A few generalizations can be made in terms of the clinical evaluation of autoimmune disorders of the eye. First, the pace of the evaluation depends on the perceived potential of a life-threatening or vision-threatening outcome. Most ocular disorders are not life threatening, but many are vision threatening, including irreversible injury to the retina and optic nerve. Second, when signs of inflammation dominate the clinical presentation, it necessitates the expeditious exclusion of infectious disease, since infections are potentially curable and will often worsen if inadvertently treated as a solely immune-mediated pathology. Third, a number of drugs have been causally associated with ocular inflammation. Such drug-induced complications are easily overlooked if not specifically screened for.

1.12 SUMMARY

The eye serves as a classic example of regional immunity, as the microenvironment of the eye can alter portions of the immune arc. The immunologic microenvironment of the eye, however, is not a singular entity but could represent as many as five. From a historical perspective, the eye provided the first compelling evidence that human autoimmune disease existed in the descriptions of sympathetic ophthalmia. Like many biological hypotheses, basic science and laboratory technology had to catch up for them to be meaningfully tested. During this protracted interval, another exceptional feature of the eye was discovered – its tolerance to allograph transplants. The concept of immune tolerance thus matured through research into the ocular microenvironments that permits self-antigen sequestration during embryogenesis and anatomical isolation after birth. Given that the eye has been granted so many immunologic privileges, it still bears a substantial burden of autoimmune disease. The molecular elucidation of noninfectious ocular inflammation is leading to targeted therapies that will be able to effect remediation through the neutralization of pro-inflammatory pathways or the enhancement of regulatory ones.

REFERENCES

1. Theofilooulos AN. Molecular pathology of autoimmune disease: an overview. In: Theofilopoulos AN, Bona CA, eds, *The molecular pathology of autoimmune diseases*, 2nd edn. New York: Taylor & Francis, 2002:1–16.
2. Silverstein AM. *A history of immunology*. San Diego: Academic Press, 1989:169–175.
3. Albert DM, Diaz-Rohena R. A historical review of sympathetic ophthalmia and its epidemiology. *Surv Ophthalmol*. 1989;34(1):1–4.
4. Medawar PB. A second study of the behaviour and fate of skin homografts in rabbits: a report to the war wounds committee of the medical research council. *J Anat*. 1945;79:159–176.
5. Srinivasan BD, Jakobiec FA, Iwamoto T. Conjunctiva. In: Duane TD, Jaeger EA, eds, *Biomedical foundations of ophthalmology*, volume 1, chapter 29. Philadelphia: Harper & Row, 1986:1–28.
6. Mirchess AK, Schechter JE. Immune mechanisms of dry-eye disease. In: Levin LA, Albert DM, eds, *Ocular disease: mechanisms and management*. Philadelphia: Saunders, 2010:114–122.

7. Knop E, Knop N. Influence of the eye-associated lymphoid tissue (EALT) on inflammatory ocular surface disease. *Ocul Surf.* 2005 Oct.;3(Suppl 4):S180–S186.
8. Medawar PB. Immunity to homologous grafted skin. II. The fate of skin homographs transplanted to the brain, to subcutaneous tissue, and to the anterior chamber of the eye. *Br J Exp Pathol.* 1948;29(1):58–69.
9. Saban DR, Dastjerdi DH, Dana R. Corneal graft rejection. In: Levin LA, Albert DM, eds, *Ocular disease: mechanisms and management.* Philadelphia: Saunders, 2010:56–63.
10. Patterson CA. The lens. In: Hart WM Jr, ed, *Adler's physiology of the eye,* 9th edn. St Louis: Mosby; 1992:348–390.
11. Fine BS, Yanoff M. *Ocular histology: a text and atlas,* 2nd edn. Hagerstown: Harper & Row, 1979:59–128.
12. Nicholls JG, Martin AR, Wallace BG, et al. *From neuron to brain,* 4th edn. Sunderland: Sinauer Associates, 2001:150–151.
13. Web JG. The kallikrein/kinin system in ocular function. *J Ocul Pharmacol Ther.* 2011;27(6):539–543.
14. Silverstein AM. *A history of immunology.* San Diego: Academic Press, 1989:176–179.
15. Wasson T. *Nobel prize winners: an H. W. Wilson biographic dictionary.* New York: HW Wilson Company, 1987:170–172, 686–689.
16. Rose NR, Mackay IR. Prospectus: the road to autoimmune disease. In: Rose NR, Mackay IR, eds, *The autoimmune diseases,* 4th edn. Amsterdam: Elsevier Academic Press, 2002:xix–xxv.
17. Zinkernagel RM, Doherty PC. Functional heterogeneity of lymphocytic choriomeningitis virus-specific T lymphocytes. I. Identification of effector and memory subsets. *J Exp Med.* 1975;141:866–881.
18. Zinkernagel RM, Doherty PC. MHC-restricted cytotoxic T cells: studies on the biological role of polymorphic major transplantation antigens determining T-cell restriction-specificity, function, and responsiveness. *Adv Immunol.* 1979;27:51–177.
19. Zinkernagel RM, Doherty PC. The discovery of MHC restriction. *Immunol Today.* 1997;18:14–17.
20. Yeh S, Li Z, Nussenblatt RB. Immunologic mechanisms of uveitis. In: Levin LA, Albert DM, eds, *Ocular disease: mechanisms and management.* Philadelphia: Saunders, 2010:619–627.
21. Balamurugan S, Das D, Hasanreisoglu M, et al. Interleukins and cytokine biomarkers in uveitis. *Indian J Ophthalmol.* 2020;68(9):1750–1763.
22. Weinstein JE, Pepple KL. Cytokines in uveitis. *Curr Opin Ophthamol.* 2018;29(3):267–274.
23. Kaplan HJ, Streilein JW. Immune response to immunization via the anterior chamber of the eye: I F1 lymphocytes induced immune deviation. *J Immunol.* 1977;118:809–814.
24. Streilein JW. Anterior chamber associated immune deviation: the privilege of immunity in the eye. *Surv Ophthalmol.* 1990;35:67–73.
25. Cursiefen C, Chen L, Saint-Geniez M, et al. Nonvascular VEGF receptor 3 expression by corneal epithelium maintains avascularity and vision. *Proc Natl Acad Sci USA.* 2006;103:11405–11410.
26. Albini T, Rao NA. Immunologic processes in disease. In: Garner A, Klintworth GK, eds, *Pathobiology of ocular disease,* 3rd edn. New York: Inform Healthcare, 2008:47–67.
27. Elner VM, Demirci H, Elner SG. Apoptosis. In: Garner A, Klintworth GK, eds, *Pathobiology of ocular disease,* 3rd edn. New York: Inform Healthcare, 2008:29–46.
28. Keino H, Horie S, Sugita S. Immune privilege and eye-derived T-regulatory cells. *J Immun Res.* 2018;1–12.
29. Hori J, Yamaguchi T, Keino H, et al. Immune privilege in corneal transplant. *Prog Retina Eye Res.* 2019;72:1–24.
30. Yamagami S, Dana MR. The critical role of lymph nodes in corneal alloimmunization and graft rejection. *Invest Ophthalmol Vis Sci.* 2001;42:1293–1298.
31. Lubin JR, Albert DM, Weinstein M. Sixty-five years of sympathetic ophthalmia: a clinicopathologic review of 105 cases (1913–1978). *Ophthalmology.* 1980;87:109–121.
32. Kumaradas M, Rao NA. Sympathetic ophthalmia. In: Levin LA, Albert DM, eds, *Ocular disease: mechanisms and management.* Philadelphia: Saunders, 2010:635–641.
33. Tsai JH, Rao NA. Intraocular manifestation of immune disorders. In: Garner A, Klintworth GK, eds, *Pathobiology of ocular disease,* 3rd edn. New York: Inform Healthcare, 2008:72–78.
34. Margo CE, Harman LE. Autoimmune disease: conceptual history and contributions of ocular immunology. *Surv Opththalmol.* 2016;61(5):680–688.
35. Verhoeff FH, Lemoine AN. Endophthalmitis phacoanaphylatica. *Am J Ophthalmol.* 1922;5: 737–746.
36. Marak GE, Jr. Phacoanaphylatic endophthalmitis. *Surv Ophthalmol.* 1992;36:325–339.

37. Nussenblass RB, Whitcup SM, Palestine AG. *Uveitis: fundamental and clinical practice*, 2nd edn. St Louis: Mosby, 1996:312–324.

38. Yang P, Zhong Y, Du L, et al. Development and evaluation of diagnostic criteria for Vogt-Koyanagi-Harada disease. *JAMA Ophthalmol*. 2018;136(9):1025–1031.

39. El-Asrar AM, Damme JV, Struyl S, et al. New perspective on the immunopathogenesis and treatment of uveitis associated with Vogt-Koyanagi-Harada disease. *Frontiers Med*. Nov. 2021. doi:10.3389/fmed.2021.705796.

40. Sugita S, Takase H, Taguchi C, et al. Ocular infiltrating CD4+ T cells from patients with Vogt-Koyanagi-Harada disease recognized human melanocytes antigens. *Invest Ophthalmol Vis Sci*. 2006;47(6):2547–2554.

41. Levy-Clarke GA, Leila L, Kump LI, et al. Ocular disease. In: Rose NR, Mackay IR, eds, *The autoimmune diseases*, 4th edn. Amsterdam: Elsevier Academic Press, 2002:669–679.

42. Tauber J. Autoimmune diseases affecting the ocular surface. In: Holland EJ, Mannis MJ, eds, *Ocular surface disease medical and surgical management*. New York: Springer, 2002:113–127.

43. Gery I, Nussenblatt RB, Chan CC, et al. Autoimmune disease of the eye. In: Theofilopoulos AN, Bona CA, eds, *The molecular pathology of autoimmune diseases*, 2nd edn. CRC Press; 2002:978–998.

44. Nieto-Aristizabal I, Mera JJ, Giraldo JD, et al. From ocular immune privilege to primary auto-immune disease of the eye. *Autoimmun Rev*. 2022;21(8):103–122.

2 Approach to the Patient with Ophthalmologic Manifestations of Rheumatic Disease

Amit Reddy, John Gonzalez, and Jason Kolfenbach

2.1 THE OPHTHALMOLOGIST'S EVALUATION

The initial approach to a patient with ocular inflammation is typically centered around a few important characterizations: (a) understanding the onset, course, and duration of the disease; (b) evaluating the anatomical site(s) of inflammation; (c) grading the level of inflammation; and (d) determining the presence of any coexisting systemic diseases (Table 2.1). The goals of this approach are to produce a working diagnosis – or at a minimum a categorization of disease (particularly distinguishing infectious from noninfectious causes of ocular inflammation) – to guide subsequent laboratory and radiographic testing, and allow for selection of appropriate initial therapies.

As in all fields of medicine, a thorough history and review of systems (ROS) is the first step in reaching a correct diagnosis in ocular inflammatory disease. The Standardization of Uveitis Nomenclature (SUN) Working Group established consensus definitions for commonly used descriptors of uveitis.[1] While meant to be applied specifically to intraocular inflammation or uveitis, these definitions are often extrapolated to external ocular inflammation, such as scleritis, as well. Within the SUN Working Group's report, the onset of disease is defined as sudden or insidious based on the pattern of the patient's subjective symptoms. The duration is defined as limited if ongoing for less than or equal to 3 months and persistent if greater than 3 months. Finally, the course of the disease is divided into three potential patterns: acute (sudden onset with limited duration), recurrent (multiple episodes that are separated by at least 3 months without treatment), and chronic (inflammation that relapses in less than 3 months after discontinuing treatment).

After obtaining this history along with a pertinent ROS, ophthalmic examination should be performed in order to accurately classify the site or sites of inflammation. Proceeding from anterior to posterior, the external exam can reveal evidence of **orbital inflammation**. This typically manifests as proptosis, pain and limitation in extraocular motility that may cause binocular diplopia, edema of the periorbital soft tissues, and chemosis.[2]

Examination next of the **conjunctiva** may reveal secondary injection in the setting of active ocular inflammation. Careful evaluation of the fornices and eyelids can reveal symblepharon and forniceal shortening, which could suggest the presence of an underlying cicatrizing disease such as ocular cicatricial pemphigoid.[3]

The **episclera** and **sclera** are typically examined next. Inflammation of these structures can be difficult to differentiate, but distinguishing these entities is crucial because they have differing prognoses, treatments, and potential systemic disease associations. Classically, episcleritis presents with milder symptoms of ocular irritation, whereas scleritis causes a severe, boring pain that can wake the patient from sleep. Because episcleritis involves more superficial blood vessels, the injection will have a pink to red coloration under natural light, and the injection will blanch after application of topical phenylephrine. Scleritis, in contrast, will typically display a violaceous hue and will not blanch with phenylephrine.[4] Both episcleritis and scleritis were classified in a seminal paper by Watson and Hayreh in 1976 – episcleritis into simple and nodular, scleritis into anterior and posterior based on the presence of inflammation relative to the location of rectus muscle insertion points. Anterior scleritis was then further sub-classified into diffuse, nodular, and necrotizing.[5]

A thorough **corneal exam** can also identify inflammatory disease. Peripheral ulcerative keratitis, for example, is an inflammatory process of the peripheral cornea that classically causes a crescentic area of corneal thinning with an overlying epithelial defect, occasionally adjacent to an area of scleritis.[6,7] The cornea should also be examined for keratic precipitates, which are nonspecific focal inflammatory deposits on the corneal endothelium, and corneal edema. Epithelial dendritiform lesions can also be seen and are most commonly secondary to herpetic infection.[8]

An **intraocular exam** is then performed, with evaluation of the anterior chamber, vitreous, retina, and choroid for signs of inflammation. The SUN Working Group classified uveitis into four anatomic groups based on the primary site of inflammation: *anterior uveitis* when the anterior chamber is the primary site, *intermediate uveitis* when the vitreous is the primary site, *posterior uveitis* when the retina or choroid is the primary site, and *panuveitis* when there is inflammation in all anatomical sites (Figure 2.1, Table 2.1).[9] The SUN Working Group also provided a precise grading scale for anterior chamber inflammation, based on both anterior chamber cells and anterior chamber flare. Cell

DOI: 10.1201/9781003453710-2

Table 2.1 Rheumatic Conditions* Associated with Ocular Inflammation by Anatomic Site

Orbital inflammatory disease (OID)	■ ANCA-associated vasculitis (GPA > EGPA > MPA) ■ Sarcoidosis ■ IgG4-related disease ■ Thyroid-eye disease
Episclera/Sclera	■ Rheumatoid arthritis ■ ANCA-associated vasculitis (GPA most commonly) ■ Relapsing polychondritis ■ IBD-associated ■ Systemic lupus erythematosus ■ SpA
Uveitis ■ Anterior	■ HLA-B27associated ■ SpA ■ TINU (tubulointerstitial nephritis with uveitis) ■ Behçet's disease ■ Juvenile idiopathic arthritis (JIA) ■ Sarcoidosis ■ IBD-associated
■ Intermediate	■ Pars planitis (idiopathic) ■ Sarcoidosis ■ Multiple sclerosis ■ Behçet's disease
■ Posterior	■ Behçet's disease ■ Sarcoidosis ■ SpA (non-HLA-B27-associated, such as PsA, IBD) ■ VKH disease
■ Panuveitis	■ VKH disease ■ Behçet's disease ■ Sarcoidosis

* Table lists the most common rheumatic conditions associated with ocular inflammation at the anatomic site and is not exhaustive. Importantly, non-rheumatic etiologies (viral, bacterial, fungal, malignant, and others) can cause similar presentations and should be evaluated for during the initial ophthalmology evaluation.

Abbreviations: ANCA: antineutrophil cytoplasmic antibody; GPA: granulomatosis with polyangiitis; EGPA: eosinophilic granulomatosis with polyangiitis; MPA: microscopic polyangiitis; IBD: inflammatory bowel disease; SpA: spondyloarthritis; VKH: Vogt–Koyanagi–Harada.

grading is based on the number of white blood cells seen in the anterior chamber through a field defined by a 1 × 1 millimeter slit beam, with grading from 0 to 4+. For example, 2+ anterior chamber cell corresponds to 16 to 25 such cells per field. Flare occurs due to exudation of protein into the anterior chamber, leading to reflection of light and a subsequent "hazy" view to the iris and lens. No similar consensus was reached for the grading of vitreous cells. A prior grading system was kept for vitreous haze, which was based on standardized photographs.[10] Interobserver agreement within one grade for both anterior chamber cell and vitreous haze was found to be excellent.[11]

Particularly for inflammation involving the posterior segment, adjunctive in-clinic imaging technologies have become indispensable in aiding diagnosis and monitoring disease activity. Ocular coherence tomography (OCT) is a non-invasive modality similar to ultrasonography, but it utilizes light instead of sound waves, providing micrometer-level imaging resolution (Figure 2.2).[12] OCT scans through the macula are invaluable in managing common structural complications of uveitis such as epiretinal membrane and cystoid macular edema (CME) (Figure 2.3). CME is present in up to 40% of patients with uveitis and is a leading cause of vision loss in this disease.[13]

Invasive imaging tests, particularly fluorescein angiography (FA) (Figure 2.4) and indocyanine green angiography (ICGA) (Figure 2.5), also provide extremely useful information in the evaluation of uveitis. FA involves intravenous injection of sodium fluorescein followed by retinal photography. Ultra-widefield retinal cameras are able to capture both the central and much of the peripheral retina in one image (Figure 2.6). In addition to showing CME, FA allows for evaluation of retinal vascular inflammation (Figure 2.7), retinal non-perfusion, and neovascularization. Retinal photography

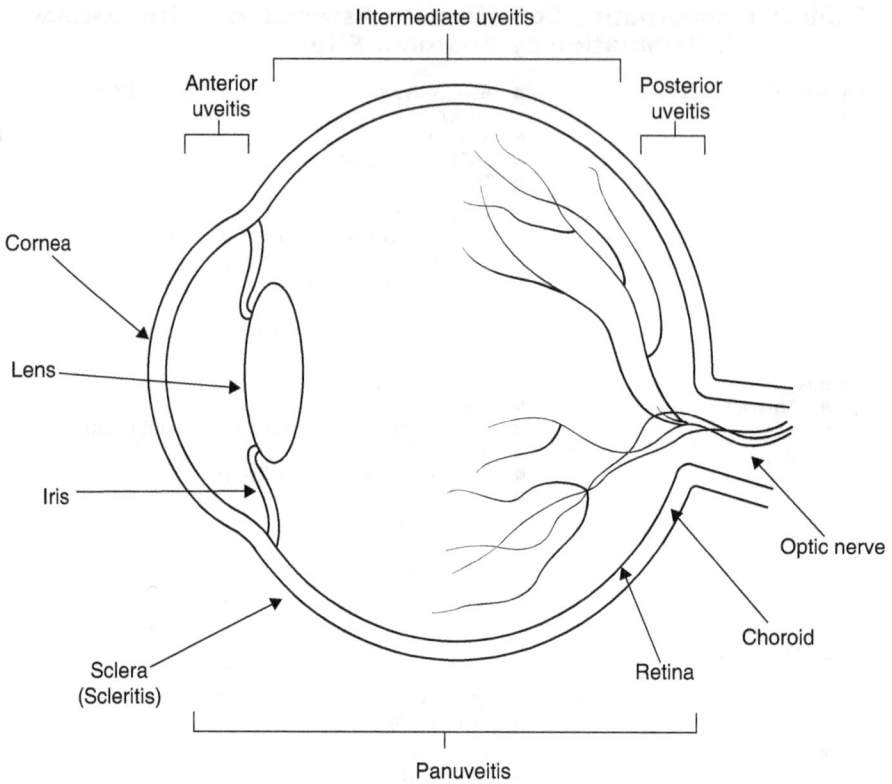

Figure 2.1 Cross-sectional schematic of an eyeball, indicating the anatomic locations of anterior, intermediate, posterior, and panuveitis.

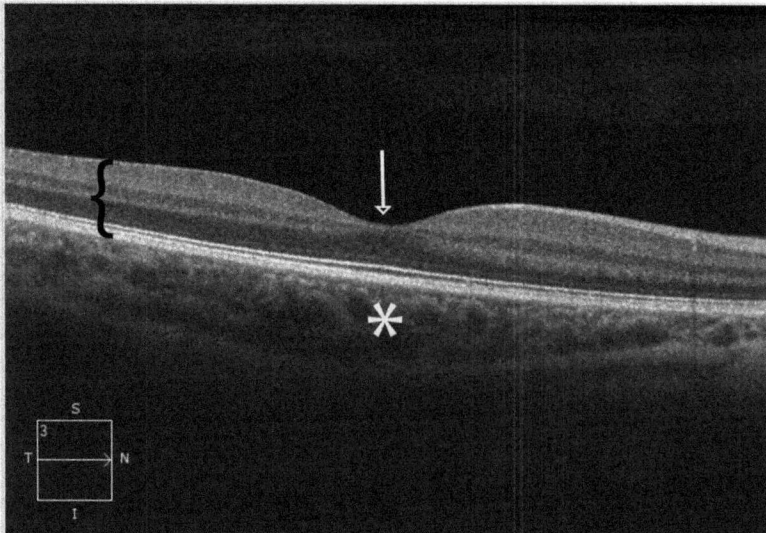

Figure 2.2 Example of a normal ocular coherence tomograph scan through the macula of the right eye, demonstrating a normal foveal contour (white arrow). The bracket displays the extent of the retina, and the asterisk is within the choroid.

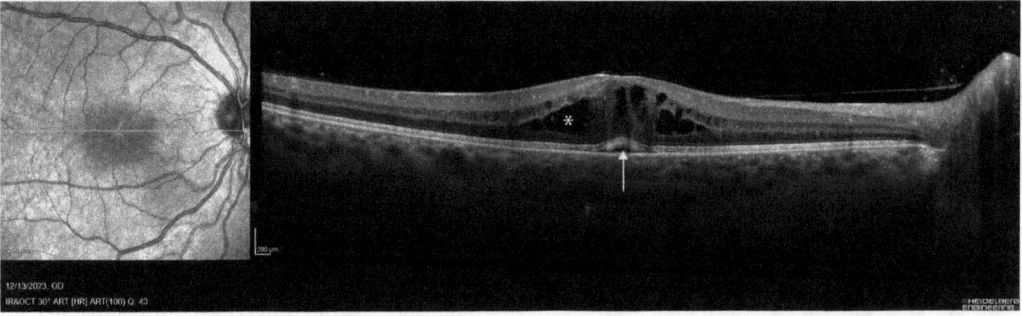

Figure 2.3 Ocular coherence tomography through the macula of the right eye in a patient with chronic panuveitis showing cystoid spaces (asterisk) and subretinal fluid (arrow), consistent with cystoid macular edema.

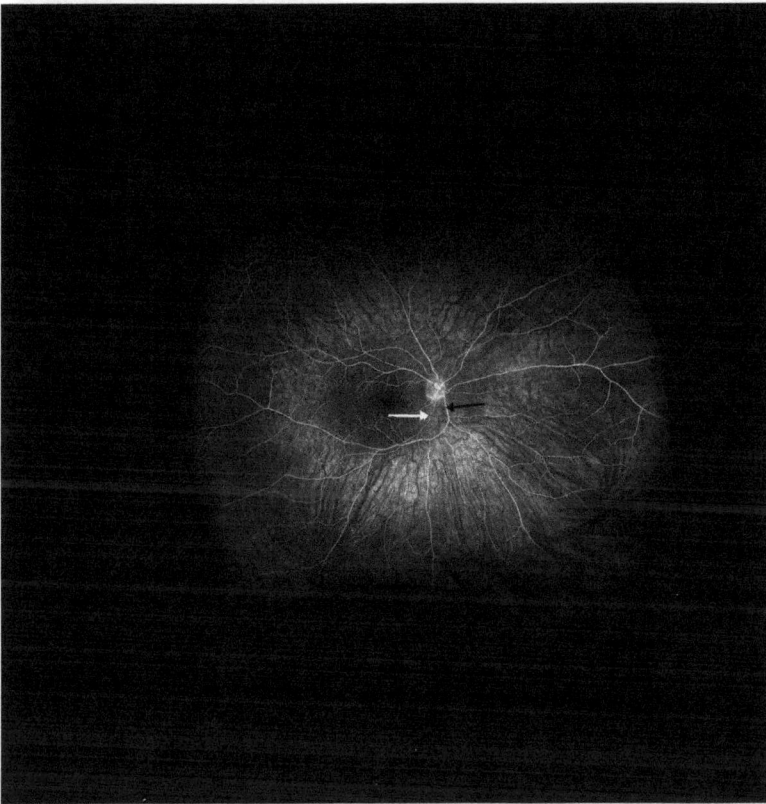

Figure 2.4 Example of a normal fluorescein angiogram, displaying normal filling without leakage in both the retinal veins (black arrow) and retinal arterioles (white arrow).

following injection of indocyanine green provides additional information on the choroid specifically, which can be useful in conditions such as birdshot chorioretinopathy (Figure 2.8).[14]

The initial evaluation for a patient with ocular inflammation should be driven by the patient's history and ROS. All patients should undergo serologic testing for syphilis and lung imaging (typically chest radiograph) to evaluate for pulmonary sarcoidosis and screen for exposure to tuberculosis. Additional testing may then be pursued according to the disease phenotype of each specific patient – for example, HLA-B27 testing would be beneficial in a patient with acute, unilateral anterior

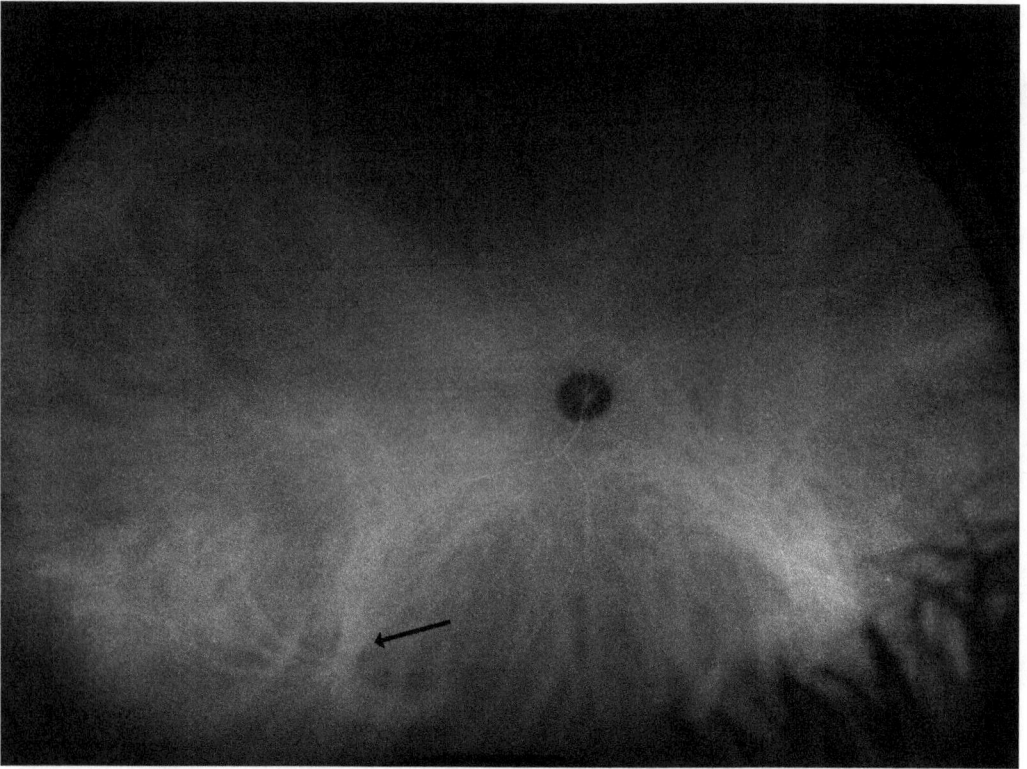

Figure 2.5 Example of a normal indocyanine green angiogram. The black arrow is pointing to an example of a choroidal vessel leading to a draining vortex vein.

uveitis. Similarly, antibody testing for rheumatoid arthritis and antineutrophilic cytoplasmic antibody (ANCA)-associated vasculitis would be reasonable in patients presenting with scleritis due to high rates of concurrent systemic inflammatory disease.[15]

Data collected from the exam and imaging, along with the results of systemic testing, are then used to establish a specific ocular inflammatory disease diagnosis. To assist in standardizing these diagnoses, the SUN Working Group utilized machine learning to develop classification criteria for 25 common uveitic diseases.[16] It is important to note that despite appropriate history, ROS, and testing, the majority of patients with presumed immune-mediated ocular inflammation will not have clear evidence for a systemic disease process and are considered to have idiopathic or unclassified disease.

2.2 DIFFERENTIAL DIAGNOSIS AND RULING OUT COMPETING DIAGNOSES (INFECTION, MALIGNANCY, AND OTHER MASQUERADE SYNDROMES)

Uveitis specialists must first determine whether ocular inflammation is infectious or noninfectious/autoimmune/autoinflammatory in nature. This is important because the treatment paradigms are distinctly different: infectious processes are managed with antimicrobial therapy, whereas noninfectious/autoinflammatory processes are managed with immunosuppression (whether local in the form of topical or regional corticosteroids, systemic corticosteroids, or steroid-sparing immunosuppression).

Even in patients with a known rheumatologic disease (such as Behçet's disease or an HLA-B27 seronegative spondyloarthropathy), the first presentation of uveitis is approached by methodically determining whether an infectious or noninfectious process is at play. Uveitis-directed testing is mandated in all patients, and assumptions are never made. The initial development of a differential diagnosis occurs before the patient is even examined. A thorough review of systems, past medical history, social history (which includes a thorough review of sexual and illicit substance histories), and all medications (not only ocular medications but *all* medications) is gathered. For example,

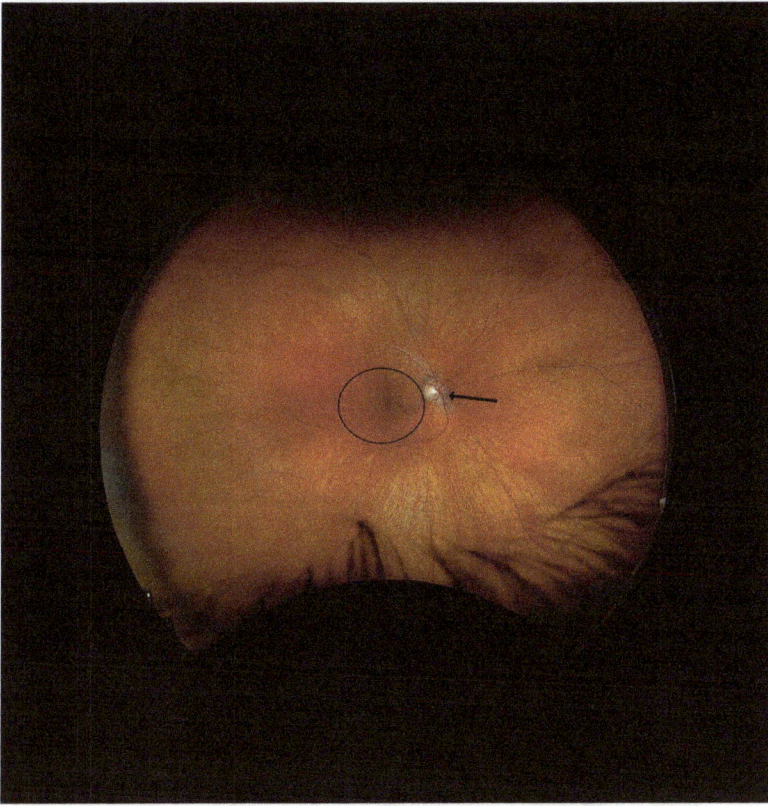

Figure 2.6 Example of a normal color photograph of the retina, including the macula (encompassed within the ellipse) and optic nerve head (black arrow).

some medications are known to be associated with ocular inflammation, and prior sexual activity is a risk factor for syphilis.[17] Syphilis and tuberculosis are infectious processes that can mimic nearly any type of inflammation and should be tested for prior to use of peri/intraocular or systemic corticosteroids.

The next step in refining the differential diagnosis is identifying the anatomical location of inflammation. Using the SUN criteria, intraocular inflammation may present as anterior, intermediate, posterior, or panuveitis. Inflammation of the sclera may present as an anterior scleritis or posterior scleritis. Unlike the eye itself (including the sclera and intraocular structures), inflammation in the orbit is more challenging to evaluate clinically as it is precluded from direct observation. However, reduced extraocular motility, proptosis (or bulging) of the eye, abnormalities in pupillary constriction (an afferent pupillary defect), vision that is out of proportion worse to clinical exam, or inflammation of adnexal structures (such as the lacrimal gland or lacrimal sac) may direct a uveitis specialist to obtain neuroimaging with a focus on the orbit to identify orbital inflammation or inflammation or compression of the optic nerve, which travels through the orbit.

For intraocular inflammation presenting as an anterior uveitis, the next clinically important feature in refinement of the differential diagnosis is determining if there are keratic precipitates (cellular deposits on the corneal epithelium) and, if so, what their shape is. Small, round as well as larger (so-called mutton fat or granulomatous) precipitates localized to the inferior aspect of the cornea may be more compatible with a noninfectious process. However, keratic precipitates that are diffuse and/or have a star-shaped, or stellate, appearance may be seen in viral infections (particularly herpetic and rubella). Atrophy of the iris and/or elevated intraocular pressure during active inflammation are additional suggestive clues of a possible viral etiology.[18] In such a case, an anterior chamber paracentesis may be considered with directed polymerase chain reaction (PCR) testing for herpes simplex virus (HSV), varicella zoster virus (VZV), and cytomegalovirus (CMV).[19] If examination of the anterior chamber finds a hypopyon, a robust accumulation of inflammatory cells toward the

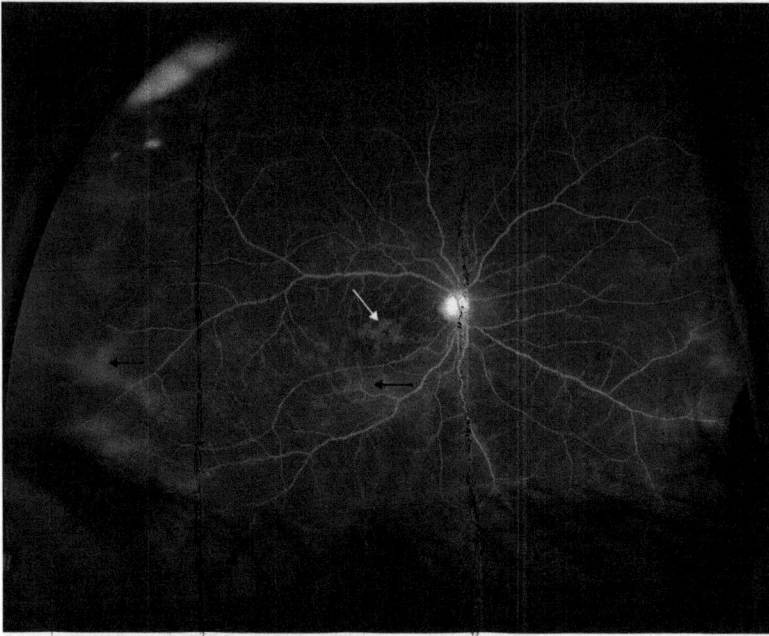

Figure 2.7 Fluorescein angiography of the same patient as Figure 2.3 showing cystoid macular edema (white arrow) and peripheral retinal vascular leakage (black arrows).

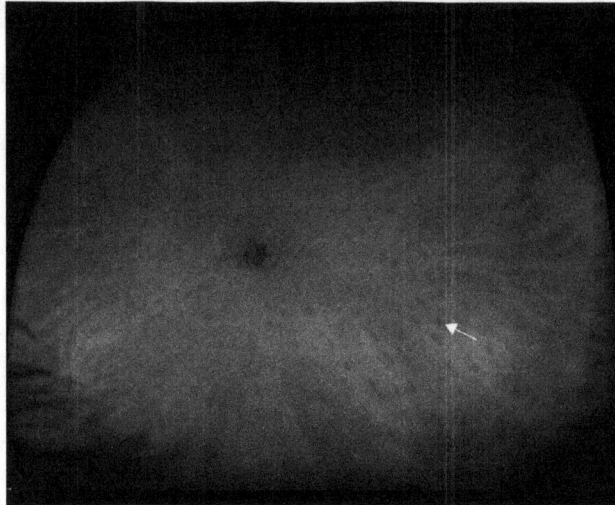

Figure 2.8 Indocyanine green angiography of a patient with birdshot chorioretinopathy showing scattered hypocyanescent spots (white arrow).

bottom of the anterior chamber, a noninfectious etiology, specifically an HLA-B27-related seronegative spondyloarthropathy or Behçet's disease, may be suspected.[20] However, if there is heme mixed in with the hypopyon or the hypopyon is not located exclusively inferiorly (which typically should occur by virtue of gravity), a leukemic masquerade may be suspected.[21, 22]

Intermediate uveitis, inflammation in the vitreous and far peripheral retina, including the area known as the pars plana, may be compatible with sarcoidosis or multiple sclerosis. While nearly all patients with new-onset uveitis receive chest radiography (typically chest X-ray, but, in select suspicious cases, high-resolution computed tomographic scan of the chest), neuroimaging is not routinely performed to "rule out" multiple sclerosis unless there are accompanying neurologic symptoms or a compatible history.[23] However, patients with intermediate uveitis who require anti-tumor necrosis factor (TNF) inhibitor therapy should undergo MRI of the brain even without neurologic symptoms due to the association between intermediate uveitis and multiple sclerosis and the potential for worsening demyelinating disease with TNF inhibitors.[24, 25] Intermediate uveitis may also have infectious causes with examination findings that can be suggestive. For example, inflammation that presents in the vitreous as fluffy balls raises suspicion for a fungal infection, a form of endophthalmitis (an intraocular infection with an intense associated inflammatory response).[26] Endophthalmitis can be endogenous (systemic infection source with hematogenous spread) or exogenous (secondary to intraocular surgery or trauma). Similarly, masquerades may present as intermediate uveitis. Inflammatory cells that accumulate as sheets of cells in the vitreous (rather than randomly or evenly distributed within the vitreous) raises suspicion for a lymphoproliferative process, in particular, vitreoretinal lymphoma, a subset of central nervous system (CNS) lymphoma. In this setting, vitreous biopsy for histological and molecular evaluation for a lymphoproliferative disorder as well as MRI with gadolinium of the brain to evaluate for CNS lesions is mandated.

Posterior uveitis encompasses inflammation in the retina and choroid and can also have infectious, autoimmune and masqueraders underlying the presentation. Inflammation presenting with retinal hemorrhages and whitening of the retina (termed a "retinitis") raises suspicion for a viral process (typically herpetic). Behçet's disease may present with such features as well, but a viral necrotizing retinitis must be ruled out first before a noninfectious process like Behçet's disease is invoked. Indeed, treatment for a necrotizing viral retinitis is commenced even before PCR results of ocular fluid evaluating for HSV, VZV, or CMV return, given the risk of significant ocular and visual morbidity associated with such an infection.[27] Retinal vasculopathy or choroidopathy, which is evaluated with intravenous fluorescein angiography, indocyanine green, and photographic imaging of the retina, can identify features compatible with systemic lupus erythematosus and ocular limited inflammatory syndromes such as birdshot chorioretinopathy.[28] In the setting of retinal hemorrhages, including those that are white-centered, a leukemic process may be more likely.[29] For inflammation presenting as a panuveitis, conditions such as sarcoidosis and Behçet's disease should be considered.

In essentially all cases of new-onset uveitis, tuberculosis and syphilis are tested. Both conditions can present as almost any type of inflammation and in any part of the eye. Syphilis is evaluated by using a treponemal-specific test (such as Treponemal antibody) and a treponemal-nonspecific test (such as the rapid plasmin reagin). The reason both types of syphilis-related tests are performed is because of the possibility of the prozone effect or the possibility of incompletely treated syphilis (particularly since ocular syphilis requires CNS treatment).[30, 31] Since uveitis specialists may use local or systemic corticosteroids to treat inflammation, doing so in an infectious process could be potentially blinding without appropriate antimicrobial therapy in place first.

Similar to uveitis, scleritis and orbital inflammatory disease may have both infectious and noninfectious/autoimmune etiologies. Zoster-related scleritis should be considered given a history of shingles in the relevant V1 dermatome. A history of ocular surgery (such as glaucoma surgery or pterygium excision) in conjunction with fluctuant or purulent material involving the sclera would be highly suspicious for an infectious scleritis and requires evaluation for bacterial or fungal causes. The most common rheumatologic diseases manifesting with scleritis include rheumatoid arthritis and antineutrophil cytoplasmic antibody (ANCA)-associated vasculitides (such as granulomatosis with polyangiitis).[32, 33] Additionally, orbital inflammation can occur in association with ANCA-associated vasculitides, sarcoidosis, and IgG4-related disease. Without a history of trauma or abutting sinus-associated infections, orbital infections are less likely.

It is important to note that once infections have been ruled out or are felt to be very unlikely and if leukemic/lymphoproliferative disorders do not fit the clinical presentation, the underlying condition in the case of uveitis, scleritis, or orbital inflammation is considered noninfectious in nature, meaning autoimmune/autoinflammatory. In approximately half of such cases, the patient may not have a systemic rheumatologic condition/autoimmune condition. Nevertheless, depending on the anatomical location of inflammation and severity, such patients are still managed with local or topical corticosteroids and, in cases of chronic, sight-threatening inflammation, with steroid-sparing immunosuppression.[34]

2.3 THE RHEUMATOLOGIST'S EVALUATION

A general understanding of ocular anatomy and inflammatory eye disease is also important to practicing rheumatologists. Rheumatologists may see patients in clinic with rheumatic disease who develop vision complaints or ocular pain. They may also receive requests for consultation in patients with ocular inflammation to determine if there is an associated underlying systemic auto-immune disease. Lastly, a rheumatologist may be asked to help guide the management of immuno-suppressive medications in a patient with idiopathic autoimmune ocular disease. In each of these scenarios, background knowledge on anatomy, conditions commonly affecting the eye, and tools used in ophthalmology to identify and monitor levels of inflammation can help facilitate communi-cation between specialists and optimize patient care.

In patients with rheumatic disease presenting with ocular symptoms, a history remains the first step in evaluation. Questions regarding ocular pain, redness, changes in vision, discharge, or pho-tophobia can be helpful. Asking about contact lens use can be important, as inappropriate use can lead to ocular irritation and elevated risk of infection. Allergic and viral etiologies remain common reasons for presentation with a red, irritated eye, and a good history can help separate those from more serious causes. As outlined in the preceding section, obtaining a detailed history regarding laterality (unilateral vs. bilateral), onset (acute vs. chronic), and course (recurrent or not) can be helpful in forming an initial differential diagnosis. Finally, review of the medication list can be important to identify adverse reactions as a potential cause (bisphosphonates, immune checkpoint inhibitors, mitogen-activated extracellular signal-regulated kinase [MEK] and BRAF inhibitors).

Rheumatologists lack access and expertise in the use of sophisticated tools for the examination of the eye, but useful information from the physical exam can still be obtained. Information on **visual acuity** can be ascertained by asking a patient to read small print at 12 inches away. An evaluation of the **external ocular structures** should be carried out to inspect for lid swelling, blepharitis, propto-sis, or lacrimal gland swelling. The presence of purulent discharge can be an indicator of underlying infectious etiology, while watery discharge may be supportive of an allergic cause. Documentation of ocular injection, while noting the specific location of involvement, can be important. **Conjunctival injection** often results in diffuse ocular redness involving the bulbar and palpebral surfaces. In con-trast, **scleritis** may present with sectoral redness with more discrete borders and a violaceous hue. Erythema focused at the limbus (**ciliary flush**) can be indicative of more serious etiologies such as anterior uveitis, keratitis, or acute angle closure glaucoma. **Pupillary** size, shape, and response to light should be documented, along with an evaluation of the **cornea** for the presence of opacities or other gross abnormalities. Finally, a **fundoscopic exam** can be carried out to identify signs of retinal ischemia or abnormalities at the optic disc and peripapillary retinal vasculature. In summary, even in situations in which access to a direct ophthalmoscope is not available, important information can be obtained from the physical exam to help the rheumatologist formulate a differential diagnosis and communicate with colleagues in ophthalmology.

The information gathered from the history and exam is useful not only for developing a differ-ential diagnosis but also in determining disease severity and speed of referral to ophthalmology. Severe pain with an inability to open the eye may suggest a corneal injury that should be evaluated acutely by ophthalmology. Similarly, sudden vision loss, the presence of hypopyon (layered white blood cells in the anterior chamber) or hyphema (blood in the anterior chamber), and new cor-neal opacities or haze, all represent urgent conditions that require same-day consultation with an ophthalmologist. In contrast, many issues affecting the conjunctiva and lids, including blepharitis, can be handled by primary care and rheumatology or referred to ophthalmology non-urgently for consultation.

Rheumatologists may also be asked to see patients with new-onset ocular inflammation to evalu-ate for the presence of an underlying systemic autoimmune condition. When communicating with colleagues in ophthalmology, obtaining the following information can be helpful:

a. Anatomic location of inflammation (orbital inflammatory disease, conjunctivitis, episcleritis, scleritis, anterior uveitis, intermediate uveitis, posterior uveitis, panuveitis)

b. Information on laterality, onset, and course (as described earlier)

c. Initial treatment response

d. Determining level of concern (or testing done to evaluate) for infectious causes or other masquerade syndromes

This information, alongside a careful history and physical exam for extra-ocular disease by the rheumatologist, can result in a prioritized differential diagnosis. Narrowing the differential diagnosis and focusing on the most likely etiologies is important, as the list of rheumatic conditions that can be associated with ocular inflammation is quite large. Indiscriminate testing (a shotgun testing approach) for all rheumatic conditions is not only wasteful but increases the odds of false-positive test results that can derail the diagnostic process. Several rheumatic conditions have a propensity to involve specific anatomic sites of the eye (Table 2.1), which can be helpful in directing a targeted evaluation plan.

Systemic autoimmune conditions can also be associated with additional ocular presentations such as optic neuritis (Sjögren's disease, systemic lupus erythematosus), arteritic anterior ischemic optic neuropathy (giant cell arteritis), retinal vasculitis (Takayasu arteritis, Behçet's disease, sarcoidosis), and occlusive vasculopathy (Susac syndrome, antiphospholipid antibody syndrome). Keratoconjunctivitis sicca (dry eye) can present as a feature of many systemic autoimmune conditions, most notably Sjögren's disease, and can result in corneal pathology and associated conjunctival irritation, which may present as a painful, red eye to the clinician. These conditions, along with their recommended evaluation and management plans, will be covered in greater depth in the chapters that follow.

2.4 SUMMARY

This chapter provides an overview of the approach to the evaluation of ocular inflammatory conditions from the perspective of both an ophthalmologist and a rheumatologist. The ophthalmologist's evaluation focuses on characterizing the onset, course, and duration of the disease, identifying the anatomical site(s) of inflammation, grading the level of inflammation, and determining the presence of any coexisting systemic diseases. This approach helps establish a differential diagnosis, guides subsequent relevant and directed testing, and allows for the selection of appropriate initial therapies. The rheumatologist's evaluation involves understanding the basics of ocular anatomy and recognizing common ocular manifestations of rheumatic diseases, which allows for effective communication with ophthalmologists. For both specialists, narrowing the differential diagnosis is important, which allows for performing the appropriate diagnostic testing. Collaboration between ophthalmologists and rheumatologists is essential for optimizing patient care, as ocular inflammation may be the first manifestation of a systemic illness or can occur in the setting of an established rheumatic disease.

REFERENCES

1. Kolfenbach JR, Palestine AG. *Autoimmune eye and ear disorders*. Philadelphia, PA: Elsevier, 2020.
2. Rosenbaum JT, Dick AD. The eyes have it: a rheumatologist's view of uveitis. *Arthritis Rheumatol.* 2018;70(10):1533–1543.
3. Corbitt K, Nowatzky J. Inflammatory eye disease for rheumatologists. *Curr Opin Rheumatol.* 2023;35(3):201–212.
4. Akpek EK, Thorne JE, Qazi FA, et al. Evaluation of patients with scleritis for systemic disease. *Ophthalmology.* 2004;111(3):501–506.
5. Jakob E, Reuland MS, Mackensen F, et al. Uveitis subtypes in a German interdisciplinary uveitis center – analysis of 1916 patients. *J Rheumatol.* 2009;36(1):127–136.
6. Choi RY, Rivera-Grana E, Rosenbaum JT. Reclassifying idiopathic uveitis: lessons from a tertiary uveitis center. *Am J Ophthalmol.* 2019;198:193–199.
7. Jabs DA, Nussenblatt RB, Rosenbaum JT, et al. Standardization of uveitis nomenclature for reporting clinical data: results of the first international workshop. *Am J Ophthalmol.* 2005;140(3):509–516.
8. Lee MJ, Planck SR, Choi D, et al. Non-specific orbital inflammation: current understanding and unmet needs. *Prog Retin Eye Res.* 2021;81:100885.
9. Wang K, Seitzman G, Gonzales JA. Ocular cicatricial pemphigoid. *Curr Opin Ophthalmol.* 2018;29(6):543–551.
10. Berchicci L, Miserocchi E, Di Nicola M, et al. Clinical features of patients with episcleritis and scleritis in an Italian tertiary care referral center. *Eur J Ophthalmol.* 2014;24(3):293–298.
11. Watson PG, Hayreh SS. Scleritis and episcleritis. *Br J Ophthalmol.* 1976;60(3):163–191.
12. Cao Y, Zhang W, Wu J, et al. Peripheral ulcerative keratitis associated with autoimmune disease: pathogenesis and treatment. *J Ophthalmol.* 2017;2017:7298026.
13. Reddy AK, Kolfenbach JR, Palestine AG. Ocular manifestations of rheumatoid arthritis. *Curr Opin Ophthalmol.* 2022;33(6):551–556.
14. Lobo AM, Agelidis AM, Shukla D. Pathogenesis of herpes simplex keratitis: the host cell response and ocular surface sequelae to infection and inflammation. *Ocul Surf.* 2019;17(1):40–49.
15. Nussenblatt RB, Palestine AG, Chan CC, et al. Standardization of vitreal inflammatory activity in intermediate and posterior uveitis. *Ophthalmology.* 1985;92(4):467–471.

16. Kempen JH, Ganesh SK, Sangwan VS, et al. Interobserver agreement in grading activity and site of inflammation in eyes of patients with uveitis. *Am J Ophthalmol.* 2008;146(6):813–818.e811.
17. Wojtkowski M, Bajraszewski T, Gorczynska I, et al. Ophthalmic imaging by spectral optical coherence tomography. *Am J Ophthalmol.* 2004;138(3):412–419.
18. Multicenter Uveitis Steroid Treatment Trial Research Group, Kempen JH, Altaweel MM, et al. The multicenter uveitis steroid treatment trial: rationale, design, and baseline characteristics. *Am J Ophthalmol.* 2010;149(4):550–561.e510.
19. Schachat AP. *Ryan's retina*, 6th edn. Edinburgh; New York: Elsevier, 2018.
20. Smith JR, Mackensen F, Rosenbaum JT. Therapy insight: scleritis and its relationship to systemic autoimmune disease. *Nat Clin Pract Rheumatol.* 2007;3(4):219–226.
21. Standardization of Uveitis Nomenclature Working Group. Development of classification criteria for the uveitides. *Am J Ophthalmol.* 2021;228:96–105.
22. Moorthy RS, Moorthy MS, Cunningham ET, Jr. Drug-induced uveitis. *Curr Opin Ophthalmol.* 2018;29(6):588–603.
23. Babu K, Konana VK, Ganesh SK, et al. Viral anterior uveitis. *Indian J Ophthalmol.* 2020;68(9): 1764–1773.
24. Anwar Z, Galor A, Albini TA, et al. The diagnostic utility of anterior chamber paracentesis with polymerase chain reaction in anterior uveitis. *Am J Ophthalmol.* 2013;155(5):781–786.
25. Ramsay A, Lightman S. Hypopyon uveitis. *Surv Ophthalmol.* 2001;46(1):1–18.
26. Gruenewald RL, Perry MC, Henry PH. Leukemic iritis with hypopyon. *Cancer.* 1979;44(4):1511–1513.
27. Abramson DH, Wachtel A, Watson CW, et al. Leukemic hypopyon. *J Pediatr Ophthalmol Strabismus.* 1981;18(3):42–44.
28. Petrushkin H, Kidd D, Pavesio C. Intermediate uveitis and multiple sclerosis: to scan or not to scan. *Br J Ophthalmol.* 2015;99(12):1591–1593.
29. Kouwenberg CV, Koopman-Kalinina Ayuso V, de Boer JH. Clinical benefits and potential risks of adalimumab in non-JIA chronic paediatric uveitis. *Acta Ophthalmol.* 2022;100(4):e994–e1001.
30. Bosch X, Saiz A, Ramos-Casals M. Monoclonal antibody therapy-associated neurological disorders. *Nat Rev Neurol.* 2011;7(3):165–172.
31. Durand ML. Bacterial and fungal endophthalmitis. *Clin Microbiol Rev.* 2017;30(3):597–613.
32. Schoenberger SD, Kim SJ, Thorne JE, et al. Diagnosis and treatment of acute retinal necrosis: a report by the American academy of ophthalmology. *Ophthalmology.* 2017;124(3):382–392.
33. Preble JM, Silpa-Archa S, Foster CS. Ocular involvement in systemic lupus erythematosus. *Curr Opin Ophthalmol.* 2015;26(6):540–545.
34. Jackson N, Reddy SC, Hishamuddin M, et al. Retinal findings in adult leukaemia: correlation with leukocytosis. *Clin Lab Haematol.* 1996;18(2):105–109.
35. Hunter EF, Adams MR, Orrison LH, et al. Problems affecting performance of the fluorescent treponemal antibody-absorption test for syphilis. *J Clin Microbiol.* 1979;9(2):163–166.
36. Berkowitz K, Baxi L, Fox HE. False-negative syphilis screening: the prozone phenomenon, nonimmune hydrops, and diagnosis of syphilis during pregnancy. *Am J Obstet Gynecol.* 1990;163(3):975–977.
37. Wakefield D, Di Girolamo N, Thurau S, Wildner G, McCluskey P. Scleritis: immunopathogenesis and molecular basis for therapy. *Prog Retin Eye Res.* 2013;35:44–62.
38. Junek ML, Zhao L, Garner S, et al. Ocular manifestations of ANCA-associated vasculitis. *Rheumatology (Oxford).* 2023;62(7):2517–2524.
39. Jabs DA. Immunosuppression for the uveitides. *Ophthalmology.* 2018;125(2):193–202.

3 Ocular Manifestations of Rheumatoid Arthritis

Prarthana Jain, Beth L. Jonas, and Karen R. Armbrust

3.1 RHEUMATOID ARTHRITIS

Rheumatoid arthritis (RA) is a chronic symmetric inflammatory polyarthritis that affects up to 1% of the population worldwide, with a peak incidence in the seventh decade of life. Risk factors for the disease include female gender, genetics, and certain environmental factors. RA is 2 to 3 times more common in women than men, although the underlying reason for this is not yet understood. Genetic factors may be responsible for up to 60% of the risk for RA in patients who are anti-cyclic citrullinated peptide (CCP) antibody positive.[1] HLA DRB1 is strongly implicated in both the onset of seropositive RA and the severity of the disease.[2, 3] Disease-associated HLA DR alleles contain a common amino acid sequence in the binding groove of the molecule, the so-called shared epitope. Smoking increases the risk of RA in a dose-dependent fashion, particularly in patients who are positive for the CCP antibody or who have the shared epitope,[4] and smokers may be less likely to respond to disease-modifying therapies.[5]

In early RA, symptoms typically begin in the small joints of the hands and feet, and over time, other joints may become involved.[6] Stiffness, which improves with joint movement, is usually the earliest sign of disease, with pain and swelling following soon after. In the hands, the wrists, MCPs and PIPs are typically involved with sparing of the DIPs. In the feet, involvement of the MTPs predominates. After the hands and feet, the most common joints involved are the elbows, shoulders, ankles, knees, and hips. If the disease is not adequately treated, inflamed synovium may result in damage in adjacent bone and cartilage, leading to malalignment, subluxation, and resultant joint dysfunction.

In RA, more advanced disease and seropositivity are associated with extra-articular features and a poorer prognosis. The skin and eye are the most common organs involved aside from the joints. Subcutaneous nodules may occur in many locations, but they are classically described on the extensor surfaces of the forearm just distal to the elbow joint and over the dorsum of the hands. Histologically, rheumatoid nodules are characterized by a central area of necrosis surrounded by palisading macrophages and lymphocytes.[7] Up to one-third of patients with RA have secondary Sjögren syndrome with xerostomia and/or keratoconjunctivitis.[8] Some patients may develop episcleritis or scleritis, the latter of which can be sight threatening.

Major organ involvement has been described in the lungs (pleurisy and interstitial lung disease), the heart (pericarditis, premature atherosclerotic disease), the vasculature (small-vessel vasculitis), and the nervous system (compressive neuropathies and mononeuritis due to vasculitis).[9] Anemia of chronic inflammation and thrombocytosis are common hematologic abnormalities, and RA is also associated with an increased risk of hematologic malignancies. Cardiovascular disease is the leading cause of premature death in patients with RA. Chronic systemic inflammation is thought to be the underlying basis of this risk.[10]

On physical examination, inflamed joints are tender and swollen and often have a reduced range of motion. The joints may have overlying erythema and palpable warmth. Palpation of inflamed joints demonstrates swelling that is soft or boggy. This contrasts with palpation of the joints in OA, which tends to be harder and bony. In more advanced disease, there may be stigmata of joint damage such as ulnar deviation of the digits, swan neck deformities, or boutonniere deformity. In the feet, erosion of the MTPs may lead to lateral drift of the toes or plantar subluxation of the metatarsal heads. Advanced disease of the midfoot may cause collapse and chronic tarsal malalignment. A complete physical examination of a patient with RA should include both a comprehensive joint evaluation and careful attention to possible extra-articular features, including assessment of the skin, eyes, lungs, nervous system, and heart.

3.2 CLASSIFICATION CRITERIA FOR RA

There are no diagnostic criteria for RA, but the 2010 ACR/EULAR classification criteria, which include both clinical and serological data, may help inform the workup for any patient with at least one swollen joint without a known explanation (Table 3.1).[11] Radiographs of the hands and feet are useful to assess for periarticular osteopenia, which suggests inflammatory joint disease or joint space narrowing, indicating loss of cartilage. The radiologic hallmark of RA is the presence of marginal erosions, where erosions are found at the margin of the joint space (in contrast to the central erosions seen in osteoarthritis). In late disease, malalignment and joint subluxation may be evident.

DOI: 10.1201/9781003453710-3

Table 3.1 ACR/EULAR Classification Criteria for Rheumatoid Arthritis

		Points
Joint Involvement	1 large joint	0
	2–10 large joints	1
	1–3 small joints	2
	4–10 small joints	3
	> 10 joints (with at least 1 small joint)	5
Serology	Negative RF and negative CCP	0
	Low positive RF or CCP	2
	High positive RF or CCP	3
Acute Phase Reactants	Normal CRP and WESR	0
	Abnormal CRP or WESR	1
Duration of Symptoms	< 6 weeks	0
	≥ 6 weeks	1

Note: A score of ≥ 6/10 is needed for classification of a patient as having definite RA.
Abbreviations: RF – rheumatoid factor; CCP – cyclic citrullinated peptide; CRP – C reactive protein; WESR – Westergren erythrocyte sedimentation rate.

3.3 MANAGEMENT OF RA

In patients with RA, affected joints may be damaged or destroyed if inflammation persists. Therefore, early recognition of active disease and measures to quickly achieve control of joint inflammation, with the goal of remission or low disease activity, is central to modifying disease outcomes. Per the 2021 ACR treatment guidelines, all patients with RA should be initiated on a disease-modifying anti-rheumatic drug (DMARD) as soon as possible following diagnosis, as better outcomes are achieved with early initiation of these drugs.[12] Glucocorticoids and non-steroidal anti-inflammatory drugs (NSAIDs) should only be used as adjunctive agents and preferably on a temporary basis while waiting for the full effect of DMARDs. Conventional DMARDs (cDMARDs) include drugs like methotrexate, sulfasalazine, hydroxychloroquine, and leflunomide. In RA patients with low disease activity, hydroxychloroquine is conditionally recommended over other cDMARDs; however, sulfasalazine, methotrexate, and leflunomide also may be used. In patients with moderate to severe RA, methotrexate is recommended as the initial DMARD of choice. Typically, oral methotrexate is started at a dose of 15 mg per week and increased as required for disease control, to a maximum dose of 20 to 25 mg per week, while monitoring for intolerance and drug toxicity. Patients should be re-evaluated in 3 to 4 months to monitor for effectiveness. In those who fail to achieve low disease activity or remission, switching to subcutaneous methotrexate (which has higher bioavailability) is recommended.

If still not at target after 3 to 6 months despite the use of maximally tolerated methotrexate, a biologic DMARD (bDMARD) or targeted synthetic DMARD (tsDMARD) may be added, or triple therapy (with methotrexate, hydroxychloroquine, and sulfasalazine) may be pursued. Options for bDMARDs include tumor necrosis factor alpha (TNF-α) inhibitors (such as etanercept, adalimumab, infliximab, golimumab, certolizumab), T cell costimulatory inhibitor (abatacept), interleukin-6 (IL-6) receptor inhibitors (tocilizumab, sarilumab), and anti-CD 20 therapies (rituximab). Options for tsDMARDs include Janus kinase (JAK) inhibitors (such as tofacitinib, baricitinib, and upadacitinib). The choice of bDMARD or tsDMARD may depend on patient preference regarding route and frequency of drug administration, presence of comorbidities, and cost barriers to drug access. In patients resistant to treatment with a bDMARD or tsDMARD, we typically switch to an alternate class of bDMARD or tsDMARD. Non-pharmacologic measures, such as patient education, physical and occupational therapy, and psychosocial interventions should be used in addition to drug therapy.

3.4 DRY EYE SYNDROME

Dry eye syndrome, or keratoconjunctivitis sicca, is the most common ocular disease reported in patients with rheumatoid arthritis, with a pooled prevalence of 16% (95% confidence interval 11% to 20%) in a meta-analysis of ocular involvement in rheumatoid arthritis.[13] Dry eye syndrome is a multifactorial disease that may involve ocular surface inflammation and/or damage, tear film instability and/or hyperosmolarity, and neurosensory abnormalities, but the key underlying element is thought to be loss of tear film homeostasis.[14] Patients with dry eye syndrome typically report ocular discomfort and/or visual disruption, and their symptoms often fluctuate. Common diagnostic testing in dry eye syndrome includes grading conjunctival hyperemia to assess ocular surface inflammation, staining the ocular surface to assess ocular surface damage, measuring tear breakup time to assess tear film stability, and tear meniscus assessment or Schirmer testing to quantitate tear film volume.[15]

Initial treatments for dry eye syndrome include humidifying the patient's environment, instilling lubricating eye drops and ointments, and eyelid warm compresses/hygiene.[16] If these treatments are insufficient, next-line treatments include cyclosporine eye drops, tacrolimus eye drops or ointment, lifitegrast eye drops, short courses of topical corticosteroids, and punctal occlusion. Autologous serum tears may be particularly helpful for neurotrophic keratitis. In severe cases of dry eye syndrome, amniotic membrane grafting and eyelid surgery to repair abnormal eyelid position or narrow the palpebral fissure may be performed. For additional information on the evaluation and treatment of dry eye syndrome, please refer to Chapter 10 (Ophthalmologic Involvement in Sjögren's Disease).

3.5 EPISCLERITIS

Episcleritis describes inflammation of the episclera, a tissue layer located between the superficial conjunctiva and deeper sclera within the wall of the eye. RA is a common comorbid condition in patients with episcleritis.[17, 18] Prevalence of episcleritis in patients with rheumatoid arthritis ranges from 1% to 25%, depending on the study population.[13, 19] Presentation of episcleritis is characterized by rapid onset of ocular redness that may be painless or associated with ocular discomfort, which is typically mild if present.[20] In contrast to scleritis, the inflamed vessels in episcleritis tend to be mobile, have a salmon-pink rather than violaceous hue in natural light, and blanch following administration of 10% phenylephrine eye drops (Figure 3.1). The clinical course of episcleritis often is self-limited, and complications are rare, so mild cases of episcleritis may be observed without treatment. Lubricating eye drops or short courses of topical corticosteroids or oral NSAIDs may be prescribed to reduce ocular redness and discomfort.

3.6 SCLERITIS

3.6.1 Introduction

Scleritis is a rare, usually painful inflammation of the sclera, which may lead to vision loss or blindness.[20] While episcleritis is a generally benign condition with a self-limited course, scleritis may be more serious and include ocular complications such as scleral thinning, corneal thinning, and ulceration, glaucoma, cataract, and uveitis.[21, 22] Therefore, the distinction between the two and therapeutic implications are of utmost importance. Scleritis is considered rare, although the true worldwide incidence and prevalence is not known. In the United Kingdom, the incidence rate was estimated

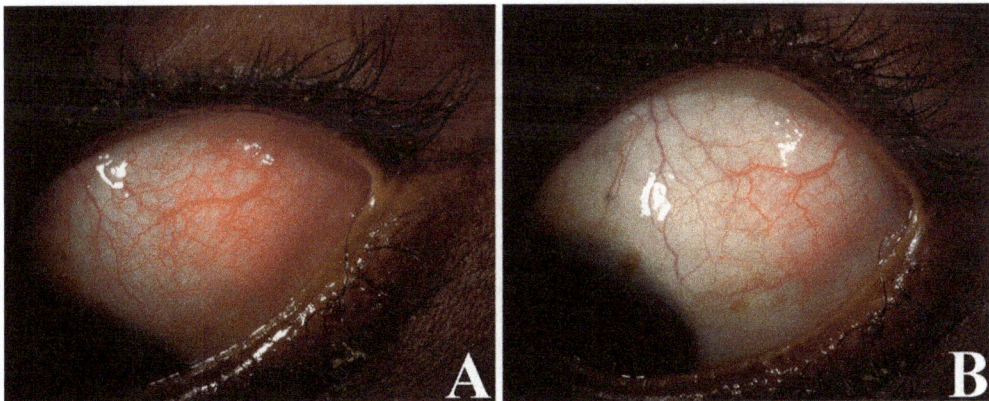

Figure 3.1 Episcleritis. Inflammation of episcleral vessels generating a reddish hue (A) with blanching after instillation of topical phenylephrine (B).

to be 4.23 per 100,000 person years in 1997, but the rate declined to 2.79 in 2018.[23] Other population studies have noted varied estimates, with an incidence rate of 4.1 per 1000,000 person years of scleritis in the Hawaiian population and 1 per 100,000 person years in metropolitan Melbourne, Australia.[24, 25] Scleritis typically affects middle-aged patients, aged 47 to 60 years, and is more common in women, with a 60% to 70% female predominance.[18, 26, 27] Causes of scleritis can be variable, but up to 30% to 50% of cases are associated with systemic autoimmune diseases,[17, 18, 28, 29] including RA, granulomatosis with polyangiitis (GPA), relapsing polychondritis (RP), and systemic lupus erythematosus (SLE), with rheumatoid arthritis being the most common associated systemic disease. Less commonly reported is scleritis from other causes, including local or systemic infections, medications, trauma, surgery, radiation, or malignancy.

3.6.2 Classification Systems

Scleritis continues to be classified according to the classification system proposed by Watson and Hayreh in 1976.[17] This system is based primarily on the anatomic site, etiology, and clinical appearance of inflammation at initial presentation. Scleritis is classified as either anterior or posterior, where anterior scleritis is defined as scleral inflammation located anterior to the insertion of the extraocular muscles. Anterior scleritis is further subdivided into diffuse, nodular, necrotizing with inflammation, and necrotizing without inflammation (also known as scleromalacia perforans).[17]

3.6.3 Association with Autoimmune Diseases

Up to half of patients diagnosed with scleritis may have or go on to develop an underlying autoimmune disease. It is also estimated that in around 15% to 59% of patients with scleritis, scleritis may be the first manifestation of an underlying systemic autoimmune disease.[30-32] Therefore, it is important to exclude multisystem disease at presentation and control any underlying systemic disease, as this has the beneficial effect of also controlling ocular inflammation. RA is the most common rheumatic condition associated with scleritis, followed by GPA.[17, 18, 31] Scleritis is also associated with Behçet's disease, Sjögren's syndrome, spondyloarthritis (SpA), SLE, RP, and less commonly inflammatory bowel disease (IBD), sarcoidosis, Takayasu arteritis, polyarteritis nodosa (PAN), temporal arteritis, and Cogan's syndrome.[23, 31, 33] Scleritis in patients with SpA and SLE is usually benign and self-limited, while scleritis in patients with RA and RP ranges from mild to severe.[31] Scleritis in the setting of GPA is more likely to be severe, necrotizing, and associated with permanent vision loss.[21, 31, 32] In contrast to RA-associated scleritis, which has an insidious nature of progression, GPA-associated scleritis tends to progress rapidly.[31, 32, 34] Patients with scleritis associated with RA are more likely to have a known diagnosis of RA prior to their first episode of scleritis, while scleritis is more likely to be the presenting sign of GPA.[35, 36] Anterior necrotizing scleritis without inflammation (also known as scleromalacia perforans) occurs almost exclusively in RA.[37]

3.6.4 Pathophysiology

There are few studies of the histopathologic features of scleritis. This is mainly because scleral biopsy is not necessary to make a diagnosis, and in some cases, biopsy of an inflamed sclera may lead to complications including globe perforation or induction of scleral necrosis.[38] Therefore, most of the limited evidence arises from severe and end-stage cases of scleritis after the eye is enucleated. A clinic-pathologic study by Rao and colleagues outlines various patterns of scleral inflammation observed in both idiopathic scleritis and autoimmune-associated scleritis. In idiopathic scleritis, pathology from scleral biopsy revealed chronic inflammatory infiltration, consisting of macrophages, T cells, and B cells, with minimal necrosis. In contrast, in RA-associated and ANCA-associated scleritis, scleral tissue had features of granulomatous inflammation with areas of tissue necrosis.[39] The necrotic areas were predominantly surrounded by CD20+ B cells and + plasma cells and sometimes associated with vasculitis.[39, 40] A subsequent study that evaluated scleral biopsies from 25 patients with necrotizing scleritis and 5 with recurrent non-necrotizing scleritis reported similar results, with histopathologic evidence of vasculitis, fibrinoid necrosis, neutrophil invasion, and immune complex deposition in vascular walls.[41]

Results of other immunohistochemical studies from resected sclera also suggest that local immune complex deposition, complement deposition, increased HLA-DR expression, and substantial T helper cell participation play a role in pathogenesis of scleritis in those with systemic autoimmune diseases.[41-43] Furthermore, matrix metalloproteinases, which are enzymes capable of degrading collagen, are thought to play an important role in the development of necrosis. The pro-inflammatory cytokine TNF-α is a potent inducer of MMP production and was found at elevated levels in tear fluid of patients with necrotizing scleritis, suggesting that TNF-α also plays a role.[44]

3.6.5 Presentation

Diffuse and nodular anterior scleritis, which are the most common forms of scleritis, usually present with severe, unremitting ocular and periocular pain that may radiate to the ear, scalp, face, or jaw. This pain is usually dull in character, exacerbated by globe palpation and/or eye movement, and may worsen at night or in the early morning. The pain may be so severe that it interferes with sleep or daily activities. Patients also may report headache, ocular redness, lacrimation, and sometimes photophobia.[22, 45] With necrotizing scleritis, patients may notice a black-blue hue to the color of their sclera, which is a result of the melanocyte-laden choroidal layer of the eye becoming visible through the thinned sclera.[45] Necrotizing anterior scleritis with inflammation typically presents with severe ocular pain and redness that worsens over days to weeks, usually with tenderness to palpation over the globe. Scleromalacia perforans, on the other hand, may be characterized by an absence of pain and erythema. The absence of these overt inflammatory symptoms is thought to be a result of severe disease, leading to tissue necrosis and subsequent loss of peripheral innervation, which leads to a paradoxical reduction of symptoms. An enlarging dark patch without erythema on the sclera is concerning for scleromalacia perforans, which is predominantly seen in elderly female patients with long-standing RA.

3.7 CLINICAL SIGNS

3.7.1 Diffuse Anterior Scleritis

Anterior scleritis is the most common form of scleral inflammation and tends to present bilaterally.[17] It is characterized by involvement of the anterior sclera with edema and dilation of the deep episcleral vascular plexus.[46] It may be localized to one portion of the sclera or may involve the entire anterior sclera. Corneal thinning, infiltrates, or stromal keratitis may be present, although corneal ulceration is more likely to present with necrotizing disease.[47] Slit lamp examination reveals edema

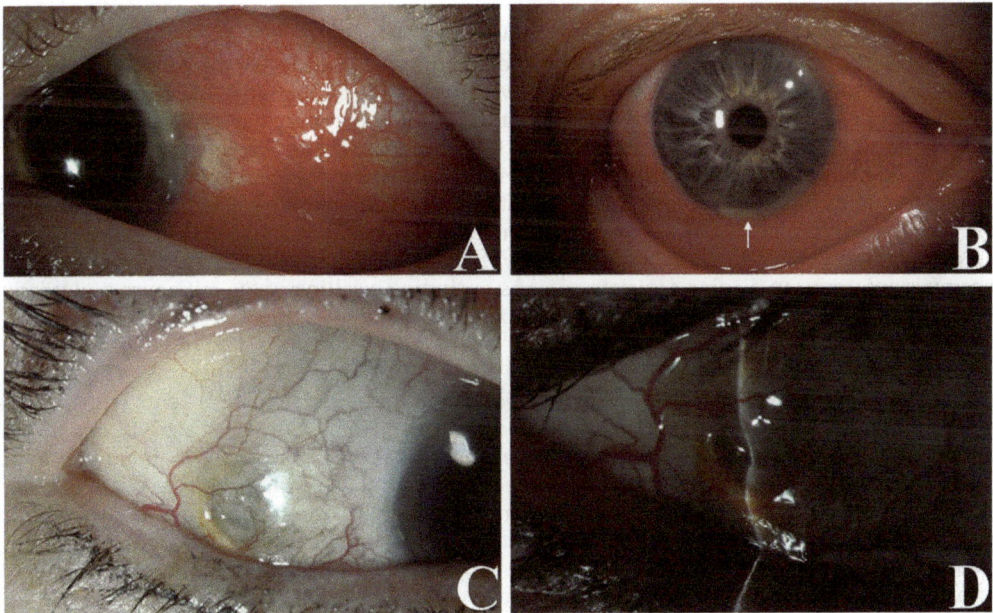

Figure 3.2 Anterior scleritis. Diffuse anterior scleritis with scleral injection that persists after instillation of topical phenylephrine (A). Sclerokeratitis (B) with associated keratitis indicated by arrow. Scleromalacia perforans (C, D): Focal patch of scleral thinning without associated eye pain or redness (C); slit beam shows degree of scleral thinning (D).

and dilated blood vessels of the sclera and episclera, giving rise to the blue-red (violaceous) color, which persists despite instillation of topical phenylephrine (Figure 3.2).

3.7.2 Nodular Anterior Scleritis

Nodular anterior scleritis is characterized by a localized area of edema in the sclera, which results in distinct nodules. It is more likely to present unilaterally compared to diffuse anterior scleritis. The nodules can be singular or multiple, are usually immobile, and are tender to palpation. However, there is no evidence of capillary closure or scleral necrosis.[22] It is considered intermediate in severity between diffuse scleritis and necrotizing disease.[48]

3.7.3 Necrotizing Anterior Scleritis

Necrotizing anterior scleritis is the most severe form of scleral inflammation and may lead to permanent vision loss.[48] The involvement of the sclera is characterized by vasculitis and closure of the episcleral vascular network, which results in visible areas of capillary non-perfusion, which is evident during ocular examination (slit lamp examination and ophthalmoscopy). Infarction and tissue necrosis of the affected sclera is also present.[22] Necrosis can range from subtle to obvious and may be localized or generalized. It can advance rapidly, potentially exposing the choroid. Often, the inflammation extends to affect the cornea, the ciliary body, and the trabecular meshwork, leading to peripheral ulcerative keratitis, anterior uveitis, and elevated intraocular pressure.[49] This elevated pressure may contribute to the formation of a staphyloma, or an outpouching in the wall of the globe.

3.7.4 Necrotizing Anterior Scleritis without Inflammation (Scleromalacia Perforans)

Scleromalacia perforans has become an exceedingly rare variant of necrotizing anterior scleritis. It results from an obliterative arteritis affecting the deep episcleral vascular plexus.[50, 51] It does not manifest with the typical signs or symptoms of necrotizing scleritis described earlier. It may be asymptomatic or cause blurred vision due to significant astigmatism from scleral thinning. The sclera can take on a parchment-white appearance and become avascular and thinned (Figure 3.2). If intraocular pressure increases, there may be exposure of the choroid and formation of a staphyloma. There is typically no involvement of the cornea except for limited peripheral corneal thinning.[22] Scleromalacia perforans most commonly occurs in older female patients with long-standing RA.

3.7.5 Posterior Scleritis

Posterior scleritis is characterized by inflammation behind the insertion of the rectus muscles. The clinical presentation of posterior scleritis can be variable and therefore may pose a diagnostic challenge. Posterior scleritis may be an isolated diagnosis, or it may occur in association with anterior scleritis, which is seen in about a third of patients. Pain is usually a presenting feature, and blurry vision is common. In those with associated anterior scleritis, the eye may be red. When posterior scleritis occurs in isolation, the eye may be white. Ocular ultrasound remains the primary diagnostic tool for identifying thickening of the sclero-choroidal complex (typically exceeding 1.7 mm) and demonstrating the pathognomonic T sign (Figure 3.3). The posterior segment may be normal in appearance, or it can display a variety of signs, including swelling of the optic nerve, exudative retinal detachment, choroidal folds, and/or choroidal detachment.

3.7.6 Workup in Patients with Scleritis

History, along with physical examination, is important in the assessment of patients with scleritis. In patients with known RA, the physical exam should include assessing for activity of articular disease, including evaluating for tender and swollen joints as well as range of motion of all upper and lower extremity joints. Since scleritis is more common in those with seropositive RA, in whom extra-articular manifestations are more common, special attention must be paid to the presence or absence of other extra-articular manifestations (such as rheumatoid nodules, interstitial lung disease, vasculitis, etc.). In patients presenting with scleritis without known systemic rheumatic disease, the evaluation consists of blood tests to evaluate for underlying systemic disease and inflammation. Autoimmune serologies, such as rheumatoid factor (RF), anti-CCP antibody, antinuclear antibodies (ANA), and antineutrophil cytoplasmic antibodies (ANCA), should be checked if there is suspicion for an underlying systemic autoimmune disease such as RA, SLE, and ANCA-associated vasculitis.[22, 52–56] Acute phase reactants, such as sedimentation rate (ESR) and C-reactive protein (CRP), may be elevated in those with underlying systemic disease and should be checked.

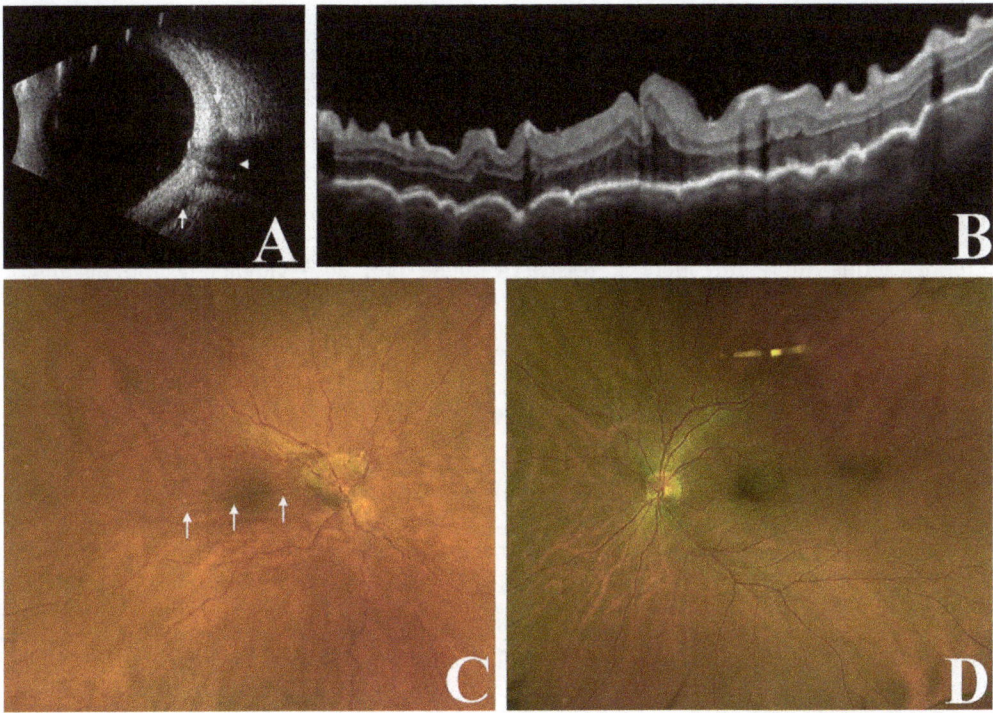

Figure 3.3 Posterior scleritis. Ultrasound showing sclero-choroidal complex thickening and T sign produced by fluid in the subtenon's space (arrows) and shadow of optic nerve head (arrowhead) (A). Choroidal folds on optical coherence tomography (B). Fundus imaging showing optic disc edema and choroidal folds (arrows indicate a prominent choroidal fold) in affected eye (C) compared to unaffected fellow eye (D).

There is a lack of evidence-based data for most laboratory tests, which often rely on clinical judgment after a thorough review of systems and physical examination. Regardless, due to the potential life-threatening complications of systemic vasculitis, all patients with scleritis should be screened for vasculitis, most often with ANCA serologies.[15] In patients with suspicion of an infectious cause of scleritis, additional testing may include rapid plasma regain (RPR), fluorescent treponemal antibody absorption test (FTA-ABS), Quantiferon-TB, and Lyme disease serologies.[52]

Imaging modalities including B-scan ultrasonography of the posterior pole can be used to confirm scleral thickening in a patient with suspected posterior scleritis.[53] Cross-sectional imaging, such as orbital computed tomography (CT) and magnetic resonance imaging (MRI), may be used to rule out alternative diagnoses or if B-scan is not conclusive. Biopsy is not typically required.

3.7.7 Course and Prognosis

Scleritis has a high likelihood for causing disease-associated morbidity. Caimmi and co-authors found that RA patients with scleritis were more symptomatic than those with episcleritis and uveitis. Patients with scleritis also often required systemic therapy, with longer time to resolution and more severe ocular sequelae compared to episcleritis.[57] Additional studies have reported similar outcomes, with a higher frequency of ocular complications in patients with scleritis compared to patients with episcleritis. In a case series of both scleritis and episcleritis at a tertiary care center, nearly 60% of patients with scleritis developed an ocular complication, compared with only 13.5% of patients with episcleritis. No patients with episcleritis had a decrease in visual acuity, compared to 15.9% of patients with scleritis. Of the subtypes of scleritis, necrotizing scleritis and posterior scleritis were more often associated with ocular complications, occurring in 91.7% and 85.7% of cases, respectively, compared to diffuse anterior scleritis and nodular anterior scleritis.[18] A US ocular registry study reported that certain demographic and clinical characteristics, such as older age, Black race, Hispanic ethnicity, and active and former smoking, as well as certain scleritis subtypes, all increased the risk of poor vision.[27] Tertiary care patients with scleritis and systemic autoimmune conditions including rheumatoid arthritis have been reported to more frequently lose vision and require treatment with steroid-sparing immunosuppressants than those with idiopathic disease.[21, 31]

3.7.8 Management

Treatment of scleritis depends on the severity of disease, extent of ocular inflammation, and presence of a systemic underlying disease. In general, patients with necrotizing anterior scleritis or posterior scleritis will require more aggressive treatment than those with non-necrotizing anterior scleritis.[18, 58] Patients with vision loss, optic nerve involvement, or a systemic inflammatory disease typically require a more intensive treatment approach as well.[58] In patients in whom an underlying systemic autoimmune disease is identified, systemic therapies are tailored to address systemic disease as well as treat the ocular inflammation.

3.8 TOPICAL CORTICOSTEROIDS

Topical corticosteroids alone often are insufficient for scleritis, as treatment of scleritis typically requires systemic therapy. Topical corticosteroids may be used as monotherapy in mild cases or in combination with oral NSAIDs, particularly for non-necrotizing anterior scleritis. However, several studies report limited success with corticosteroid eye drops alone. In a case series of non-necrotizing anterior scleritis, topical therapy with prednisolone acetate 1% led to scleritis resolution in only 47% of patients.[58] In another study, only 14.3% of patients with nodular anterior scleritis responded to topical corticosteroid monotherapy, and no cases of diffuse anterior scleritis or necrotizing scleritis responded.[18] Difluprednate 0.05%, another topical corticosteroid, has been shown to be more effective than prednisolone acetate 1%. Difluprednate is a difluorinated prednisolone derivative, and the fluorination enhances drug penetration, making it twice as potent as prednisolone acetate 1%.[59] One study noted that treatment with difluprednate alone resulted in clinical resolution of anterior scleritis in 83% of their patients, with median time to resolution of 6 weeks.[59] Patients with nodular anterior scleritis had a greater chance of resolution than those with diffuse anterior scleritis. In this study, however, there were fewer patients with an underlying systemic disease.

Most patients with scleritis and underlying rheumatic disease will require more aggressive therapy than topical corticosteroids, either to treat scleritis more effectively or to treat the underlying systemic inflammatory disease. One study showed that the addition of topical difluprednate 0.05% to systemic therapies achieved good results in patients with scleritis and a systemic inflammatory disease.[60] In this study, difluprednate was added to immunosuppressants in 65% of patients, to prednisone in 43% of patients, and NSAIDs in 25% of patients and resulted in clinical resolution of scleritis in 79.6% of patients. The median time to scleritis inactivity was 9 weeks. The results of this study support the idea that addition of difluprednate to systemic therapies is a reasonable treatment option, although monitoring of intraocular pressure for steroid-induced elevation is required.[59, 60]

3.9 ORAL NSAIDs

Oral NSAIDs can be effective monotherapy for the treatment of anterior scleritis (both diffuse and nodular subtypes) and classically are recommended as initial therapy. Jabs and colleagues found that 57% of patients with nodular anterior scleritis and 33% of patients with diffuse anterior scleritis responded to oral non-steroidal anti-inflammatory drugs.[18] Successful response to NSAIDs was associated with non-necrotizing anterior scleritis with a low degree of scleral inflammation and lack of ocular complications. Oral indomethacin, given at a dose of 25 to 75 mg three times daily, is effective, and the median duration of indomethacin treatment was 7.5 weeks. NSAIDs should ideally be continued until scleral inflammation resolves.

Data are limited, however, regarding choice of a specific NSAID over another. In clinical practice, the treatment decision is often based upon availability and side effect profile. Commonly used NSAIDs include indomethacin, ibuprofen, naproxen, piroxicam, and celecoxib.[18, 52, 61] One study found that control of scleral inflammation was achieved in 78% to 81% of scleritis patients after NSAID use and that nonselective (e.g., indomethacin, ibuprofen) and selective (e.g., celecoxib) COX inhibitors were equally efficacious.[62] In the US, ibuprofen and naproxen are available without prescription, which may allow for easier access to these medications. Co-morbidities should be considered with NSAID use, particularly in higher-risk patients with renal dysfunction or heart failure and in the elderly. The utilization of NSAIDs may be restricted by potential adverse effects and treatment ineffectiveness, particularly in patients with a high degree of scleral inflammation.

3.10 GLUCOCORTICOIDS

Systemic glucocorticoids are typically used for non-necrotizing anterior scleritis (both diffuse and nodular subtypes) after failure of oral NSAID therapy and as initial treatment for necrotizing anterior scleritis and posterior scleritis. Often, a starting dose of oral prednisone 1 mg/kg/day up to a dose of 60 to 80 mg daily is used.[63] Therapy is usually continued until the disease reaches quiescence for 1 month, after which glucocorticoids are tapered according to an individualized approach. The median duration of steroid therapy, based on one study, was estimated to be around 44 weeks. If patients do not demonstrate an appreciable improvement within 4 to 6 weeks, then an additional immunosuppressive medication may be added.[18, 63]

3.11 IMMUNOSUPPRESSIVE AGENTS

Immunosuppressants are typically considered for severe scleritis, refractory disease (when treatment with oral corticosteroids fail), or disease that recurs while tapering oral corticosteroids. Immunosuppressants may also be considered if steroid-sparing therapy is needed to minimize side effects of systemic corticosteroids.[64] Necrotizing scleritis most often required use of systemic immunosuppressive agents to reach quiescence, with 70% being reported in one study. In the same study, posterior scleritis was treated most often with oral corticosteroids (83.3%) and less commonly with immunosuppressive drugs (16.7%). There are no randomized controlled trials in scleritis regarding choice of specific immunosuppressants. For patients with idiopathic noninfectious scleritis, first-line therapies include antimetabolites such as methotrexate, with alternatives including azathioprine and mycophenolate mofetil. In patients with necrotizing scleritis, more aggressive immunosuppression such as TNF inhibitors, rituximab, or cyclophosphamide is usually required. In patients in whom an underlying systemic autoimmune disease is identified, systemic therapies are selected to address systemic disease in addition to scleritis. For rheumatoid arthritis patients, this will often include methotrexate, TNF inhibitors, and rituximab as potential therapeutics.

Methotrexate has been shown to control scleral inflammation with minimal side effects and achieve steroid-sparing results. A study by Gangaputra et al. included patients with ocular inflammatory diseases, of which 56 patients had scleritis. In this study, methotrexate was shown to lead to resolution of ocular inflammation in 56.4% of those with scleritis. Methotrexate was also shown to have corticosteroid-sparing success, defined as disease quiescence at a dose of 10 mg/day of prednisone or lower within 6 months, in 37.3% of patients.[18, 65] Other smaller studies also have evaluated the efficacy of methotrexate therapy for scleritis. A retrospective study of 17 patients on methotrexate showed that 61.9% had resolution of scleral inflammation at 3 months, and 90.5% had resolution at 12 months.[66] Therefore, methotrexate is generally recommended as first-line steroid-sparing therapy in the treatment of scleritis.

Mycophenolate mofetil, another antimetabolite, also has been used with variable efficacy.[67, 68] Daniel et al. evaluated the efficacy of mycophenolate mofetil in the treatment of patients with ocular inflammatory diseases, of which 33 had scleritis. In those with scleritis, 49% had an adequate treatment response within 6 months, and 25.5% achieved steroid-sparing success.[69] Several smaller studies have also reported successful treatment of scleritis with mycophenolate therapy.[57, 70, 71] Other studies, however, have demonstrated that mycophenolate may be less efficacious for scleritis, with lower rates of resolution of inflammation and increased likelihood of relapse. One of these studies included 85 patients with ocular inflammatory disease treated with mycophenolate after failure of methotrexate and concluded that the odds of inflammation control were lower for patients with scleritis compared to patients with other types of ocular inflammation (such as uveitis).[72] Another study of posterior scleritis patients found that mycophenolate use was associated with accelerated time to relapse.[73] Similarly, Sen and colleagues found that mycophenolate was more useful as a steroid-sparing agent in patients with controlled scleritis as maintenance therapy and not as effective in patients with active scleral inflammation requiring up titration of immunosuppression.[54, 67] Azathioprine, an anti-metabolite prodrug of 6-mercaptopurine, also has been shown to be somewhat effective, with complete control of inflammation in 20% of scleritis patients after 6 months of therapy, with ability to achieve steroid-sparing effect in 22% of patients.[74] Though less studied than methotrexate and mycophenolate, azathioprine has been shown to be beneficial in multiple other studies.[35, 75, 76]

For patients with rheumatoid arthritis, it is important to consider disease activity of the joints, as methotrexate is superior to both mycophenolate and azathioprine for control of joint disease and is the first-line treatment for articular disease in RA. Therefore, methotrexate is preferred in patients with active joint disease as well as scleritis. Mycophenolate is not effective for articular disease, and azathioprine is less effective. However, these agents may be considered in patients with scleritis when methotrexate is not effective or not tolerated.

Generally, antimetabolites are chosen as initial immunosuppressive therapy in the setting of scleritis, with subsequent transition to other agents based on disease activity, side effects, and medication toxicities. Tumor necrosis factor (TNF)-alpha inhibitors, such as infliximab and adalimumab, may be considered after antimetabolic agents in those with treatment-resistant scleritis. It is important to know that TNF inhibitors are also effective for active articular disease in RA. Several studies have examined infliximab, a chimeric human/murine monoclonal antibody to human TNFα, with good results in treatment-refractory cases.[77-79] In a small prospective study, 80% of patients with active anterior scleritis achieved quiescence on infliximab therapy, and 60% were able to successfully taper oral prednisone to < 10 mg daily.[78] Similarly, two small retrospective studies found a favorable clinical response to infliximab in all patients with refractory scleritis.[77, 79]

Evidence also supports the use of adalimumab for refractory noninfectious scleritis. A retrospective study of nine patients per group found that adalimumab plus conventional therapy (consisting of systemic glucocorticoids and other immunosuppressants) shortened time to remission, reduced flares of scleritis, and accelerated glucocorticoid withdrawal compared to conventional therapy alone.[80] Similarly, a larger retrospective study also found that adalimumab is effective for the treatment of scleritis with significant corticosteroid-sparing effect.[81] Some case reports and retrospective studies suggest that infliximab and adalimumab are superior to etanercept, which is a soluble TNF receptor fusion protein, for the treatment of scleritis. One study reported six cases in which etanercept was used for scleritis treatment, where three patients failed to improve and three had flares of scleritis during its use.[82, 83] More data is available regarding the use of infliximab and adalimumab, and these agents should be considered in the treatment algorithm for refractory cases and in systemic disease states with increased TNFα activity such as RA.

Rituximab and cyclophosphamide have both been used for refractory and severe cases of scleritis. A phase I/II randomized control trial including patients with refractory scleritis, including those with scleritis secondary to ANCA-associated vasculitis and rheumatoid arthritis, found that rituximab was effective in 75% of cases.[84] Rituximab has also been well studied and shown to be effective for articular disease from rheumatoid arthritis. Several randomized control trials demonstrate that rituximab is efficacious for achieving disease control in RA patients with active joint disease who fail to respond to other immunosuppressants.[84-87] Case reports also demonstrate its effectiveness for treatment of scleritis in those with underlying RA.[88] Therefore, rituximab may be considered in cases of refractory scleritis and patients with active joint disease from RA.

Cyclophosphamide, an alkylating agent, may be considered if there is lack of response to rituximab. One large retrospective study of patients with ocular inflammatory diseases, including 22.3% with scleritis, found that 53.3% of those with scleritis achieved complete control of inflammation, with steroid-sparing effect.[89] However, the use of cyclophosphamide is usually limited by toxicity and side effect profile. When cyclophosphamide is used, it should be used for a short period (3–6 months), after which it is replaced by an antimetabolite (such as methotrexate, azathioprine, or mycophenolate mofetil) for maintenance therapy.[22]

3.12 DURATION OF THERAPY

The duration of immunosuppression is not standardized due to the lack of studies that address the optimal duration of treatment. Usually, attempts to taper immunosuppression begin after disease quiescence is achieved for a sustained period (typically at least 12 months). For those with necrotizing scleritis, treatment may be extended for a longer period. A retrospective cohort study at four subspecialty centers found that 29.1% of patients were able to achieve disease remission, defined as lack of disease activity off systemic immunosuppressants, but that median time to remission of scleritis was 7.8 years. In this study, factors predictive of less remission of scleritis included bilateral disease and diagnosis of underlying inflammatory disease, specifically RA and GPA.[90] These results suggest that patients with underlying rheumatic disease may require a longer course of therapy, as remission is less frequently achieved when systemic inflammatory diseases are present.

3.13 PERIPHERAL ULCERATIVE KERATITIS

3.13.1 Introduction

Peripheral ulcerative keratitis (PUK) is a rare but vision-threatening ocular inflammatory disease that involves peripheral corneal thinning.[91] Disease control almost invariably requires systemic immunomodulatory treatment. PUK often occurs in patients with systemic autoimmune disease, particularly RA, and its presence may portend poor systemic disease outcomes.

3.13.1.1 Epidemiology

A population-based UK study reported the incidence of PUK to be 3.01 per million persons per year.[92] Rheumatoid arthritis is the most commonly associated systemic autoimmune disease, with 34% to 78% of PUK patients also having a diagnosis of rheumatoid arthritis.[47, 93] In a study of 34 patients with PUK refractory to conventional immunosuppressive medications, 20 (59%) also had rheumatoid arthritis.[94]

3.13.1.2 Pathophysiology

The underlying pathogenic mechanism in PUK is thought to be an imbalance between matrix metalloproteinases and tissue inhibitors of the matrix metalloproteinases in the corneal stroma.[95] The matrix metalloproteinases act as collagenases, so tipping the balance toward the matrix metalloproteinases, as is hypothesized to occur in PUK, may lead to degradation of the collagen-rich corneal stroma. Although the exact mechanisms are unknown, differences in corneal extracellular matrix arrangement, innervation, and vascularity between peripheral and central cornea may contribute to the predilection of PUK for peripheral cornea. While the central cornea is avascular, the peripheral cornea receives vascular supply from perilimbal capillaries, which may preferentially expose the peripheral cornea to inflammatory mediators and cells. Cellular and humoral immunity both are implicated in PUK pathogenesis.

3.13.1.3 Clinical Course and Prognosis

Symptoms of PUK include ocular pain, tearing, photophobia, ocular redness, and decreased vision.[37] The characteristic clinical finding in PUK is a crescentic corneal ulcer along the peripheral cornea, oriented parallel to the limbus, with an associated defect in the corneal epithelium (Figure 3.4).[96] Often, there is associated localized conjunctival and/or scleral injection. If the disease process is not arrested, the peripheral corneal tissue may progressively thin, which can lead to corneal perforation, a devastating ocular complication of PUK. The incidence of corneal perforation in patients with rheumatoid arthritis is estimated to be decreasing.[97] However, visual and systemic outcomes continue to be poor in patients with RA following corneal perforation.

3.13.1.4 Management

PUK is a rare disease, so there is a lack of definitive guidelines for disease management. Once an infectious process has been ruled out, initial treatment involves high-dose systemic glucocorticoids to arrest the inflammatory process. Early use of steroid-sparing immunomodulatory therapy is associated with better clinical outcomes, including better visual acuity and lower risk of PUK recurrence.[98, 99] Additionally, systemic immunomodulatory treatment has been shown to reduce mortality in patients with RA-associated PUK.[96, 99]

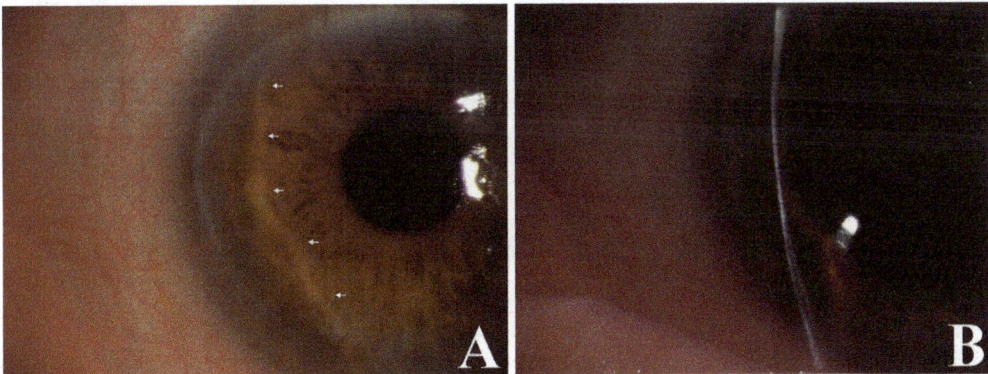

Figure 3.4 Peripheral ulcerative keratitis. Crescent-shaped peripheral corneal thinning (A) with arrows demarcating border of corneal thinning. The slit beam highlights the degree of peripheral corneal thinning (B).

Additional treatment typically includes ocular surface lubrication to promote and maintain corneal epithelial integrity as well as topical antibiotics to prevent bacterial superinfection in the setting of corneal epithelial defects. Although not an adequate substitute for systemic anti-inflammatory medication, topical cyclosporine, topical tacrolimus, and/or topical corticosteroids may help reduce inflammation in PUK.

Surgical management for active PUK is typically avoided but may be indicated in cases with impending or existing ocular perforation. Tissue adhesive and patch grafts may help maintain integrity of the globe, but complications are common following these procedures.[100–102]

3.14 RETINAL VASCULAR DISEASE

Retinal vascular disease is not a common finding associated with rheumatoid arthritis. There are rare case reports, predominantly in the older literature, describing retinal vascular findings indicative of ocular ischemia in patients with rheumatoid hyperviscosity syndrome.[103–107] Similarly, retinal vasculitis is rarely reported in patients with rheumatoid arthritis,[19, 108, 109] although subclinical retinal vascular leakage on fluorescein angiography may be more common: retinal vascular leakage was found in 18% of 60 patients with rheumatoid arthritis evaluated with fluorescein angiography.[110] However, this study was performed more than 40 years ago, so it is unclear if these findings would persist today given changes in diagnosis and management of RA. Symptoms of ocular ischemia and retinal vasculitis – including blurry vision, distorted vision, vision loss, floaters, and flashes – are nonspecific but warrant prompt ophthalmic evaluation.

3.15 SUMMARY

Rheumatoid arthritis is a chronic polyarthritis that can be complicated by scleritis, a potentially vision-threatening form of ocular inflammation. Development of a red, painful eye, acute vision changes/loss, or an enlarging blue-black scleral patch in a patient with rheumatoid arthritis warrants urgent ophthalmic consultation. Rheumatologic and ophthalmic co-management is necessary for patients with ocular manifestations of rheumatoid arthritis to ensure optimal treatment of both joint and ocular disease.

REFERENCES

1. MacGregor AJ, Snieder H, Rigby AS, et al. Characterizing the quantitative genetic contribution to rheumatoid arthritis using data from twins. *Arthritis Rheum.* 2000;43(1):30–37. doi:10.1002/1529-0131(200001)43:1<30::AID-ANR5>3.0.CO;2-B.
2. Viatte S, Plant D, Han B, et al. Association of HLA-DRB1 haplotypes with rheumatoid arthritis severity, mortality, and treatment response. *JAMA.* 2015;313(16):1645–1656. doi:10.1001/jama.2015.3435.
3. Okada Y, Wu D, Trynka G, et al. Genetics of rheumatoid arthritis contributes to biology and drug discovery. *Nature.* 2014;506(7488):376–381. doi:10.1038/nature12873.
4. Venetsanopoulou AI, Alamanos Y, Voulgari PV, et al. Epidemiology of rheumatoid arthritis: genetic and environmental influences. *Expert Rev Clin Immunol.* 2022;18(9):923–931. doi:10.1080/1744666X.2022.2106970.
5. Torrente-Segarra V, Bergstra SA, Solomon-Escoto K, et al. Is current smoking status and its relationship to anti-cyclic citrullinated peptide antibodies a predictor of worse response to biological therapies in rheumatoid arthritis patients? *Scand J Rheumatol.* 2018;47(5):360–363. doi:10.1080/03009742.2017.1418423.
6. Sparks JA. Rheumatoid arthritis. *Ann Intern Med.* 2019;170(1):ITC1–ITC16. doi:10.7326/AITC201901010.
7. Ziff M. The rheumatoid nodule. *Arthritis Rheum.* 1990;33(6):761–767. doi:10.1002/art.1780330601.
8. Conforti A, Di Cola I, Pavlych V, et al. Beyond the joints, the extra-articular manifestations in rheumatoid arthritis. *Autoimmun Rev.* 2021;20(2):102735. doi:10.1016/j.autrev.2020.102735.
9. Figus FA, Piga M, Azzolin I, et al. Rheumatoid arthritis: extra-articular manifestations and comorbidities. *Autoimmun Rev.* 2021;20(4):102776. doi:10.1016/j.autrev.2021.102776.
10. England BR, Thiele GM, Anderson DR, et al. Increased cardiovascular risk in rheumatoid arthritis: mechanisms and implications. *BMJ.* 2018;361:k1036. doi:10.1136/bmj.k1036.
11. Aletaha D, Neogi T, Silman AJ, et al. 2010 rheumatoid arthritis classification criteria: an American College of Rheumatology/European League Against Rheumatism collaborative initiative. *Arthritis Rheum.* 2010;62(9):2569–2581. doi:10.1002/art.27584.

12. Fraenkel L, Bathon JM, England BR, et al. 2021 American College of Rheumatology guideline for the treatment of rheumatoid arthritis. *Arthritis Care Res (Hoboken)*. 2021;73(7):924–939. doi:10.1002/acr.24596.
13. Turk MA, Hayworth JL, Nevskaya T, et al. Ocular manifestations in rheumatoid arthritis, connective tissue disease, and vasculitis: a systematic review and metaanalysis. *Journal of Rheumatology*. 2021;48(1):25–34. doi:10.3899/JRHEUM.190768.
14. Craig JP, Nichols KK, Akpek EK, et al. TFOS DEWS II definition and classification report. *Ocul Surf*. 2017;15(3):276–283. doi:10.1016/j.jtos.2017.05.008.
15. Wolffsohn JS, Arita R, Chalmers R, et al. TFOS DEWS II diagnostic methodology report. *Ocul Surf*. 2017;15(3):539–574. doi:10.1016/j.jtos.2017.05.001.
16. Jones L, Downie LE, Korb D, et al. TFOS DEWS II management and therapy report. *Ocul Surf*. 2017;15(3):575–628. doi:10.1016/j.jtos.2017.05.006.
17. Watson PG, Hayreh SS. Scleritis and episcleritis. *Br J Ophthalmol*. 1976;60(3):163–191. doi:10.1136/bjo.60.3.163.
18. Jabs DA, Mudun A, Dunn JP, et al. Episcleritis and scleritis: clinical features and treatment results. *Am J Ophthalmol*. 2000;130(4):469–476. doi:10.1016/s0002-9394(00)00710-8.
19. Zlatanović G, Veselinović D, Cekić S, et al. Ocular manifestation of rheumatoid arthritis-different forms and frequency. *Bosn J Basic Med Sci*. 2010;10(4):323–327. doi:10.17305/bjbms.2010.2680.
20. Whitcup SM, Sen HN. *Whitcup and Nussenblatt's uveitis fundamentals and clinic practice*, 5th edn. Elsevier Inc., 2021.
21. Wieringa WG, Wieringa JE, ten Dam-van Loon NH, et al. Visual outcome, treatment results, and prognostic factors in patients with scleritis. *Ophthalmology*. 2013;120(2):379–386. doi:10.1016/j.ophtha.2012.08.005.
22. Okhravi N, Odufuwa B, McCluskey P, et al. Scleritis. *Surv Ophthalmol*. 2005;50(4):351–363. doi:10.1016/j.survophthal.2005.04.001.
23. Braithwaite T, Adderley NJ, Subramanian A, et al. Epidemiology of scleritis in the United Kingdom from 1997 to 2018: population-based analysis of 11 million patients and association between scleritis and infectious and immune-mediated inflammatory disease. *Arthritis Rheumatol*. 2021;73(7):1267–1276. doi:10.1002/art.41709.
24. Homayounfar G, Nardone N, Borkar DS, et al. Incidence of scleritis and episcleritis: results from the Pacific ocular inflammation study. *Am J Ophthalmol*. 2013;156(4):752–758. doi:10.1016/j.ajo.2013.05.026.
25. Thong LP, Rogers S, Hart C, et al. Incidence and prevalence of episcleritis and scleritis in metropolitan Melbourne. *Invest Ophthalmol Vis Sci*. 2018;59(9):4168.
26. Daniel Diaz J, Sobol EK, Gritz DC. Treatment and management of scleral disorders. *Surv Ophthalmol*. 2016;61(6):702–717. doi:10.1016/j.survophthal.2016.06.002/.
27. Armbrust KR, Kopplin LJ. Characteristics and outcomes of patients with scleritis in the IRIS® registry (intelligent research in sight) database. *Ophthalmol Sci*. 2022;2(3):100178.
28. Vergouwen DPC, Rothova A, Berge JCT, et al. Current insights in the pathogenesis of scleritis. *Exp Eye Res*. 2020;197:108078. doi:10.1016/j.exer.2020.108078.
29. Murthy SI, Sabhapandit S, Balamurugan S, et al. Scleritis: differentiating infectious from non-infectious entities. *Indian J Ophthalmol*. 2020;68(9):1818–1828. doi:10.4103/ijo.IJO_2032_20.
30. Sainz de la Maza M, Molina N, Gonzalez-Gonzalez LA, et al. Clinical characteristics of a large cohort of patients with scleritis and episcleritis. *Ophthalmology*. 2012;119(1):43–50. doi:10.1016/j.ophtha.2011.07.013.
31. Sainz de la Maza M, Foster CS, Jabbur NS. Scleritis associated with systemic vasculitic diseases. *Ophthalmology*. 1995;102(4):687–692. doi:10.1016/s0161-6420(95)30970-0.
32. Gu J, Zhou S, Ding R, et al. Necrotizing scleritis and peripheral ulcerative keratitis associated with Wegener's granulomatosis. *Ophthalmol Ther*. 2013;2(2):99–111. doi:10.1007/s40123-013-0016-1.
33. Berkenstock MK, Carey AR. Health system wide "big data" analysis of rheumatologic conditions and scleritis. *BMC Ophthalmol*. 2021;21:14. doi:10.1186/s12886-020-01769-3.
34. Cocho L, Gonzalez-Gonzalez LA, Molina-Prat N, et al. Scleritis in patients with granulomatosis with polyangiitis (Wegener). *Br J Ophthalmol*. 2016;100(8):1062–1065. doi:10.1136/bjophthalmol-2015-307460.
35. Yoshida A, Watanabe M, Okubo A, et al. Clinical characteristics of scleritis patients with emphasized comparison of associated systemic diseases (anti-neutrophil cytoplasmic antibody-associated vasculitis and rheumatoid arthritis). *Jpn J Ophthalmol*. 2019;63(5):417–424. doi:10.1007/s10384-019-00674-7.

36. Akpek EK, Thorne JE, Qazi FA, et al. Evaluation of patients with scleritis for systemic disease. *Ophthalmology*. 2004;111(3):501–506. doi:10.1016/j.ophtha.2003.06.006.

37. Galor A, Thorne JE. Scleritis and peripheral ulcerative keratitis. *Rheum Dis Clin North Am*. 2007;33(4):835–854, vii. doi:10.1016/j.rdc.2007.08.002.

38. Wakefield D, Di Girolamo N, Thurau S, et al. Scleritis: challenges in immunopathogenesis and treatment. *Discov Med*. 2013;16(88):153–157.

39. Rao NA, Marak GE, Hidayat AA. Necrotizing scleritis: a clinico-pathologic study of 41 cases. *Ophthalmology*. 1985;92(11):1542–1549.

40. Usui Y, Parikh J, Goto H, et al. Immunopathology of necrotising scleritis. *Br J Ophthalmol*. 2008;92(3):417–419. doi:10.1136/bjo.2007.126425.

41. Fong LP, Sainz de la Maza M, Rice BA, et al. Immunopathology of scleritis. *Ophthalmology*. 1991;98(4):472–479. doi:10.1016/s0161-6420(91)32280-2.

42. Sainz de la Maza M, Foster CS. Necrotizing scleritis after ocular surgery: a clinicopathologic study. *Ophthalmology*. 1991;98(11):1720–1726. doi:10.1016/s0161-6420(91)32062-1.

43. Díaz-Valle D, Benítez del Castillo JM, Castillo A, et al. Immunologic and clinical evaluation of postsurgical necrotizing sclerocorneal ulceration. *Cornea*. 1998;17(4):371–375. doi:10.1097/00003226-199807000-00005.

44. Seo KY, Lee HK, Kim EK, et al. Expression of tumor necrosis factor alpha and matrix metalloproteinase-9 in surgically induced necrotizing scleritis. *Ophthalmic Res*. 2006;38(2):66–70. doi:10.1159/000090010.

45. Sims J. Scleritis: presentations, disease associations and management. *Postgrad Med J*. 2012;88(1046):713–718. doi:10.1136/postgradmedj-2011-130282.

46. Wilhelmus KR, Grierson I, Watson PG. Histopathologic and clinical associations of scleritis and glaucoma. *Am J Ophthalmol*. 1981;91(6):697–705. doi:10.1016/0002-9394(81)90001-5.

47. Sainz de la Maza M, Foster CS, Jabbur NS, et al. Ocular characteristics and disease associations in scleritis-associated peripheral keratopathy. *Arch Ophthalmol*. 2002;120(1):15–19. doi:10.1001/archopht.120.1.15.

48. Tuft SJ, Watson PG. Progression of scleral disease. *Ophthalmology*. 1991;98(4):467–471. doi:10.1016/s0161-6420(91)32269-3.

49. Sainz de la Maza M, Jabbur NS, Foster CS. Severity of scleritis and episcleritis. *Ophthalmology*. 1994;101(2):389–396. doi:10.1016/s0161-6420(94)31325-x.

50. Ellis OH, Holtz MJ. Scleromalacia perforans. *Calif Med*. 1953;78(1):60–63.

51. Mader TH, Stulting RD, Crosswell HH. Bilateral paralimbal scleromalacia perforans. *Am J Ophthalmol*. 1990;109(2):233–234. doi:10.1016/s0002-9394(14)75998-7.

52. Lagina A, Ramphul K. Scleritis. In: *StatPearls [Internet]*. StatPearls Publishing, 2023. https://www.ncbi.nlm.nih.gov/books/NBK499944/. Accessed 12 Oct. 2023.

53. Benson WE. Posterior scleritis. *Survey of Ophthalmology*. 1988;32(5):297–316. doi:10.1016/0039-6257(88)90093-8.

54. Benson WE, Shields JA, Tasman W, et al. Posterior scleritis: a cause of diagnostic confusion. *Arch Ophthalmol*. 1979;97(8):1482–1486. doi:10.1001/archopht.1979.01020020144012.

55. Sainz de la Maza M, Foster CS, Jabbur NS. Scleritis associated with rheumatoid arthritis and with other systemic immune-mediated diseases. *Ophthalmology*. 1994;101(7):1281–1286; discussion 1287–1288.

56. Maleki A, Ruggeri M, Colombo A, et al. B-scan ultrasonography findings in unilateral posterior scleritis. *J Curr Ophthalmol*. 2022;34(1):93–99. doi:10.4103/joco.joco_267_21.

57. Caimmi C, Crowson CS, Smith WM, et al. Clinical correlates, outcomes, and predictors of inflammatory ocular disease associated with rheumatoid arthritis in the biologic era. *J Rheumatol*. 2018;45(5):595–603. doi:10.3899/jrheum.170437.

58. McMullen M, Kovarik G, Hodge WG. Use of topical steroid therapy in the management of non-necrotizing anterior scleritis. *Can J Ophthalmol*. 1999;34(4):217–221.

59. Liberman P, Burkholder BM, Thorne JE, et al. Effectiveness of difluprednate for the treatment of anterior scleritis. *Am J Ophthalmol*. 2022;235:172–177. doi:10.1016/j.ajo.2021.09.008.

60. Liberman P, Thorne J, Burkholder B, et al. Effectiveness of difluprednate in addition to systemic therapy for the treatment of anterior scleritis. *Br J Ophthalmol*. Published online 2023 Sept. 4. doi:10.1136/bjo-2022-322841.

61. Sainz de la Maza M, Molina N, Gonzalez-Gonzalez LA, et al. Scleritis therapy. *Ophthalmology*. 2012;119(1):51–58. doi:10.1016/j.ophtha.2011.07.043.

62. Kolomeyer AM, Ragam A, Shah K, et al. Cyclo-oxygenase inhibitors in the treatment of chronic non-infectious, non-necrotizing scleritis and episcleritis. *Ocul Immunol Inflamm.* 2012;20(4):293–299. doi:10.3109/09273948.2012.689075.

63. Jabs DA. Treatment of ocular inflammation. *Ocul Immunol Inflamm.* 2004;12(3):163–168. doi:10.1080/09273940490883671.

64. Albini TA, Rao NA, Smith RE. The diagnosis and management of anterior scleritis. *Int Ophthalmol Clin.* 2005;45(2):191–204. doi:10.1097/01.iio.0000155900.64809.b2.

65. Gangaputra S, Newcomb CW, Liesegang TL, et al. Methotrexate for ocular inflammatory diseases. *Ophthalmology.* 2009;116(11):2188–98.e1. doi:10.1016/j.ophtha.2009.04.020.

66. Sands DS, Chan SCY, Gottlieb CC. Methotrexate for the treatment of noninfectious scleritis. *Can J Ophthalmol.* 2018;53(4):349–353. doi:10.1016/j.jcjo.2017.11.009.

67. Sen HN, Suhler EB, Al-Khatib SQ, et al. Mycophenolate mofetil for the treatment of scleritis. *Ophthalmology.* 2003;110(9):1750–1755. doi:10.1016/S0161-6420(03)00570-0.

68. Thorne JE, Jabs DA, Qazi FA, et al. Mycophenolate mofetil therapy for inflammatory eye disease. *Ophthalmology.* 2005;112(8):1472–1477. doi:10.1016/j.ophtha.2005.02.020.

69. Daniel E, Thorne JE, Newcomb CW, et al. Mycophenolate mofetil for ocular inflammation. *Am J Ophthalmol.* 2010;149(3):423–432.e1–e2. doi:10.1016/j.ajo.2009.09.026.

70. Kolomeyer AM, Ragam A, Shah K, et al. Mycophenolate mofetil in the treatment of chronic non-infectious, non-necrotizing scleritis. *Ocul Immunol Inflamm.* 2012;20(2):113–118. doi:10.3109/09273948.2012.655398.

71. Hwang YS, Chen HCJ, Chen KJ, et al. Enteric-coated mycophenolate sodium as a corticosteroid-sparing agent for the treatment of autoimmune scleritis. *Cornea.* 2011;30(3):260–264. doi:10.1097/ICO.0b013e3181e9af18.

72. Sobrin L, Christen W, Foster CS. Mycophenolate mofetil after methotrexate failure or intolerance in the treatment of scleritis and uveitis. *Ophthalmology.* 2008;115(8):1416–1421.e1. doi:10.1016/j.ophtha.2007.12.011.

73. Lavric A, Gonzalez-Lopez JJ, Majumder PD, et al. Posterior scleritis: analysis of epidemiology, clinical factors, and risk of recurrence in a cohort of 114 patients. *Ocul Immunol Inflamm.* 2016;24(1):6–15. doi:10.3109/09273948.2015.1005240.

74. Pasadhika S, Kempen JH, Newcomb CW, et al. Azathioprine for ocular inflammatory diseases. *Am J Ophthalmol.* 2009;148(4):500–509.e2. doi:10.1016/j.ajo.2009.05.008.

75. Kumar A, Ghose A, Biswas J, et al. Clinical profile of patients with posterior scleritis: a report from Eastern India. *Indian J Ophthalmol.* 2018;66(8):1109–1112. doi:10.4103/ijo.IJO_121_18.

76. Sainz-de-la-Maza M, Molina N, Gonzalez-Gonzalez LA, et al. Scleritis associated with relapsing polychondritis. *Br J Ophthalmol.* 2016;100(9):1290–1294. doi:10.1136/bjophthalmol-2015-306902.

77. Ahn SJ, Oh JY, Kim MK, et al. Treating refractory scleritis with infliximab. *Jpn J Ophthalmol.* 2009;53(3):286–287. doi:10.1007/s10384-008-0652-5.

78. Sen HN, Sangave A, Hammel K, et al. Infliximab for the treatment of active scleritis. *Can J Ophthalmol.* 2009;44(3):e9–e12. doi:10.3129/i09-061.

79. Doctor P, Sultan A, Syed S, et al. Infliximab for the treatment of refractory scleritis. *Br J Ophthalmol.* 2010;94(5):579–583. doi:10.1136/bjo.2008.150961.

80. Chen B, Yang S, Zhu L, et al. Adalimumab plus conventional therapy versus conventional therapy in refractory non-infectious scleritis. *J Clin Med.* 2022;11(22):6686. doi:10.3390/jcm11226686.

81. Brown JE, Thomas AS, Armbrust KR, et al. Therapeutic outcomes of non-infectious scleritis treated with tumor necrosis factor-alpha inhibitors. *Ocul Immunol Inflamm.* Published online 2023 Apr. 12:1–7. doi:10.1080/09273948.2023.2191712.

82. Smith JR, Levinson RD, Holland GN, et al. Differential efficacy of tumor necrosis factor inhibition in the management of inflammatory eye disease and associated rheumatic disease. *Arthritis Rheum.* 2001;45(3):252–257. doi:10.1002/1529-0131(200106)45:3<252::AID-ART257>3.0.CO;2-5.

83. Gaujoux-Viala C, Giampietro C, Gaujoux T, et al. Scleritis: a paradoxical effect of etanercept? Etanercept-associated inflammatory eye disease. *J Rheumatol.* 2012;39(2):233–239. doi:10.3899/jrheum.110865.

84. Suhler EB, Lim LL, Beardsley RM, et al. Rituximab therapy for refractory scleritis: results of a phase I/II dose-ranging, randomized, clinical trial. *Ophthalmology.* 2014;121(10):1885–1891. doi:10.1016/j.ophtha.2014.04.044.

85. Rubbert-Roth A, Tak PP, Zerbini C, et al. Efficacy and safety of various repeat treatment dosing regimens of rituximab in patients with active rheumatoid arthritis: results of a phase

III randomized study (MIRROR). *Rheumatology (Oxford)*. 2010;49(9):1683–1693. doi:10.1093/rheumatology/keq116.

86. Cohen SB, Emery P, Greenwald MW, et al. Rituximab for rheumatoid arthritis refractory to anti-tumor necrosis factor therapy: results of a multicenter, randomized, double-blind, placebo-controlled, phase III trial evaluating primary efficacy and safety at twenty-four weeks. *Arthritis Rheum*. 2006;54(9):2793–2806. doi:10.1002/art.22025.

87. Mease PJ, Cohen S, Gaylis NB, et al. Efficacy and safety of retreatment in patients with rheumatoid arthritis with previous inadequate response to tumor necrosis factor inhibitors: results from the SUNRISE trial. *J Rheumatol*. 2010;37(5):917–927. doi:10.3899/jrheum.090442.

88. Iaccheri B, Androudi S, Bocci EB, et al. Rituximab treatment for persistent scleritis associated with rheumatoid arthritis. *Ocul Immunol Inflamm*. 2010;18(3):223–225. doi:10.3109/09273941003739928.

89. Pujari SS, Kempen JH, Newcomb CW, et al. Cyclophosphamide for ocular inflammatory diseases. *Ophthalmology*. 2010;117(2):356–365. doi:10.1016/j.ophtha.2009.06.060.

90. Kempen JH, Pistilli M, Begum H, et al. Remission of non-infectious anterior scleritis: incidence and predictive factors. *Am J Ophthalmol*. 2021;223:377–395. doi:10.1016/j.ajo.2019.03.024.

91. Gupta Y, Kishore A, Kumari P, et al. Peripheral ulcerative keratitis. *Surv Ophthalmol*. 2021;66(6):977–998. doi:10.1016/j.survophthal.2021.02.013.

92. McKibbin M, Isaacs JD, Morrell AJ. Incidence of corneal melting in association with systemic disease in the Yorkshire Region, 1995–7. *Br J Ophthalmol*. 1999;83(8):941–943. doi:10.1136/bjo.83.8.941.

93. Tauber J, Sainz de la Maza M, Hoang-Xuan T, et al. An analysis of therapeutic decision making regarding immunosuppressive chemotherapy for peripheral ulcerative keratitis. *Cornea*. 1990;9(1):66–73.

94. Dominguez-Casas LC, Sánchez-Bilbao L, Calvo-Río V, et al. Biologic therapy in severe and refractory peripheral ulcerative keratitis (PUK): multicenter study of 34 patients. *Semin Arthritis Rheum*. 2020;50(4):608–615. doi:10.1016/j.semarthrit.2020.03.023.

95. Gupta Y, Kishore A, Kumari P, et al. Peripheral ulcerative keratitis. *Surv Ophthalmol*. 2021;66(6):977–998. doi:10.1016/j.survophthal.2021.02.013.

96. Foster CS, Forstot SL, Wilson LA. Mortality rate in rheumatoid arthritis patients developing necrotizing scleritis or peripheral ulcerative keratitis: effects of systemic immunosuppression. *Ophthalmology*. 1984;91(10):1253–1263. doi:10.1016/s0161-6420(84)34160-4.

97. Timlin HM, Hall HN, Foot B, et al. Corneal perforation from peripheral ulcerative keratopathy in patients with rheumatoid arthritis: epidemiological findings of the British ophthalmological surveillance unit. *Br J Ophthalmol*. 2018;102(9):1298–1302. doi:10.1136/bjophthalmol-2017-310671.

98. Ruiz-Lozano RE, Ramos-Davila EM, Garza-Garza LA, et al. Rheumatoid arthritis-associated peripheral ulcerative keratitis outcomes after early immunosuppressive therapy. *Br J Ophthalmol*. 2023;107(9):1246–1252. doi:10.1136/bjophthalmol-2022-321132.

99. Ogra S, Sims JL, McGhee CNJ, et al. Ocular complications and mortality in peripheral ulcerative keratitis and necrotising scleritis: the role of systemic immunosuppression. *Clin Exp Ophthalmol*. 2020;48(4):434–441. doi:10.1111/ceo.13709.

100. Bernauer W, Ficker LA, Watson PG, et al. The management of corneal perforations associated with rheumatoid arthritis: an analysis of 32 eyes. *Ophthalmology*. 1995;102(9):1325–1337. doi:10.1016/s0161-6420(95)30867-6.

101. Pleyer U, Bertelmann E, Rieck P, et al. Outcome of penetrating keratoplasty in rheumatoid arthritis. *Ophthalmologica*. 2002;216(4):249–255. doi:10.1159/000063847.

102. Sabhapandit S, Murthy SI, Sharma N, et al. Surgical management of peripheral ulcerative keratitis: update on surgical techniques and their outcome. *Clin Ophthalmol (Auckland, NZ)*. 2022;16:3547–3557. doi:10.2147/OPTH.S385782.

103. Pope RM, Fletcher MA, Mamby A, et al. Rheumatoid arthritis associated with hyperviscosity syndrome and intermediate complex formation. *Arch Intern Med*. 1975;135(2):281–285. doi:10.1001/archinte.1975.00330020085011.

104. Sarnat RL, Jampol LM. Hyperviscosity retinopathy secondary to polyclonal gammopathy in a patient with rheumatoid arthritis. *Ophthalmology*. 1986;93(1):124–127. doi:10.1016/s0161-6420(86)33782-5.

105. Rezai KA, Patel SC, Eliott D, et al. Rheumatoid hyperviscosity syndrome: reversibility of microvascular abnormalities after treatment. *Am J Ophthalmol*. 2002;134(1):130–132. doi:10.1016/s0002-9394(02)01504-0.

106. Zakzook SI, Yunus MB, Mulconrey DS. Hyperviscosity syndrome in rheumatoid arthritis with Felty's syndrome: case report and review of the literature. *Clin. Rheumatol.* 2002;21(1):82–85. doi:10.1007/s100670200020.
107. Miller JB, Baer AN. Hyperviscosity syndrome in rheumatoid arthritis. *J Rheumatol.* 2021; 48(5):788–789. doi:10.3899/jrheum.200591.
108. Matsuo T, Koyama T, Morimoto N, et al. Retinal vasculitis as a complication of rheumatoid arthritis. *Ophthalmologica.* 1990;201(4):196–200. doi:10.1159/000310151.
109. Matsuo T, Masuda I, Matsuo N. Geographic choroiditis and retinal vasculitis in rheumatoid arthritis. *Jpn J Ophthalmol.* 1998;42(1):51–55. doi:10.1016/s0021-5155(97)00102-0.
110. Giordano N, D'Ettorre M, Biasi G, et al. Retinal vasculitis in rheumatoid arthritis: an angiographic study. *Clin Exp Rheumatol.* 1990;8(2):121–125.

4 Ophthalmologic Disease in the ANCA-Associated Vasculitides

Lingling Huang, Eric Suhler, and Jason Michael Springer

4.1 INTRODUCTION

ANCA-associated vasculitis (AAV) refers to a group of necrotizing, predominantly small-vessel vasculitides with few or no immune deposits in the arterial wall.[1] Clinical phenotypes of AAV include granulomatosis with polyangiitis (GPA, formerly Wegener's granulomatosis), microscopic polyangiitis (MPA), and eosinophilic granulomatosis with polyangiitis (EGPA, formerly Churg–Strauss syndrome). Granulomatosis manifestations (e.g., retro-orbital disease) are characteristic features of GPA and EGPA, while absent in MPA. Various ocular and orbital manifestations can develop in patients with AAV. Prompt identification of sight-threatening manifestations can be critical to preventing permanent damage. Herein, we outline the common presentations, exam findings, diagnostic tests, treatment modalities, and prognosis of the broad spectrum of ocular and orbital manifestations faced by clinical practitioners exposed to patients with AAV.

4.2 OVERVIEW OF ANCA-ASSOCIATED VASCULITIS

4.2.1 Epidemiology

A 2022 meta-analysis of 25 studies estimated the global incidence of AAV to be 17.2 per million person-years (95% CI 13.3–21.6) and global pooled prevalence of 198.0 per million persons (95% CI 187.0–210.0).[2] The global incidence (per million person-years) by subtype is 9.0 for GPA,[2] 5.9 for MPA,[2] and 1.22–1.7 for EGPA.[2, 3] The predominant phenotype differs based on geographic locations. While GPA is the predominant phenotype in Northern Europe, MPA appears to be more predominant in Japan.[4] Multiple studies have suggested an increased incidence and prevalence of AAV in various geographic regions.[2] However, this may reflect improved diagnostic tests and clinical recognition over time.

The etiology of AAV is not fully delineated, but several associations have been reported in the literature. In GPA, associations have been reported with farming[5] and dwelling in rural communities.[6] Drugs with the highest association with AAV include hydralazine, propylthiouracil, thiamazole, sofosburvir, minocycline, carbimazole, mirabegron, and nintedanib.[7]

4.2.2 Diagnosis

Misdiagnosis, estimated to occur in 70% of patients with vasculitis, is one of the leading healthcare-related factors leading to prolonged delay in diagnosis.[8] While a positive antineutrophil cytoplasmic antibody (ANCA) test can be supportive, it is not sufficient or always necessary to make a diagnosis of ANCA-associated vasculitis. ANCA positivity is seen in approximately 90% of patients with GPA, close to 100% in MPA, and 40% to 50% in EGPA.[9–11] While the most typical ANCA pattern in GPA is cytoplasmic (c-ANCA) by immunofluorescence and proteinase-3 (PR3-ANCA) by EIA, approximately 20% of patients may have a perinuclear (p-ANCA) and myeloperoxidase (MPO-ANCA) pattern. Almost all ANCA-positive patients with either MPA or EGPA have a p-ANCA and MPO-ANCA pattern.[9] Whenever possible, and especially in ANCA-negative disease, a biopsy should be done to confirm the diagnosis. Almost all patients with EGPA will have significant eosinophilia, with an absolute eosinophil count over 1500/mL (off glucocorticoids), and asthma, generally of adult onset. Features distinguishing the clinical phenotype of GPA from MPA include the presence of granulomas (e.g., lungs, retro-orbital, breast, skin) and upper airway manifestations (e.g., recurrent sinusitis, otitis media). Before making a diagnosis of AAV it is important to consider diseases with similar presentations that can also cause positive ANCA serologies including endocarditis, cocaine/levamisole toxins, and drug-induced vasculitis (e.g., propylthiouracil).[12–14]

4.2.3 General Treatment Paradigms

Current treatment paradigms focus on an initially aggressive induction therapy for achievement of remission, followed by less aggressive therapies to maintain remission. The choice of induction agents is guided by the presence of severe manifestations, defined as organ or life threatening (e.g., scleritis, uveitis, nephritis, diffuse alveolar hemorrhage, etc.).[15] For severe GPA and MPA, both rituximab and cyclophosphamide, in combination with high-dose glucocorticoids, have been shown to be effective induction agents.[16, 17] Rituximab may be superior in patients presenting with relapsing disease.[16] Avacopan, a C5a receptor inhibitor, has been shown in a phase III, randomized controlled trial to be non-inferior to high-dose glucocorticoids for induction of remission in severe GPA and

DOI: 10.1201/9781003453710-4

MPA, thus minimizing the glucocorticoid burden in the population.[18] For non-severe presentations, a less aggressive approach with methotrexate is recommended over rituximab or cyclophosphamide.[15, 19] Once remission in GPA or MPA is achieved, patients are changed to a less aggressive agent for maintenance of remission, with the best support behind methotrexate, azathioprine, and rituximab.[20–22] While there are few large randomized controlled trials in EGPA, many of the same immunosuppressive therapies (e.g., cyclophosphamide, methotrexate, azathioprine) have been used in smaller studies.[23–25] Mepolizumab, an anti-interleukin 5 agent, has been shown to be effective in a phase III, randomized controlled trial, excluding patients with severe manifestations.[26] The 2021 American College of Rheumatology/Vasculitis Foundation Guideline for Management of ANCA-Associated Vasculitis provides a resource for management decisions.[15, 25, 27]

4.3 ORBITAL/OCULAR DISEASES AND EVALUATIONS IN PATIENTS WITH ANCA-ASSOCIATED VASCULITIS

Three large-scale retrospective studies revealed the overall prevalence of ophthalmologic manifestations in all forms of AAV ranges from 15.6% to 23.1%.[28–30] The literature on ophthalmologic manifestations of AAV is largely focused on GPA due to significantly higher frequency of eye involvement than other forms of AAV. We will devote the following sections to introducing the major orbital and ocular diseases in patients with GPA. However, it is critical to remember that ophthalmologic manifestations can occur in all forms of AAV, and early diagnosis with prompt treatment is essential to prevent long-term complications.

The prevalence of ophthalmologic manifestations in GPA ranges from 29% to 58%[31–34] and 8% to 16% of instances present with ophthalmologic complications as the initial manifestations.[35–38] Orbital diseases, nasolacrimal involvement, conjunctivitis/episcleritis, and scleritis are among the most common eye conditions in GPA. Posterior segment complications, including retinal vasculitis and retinal arterial or venous occlusions, have been reported but remain uncommon.[38]

4.3.1 Orbital Diseases

Various studies have shown that orbital diseases are among the most common ophthalmologic manifestations and occur in 5% to 33% of patients with GPA.[28, 31–34, 36] Orbital inflammation may develop as primary orbital granuloma, lacrimal gland involvement, diffuse infiltration secondary to sinonasal disease, or extraocular myositis. In 14% to 58% of cases, orbital involvement can be bilateral.[39–41]

4.3.1.1 Common Symptoms

In the active inflammatory phase, patients can present with decreased vision, ocular and/or periorbital pain, diplopia, proptosis, lid edema/hyperemia, eye redness, and extraocular motility restriction. Symptoms can resemble preseptal and orbital cellulitis, but the treatments are drastically different. Therefore, a thorough history and physical examination in addition to orbital imaging are critical in making the correct diagnosis and initiating appropriate treatment.

4.3.1.2 Findings and Diagnostic Testing

A comprehensive eye examination starts with checking best corrected vision, color vision, relative afferent pupillary defect, and intraocular pressure. External evaluation may reveal eyelid erythema and edema, proptosis, globe displacement, enlargement and inflammation of the lacrimal gland, strabismus in primary gaze, and ocular motility restriction. Concurrent conjunctival injection, episcleritis, or scleritis may be seen. Slit lamp biomicroscopy can identify any corneal abnormality and anterior chamber reaction. Dilated fundoscopy is essential to rule out compressive optic neuropathy, which is a common cause of vision loss. Multimodal ocular imaging (ocular coherence tomography, fluorescein angiography) can be helpful to evaluate for retinal abnormalities. Orbital imaging such as computed tomography (CT) or magnetic resonance imaging (MRI) is an essential part of evaluation to identify sinus disease, orbital mass, bony destruction, myositis, and lacrimal gland enlargement. Importantly, other etiologies such as orbital cellulitis, sarcoidosis, orbital pseudotumor, IgG-4-associated systemic disease or thyroid eye disease, which can have similar orbital presentations, should be ruled out with appropriate diagnostic testing. Early diagnosis of orbital GPA can be difficult because ANCA screening can be negative at initial presentation. Orbital biopsy is beneficial in establishing the diagnosis, which may reveal necrotizing vasculitis, small-vessel vasculitis without necrosis, granulomatous inflammation, and chronic nonspecific inflammation.

4.3.1.3 Treatments

Systemic immunosuppressive therapy is required to halt the inflammatory process and prevent tissue damage and organ dysfunction. In diseases that are limited to the orbit and not vision threatening, the mainstay of treatment is high-dose systemic glucocorticoids with concomitant methotrexate or mycophenolate mofetil. In life- or vision-threatening diseases, more intensive immunosuppressive treatment such as cyclophosphamide or rituximab is required. Certain cases may require surgical interventions including debulking surgery or orbital decompression. Dacryocystorhinostomy is a safe and effective treatment for nasolacrimal duct obstruction in patients with well-managed nasal sinus and systemic disease.[42] A multidisciplinary approach, involving rheumatologists, ophthalmologists, otorhinolaryngologists, pulmonologists, and nephrologists, is necessary to achieve the best outcomes.

4.3.1.4 Prognosis

Studies have shown that orbital GPA can remain localized without systemic progression in the long term.[41, 43] Aggressive therapy results in good outcomes, though local recurrence may occur. One study compared orbital mass with and without lacrimal gland involvement in GPA patients and found that those without lacrimal gland involvement had a less favorable visual outcome, a high rate of neighboring structure damage, a higher rate of recurrence, and more frequent systemic disease.[36]

4.3.2 Conjunctivitis, Episcleritis, and Scleritis

Eye redness, which is the most common ocular symptom in ANCA-associated vasculitis, may be caused by inflammation of the conjunctiva, episclera, or sclera.[28–30] Injection of the conjunctiva or episclera sometimes manifests as a sign of orbital inflammation. Here, we will discuss specific inflammation of the conjunctiva, episclera, or sclera in the absence of orbital inflammation.

4.3.2.1 Common Symptoms

Conjunctival disease in GPA patients can present with nonspecific symptoms such as eye redness, foreign body sensation, blurred vision, and occasionally bloody tears. Conjunctival hyperemia is commonly seen in early disease. Ulceration and necrosis may occur and can result in cicatricial changes including symblepharon, entropion, and trichiasis.[44–46] Tarsal-conjunctivital disease has been reported to be associated with higher risk of subglottic stenosis and nasolacrimal duct obstruction.[47]

Episcleritis usually presents as eye redness without severe pain or visual impairment. In contrast, scleritis can result in marked vision loss, and patients often report deep, boring pain worse at night that may wake them up from sleep. This pain may radiate to the scalp, temple, and jaw and be exacerbated by eye movements due to extraocular muscle insertions into the sclera.

Scleritis can be categorized into anterior and posterior, which have different presentations and complications. Anterior scleritis typically manifests as painful, intense hyperemia with a characteristic violet-bluish hue (Figure 4.1). It can be further subcategorized into diffuse, nodular, or necrotizing. Necrotizing scleritis is the most severe form, signified by areas of vascular infarction, scleral necrosis, and thinning with exposure of underlying choroid. It can lead to scarring, infection, and perforation in a matter of days. Importantly, scleritis may be the initial clinical manifestation of GPA and can be more severe than scleritis of other etiologies.[33, 44, 48]

4.3.2.2 Findings and Diagnostic Testing

Recurrent conjunctivitis with atypical features and cicatricial conjunctivitis should raise the suspicion for GPA, and conjunctival biopsy may offer diagnostic insights. Anterior scleritis presents with scleral edema and intense injection with a violaceous hue that is better visualized in natural light. The area of scleral inflammation is usually tender to palpation. On slit lamp biomicroscopy, inflamed scleral vessels are adherent to the sclera and cannot be moved with a cotton-tipped applicator. In comparison, inflamed episcleral vessels are more superficial and mobile. A simple but important diagnostic test is 2.5% to 10% phenylephrine trial, which can blanch the conjunctival and episcleral vessels but does not affect the deep scleral vessels (see Chapter 3, Figures 3.1 and 3.2). Posterior scleritis lacks the visible anterior scleral inflammation. The detection of posterior scleritis can be aided by B-scan ultrasonography and orbital MRI. Classic ultrasonographic features include distended optic nerve sheath, fluid in the subtenon's space (T sign), scleral and choroidal thickening (Figure 4.2). OCT, particularly with enhanced depth imaging, may reveal increased thickness of the choroid, subretinal fluid, and chorioretinal folds (Figure 4.3).

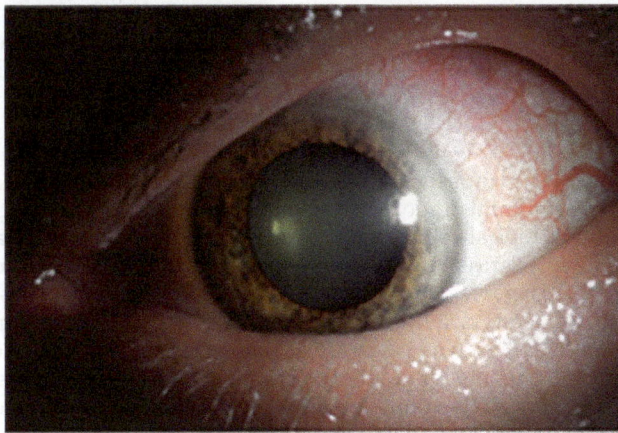

Figure 4.1 Example of anterior scleritis in a patient diagnosed with GPA. Intense sectoral scleral hyperemia with a characteristic violet-bluish hue was accompanied by superior scleral edema.

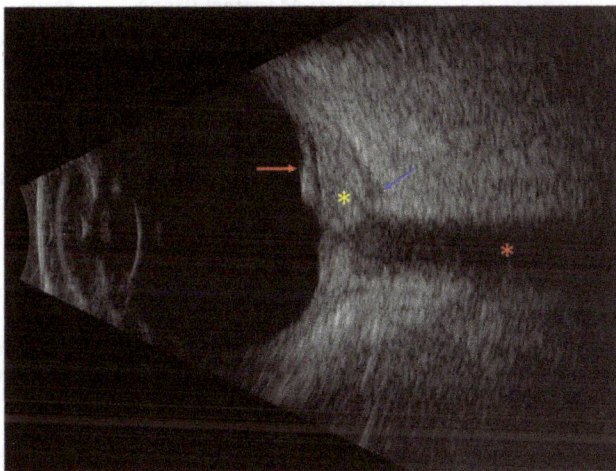

Figure 4.2 B-scan ultrasound of the left eye in a patient with GPA demonstrated a thickened posterior sclera (yellow star), positive T sign formed by fluid in the subtenon space (blue arrow) and optic nerve (red star), and macular detachment (red arrow). (Reprinted with permission: Sandhu RK, Adams T, Sibley C, et al. Granulomatosis with polyangiitis (GPA) presenting with frosted branch angiitis. *Retin Cases Brief Rep.* 2016;10(3):249–251. doi:10.1097/ICB.0000000000000242.)

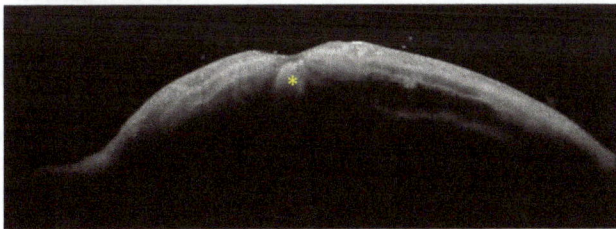

Figure 4.3 Spectral domain optical coherence tomography (OCT) of the left eye in a patient with GPA showing severe edema and subfoveal neurosensory detachment (yellow star). (Reprinted with permission: Sandhu RK, Adams T, Sibley C, et al. Granulomatosis with polyangiitis (GPA) Presenting with Frosted Branch Angiitis. *Retin Cases Brief Rep.* 2016;10(3):249–251. doi:10.1097/ICB.0000000000000242).

All patients presenting with scleritis should be evaluated for associated systemic disease, including infectious etiologies (tuberculosis, syphilis), rheumatologic diseases (rheumatoid arthritis, ANCA-associated vasculitis, sarcoidosis, HLA-B27), and occasionally malignant masquerades.

4.3.2.3 *Treatments and Prognosis*

The management of ocular manifestations in GPA typically involves addressing the underlying condition through the administration of systemic glucocorticoids and cytotoxic medications. Adjunctive treatment with topical or periocular glucocorticoids may provide additional benefits. Mild conjunctivitis and episcleritis in GPA can be managed with topical glucocorticoids. If cicatricial changes are noted, therapies may need to be escalated. Scleritis poses a potential threat to vision. In mild to moderate scleritis of other etiologies, high-potency non-steroidal anti-inflammatory drugs (NSAIDs) such as naproxen or indomethacin are often the first-line therapy. However, scleritis in GPA patients, particularly necrotizing scleritis, requires prompt initiation of aggressive immunosuppressants similar to treating organ- or vision-threatening orbital diseases. Subconjunctival triamcinolone injection has demonstrated safety and efficacy in treating noninfectious, non-necrotizing anterior scleritis.[49] Caution should be exercised in cases associated with elevated intraocular pressure or known history of steroid-responsive ocular hypertension and avoided in necrotizing disease.

4.3.3 Intraocular Manifestations

Intraocular manifestations of GPA can be classified according to anatomical locations: cornea and uveal tract including anterior chamber, vitreous, retina, and choroid.

4.3.3.1 *Common Symptoms*

Corneal involvement may be observed as an associated adjacent corneal infiltrate in active scleritis.[50] It may appear as interstitial keratitis or peripheral ulcerative keratitis.[44, 51] Exposure keratopathy can be a secondary complication from severe orbital diseases and proptosis. Patients frequently display symptoms such as pain, eye redness, reduced vision, and corneal haze. Conjunctivalization of the corneal epithelium develops because of chronic cicatricial disease.

Uveitis, which can be anterior, posterior, or panuveitis, is not a common manifestation of GPA. Inflammation in the anterior chamber or vitreous may accompany scleritis, keratitis, or active inflammation in nearby structures. Symptoms, including pain, photophobia, and conjunctival hyperemia, are similar to uveitis of other etiologies. Retinal and choroidal involvement in GPA appears to be rare. Contrary to widespread misconceptions, studies have demonstrated that individuals with systemic vasculitis seldom develop retinal vasculitis, and those with retinal vasculitis rarely suffer from systemic vasculitis.[28–30, 52] Sclerochoroidal granuloma may simulate the appearance of a uveal melanoma.[53] Compressive optic neuropathy due to orbital inflammation is an important cause of profound vision loss. Rare cases of ischemic optic neuropathy, presumably due to vasculitic involvement of arteries supplying the optic nerve, have been reported in the literature.[54, 55]

4.3.3.2 *Findings and Diagnostic Testing*

A thorough examination with slit lamp biomicroscopy and dilated fundoscopy is essential in the identification of intraocular inflammation. Anterior chamber cell and flare, as well as vitreous cell and haze, indicate active intraocular inflammation. Since uveitis is a rare manifestation in AAV, other infectious or inflammatory etiologies, such as syphilis, tuberculosis, sarcoidosis, HLA-B27-associated uveitis, Behçet's disease, etc., should be fully assessed. Clinically, retinal vasculitis is characterized by perivascular sheathing, arterial and venous occlusion, retinal whitening or ischemia, intraretinal hemorrhage, retinal neovascularization, and vitreous hemorrhage (Figure 4.4). Fluorescein angiography aids in the diagnosis of vasculitis by detecting vascular leakage, occlusion, non-perfusion, or neovascularization (Figure 4.4.). In patients undergoing immunosuppressive therapy, it is crucial to consider infectious retinitis in the differential with a compatible clinical picture, such as cytomegalovirus retinitis and toxoplasmosis. Choroidal folds, choroidal effusions, or exudative retinal detachment may be observed in association with chorioretinal granulomas or posterior scleritis. Additionally, vitreous hemorrhage can arise from neovascularization or chorioretinal/ciliary body granuloma.[56]

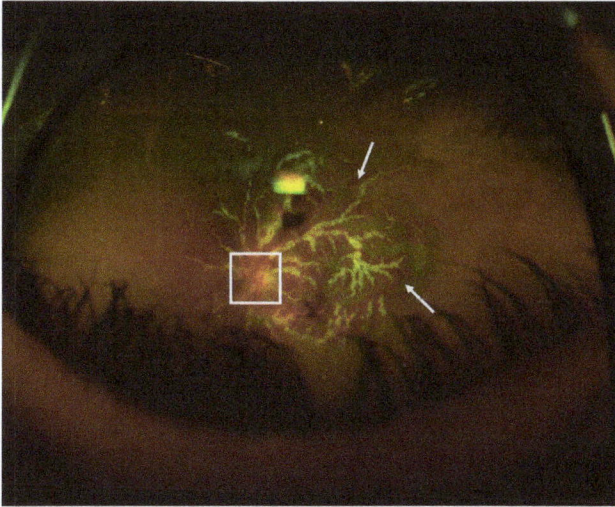

Figure 4.4 Pseudo-color fundus image of the left fundus in a patient with GPA revealed optic nerve edema (white square) and dilated venules with severe sheathing and perivascular hemorrhages (white arrows), resembling a frosted branch angiitis. (Reprinted with permission: Sandhu RK, Adams T, Sibley C, et al. Granulomatosis with polyangiitis (GPA) presenting with frosted branch angiitis. *Retin Cases Brief Rep.* 2016;10(3):249–251. doi:10.1097/ICB.0000000000000242.)

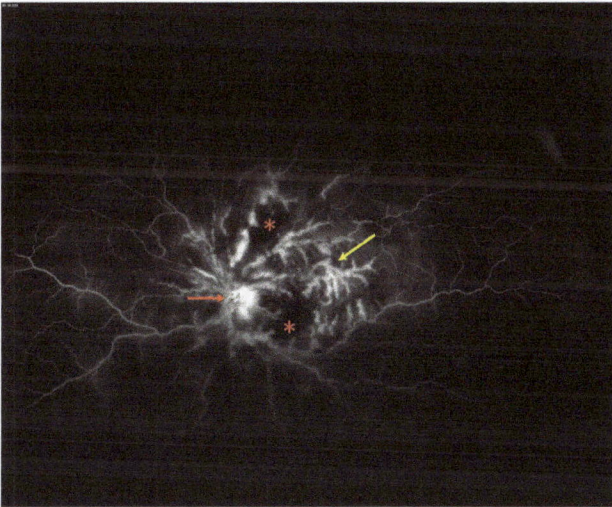

Figure 4.5 Late phase of fluorescein angiogram of the left eye in a patient with GPA showed blocking effect by retinal hemorrhage (red stars) and leakage from peripapillary (red arrow) and macular vasculature (yellow arrow), primarily the veins, consistent with retinal vasculitis. This was the same GPA patient as shown in Figure 4.4.

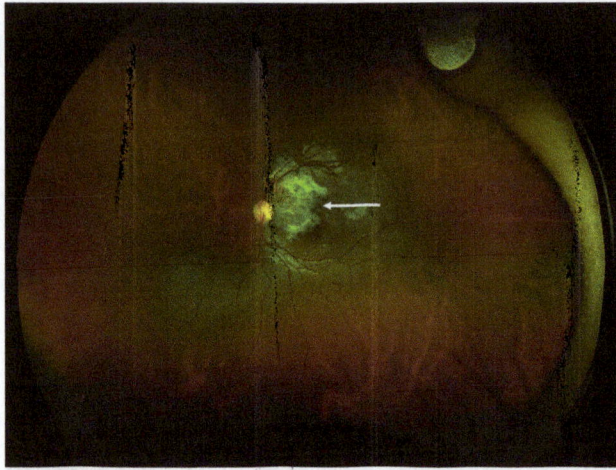

Figure 4.6 Pseudo-color fundus image demonstrated resolution of optic nerve edema and retinal vasculitis in a GPA patient after systemic treatment. The GPA patient shown in Figure 4.4 was treated with high-dose intravenous corticosteroids followed by systemic rituximab therapy weekly for 4 doses and then maintained on rituximab infusion every 6 months. Four years after the initial presentation, the systemic GPA disease as well as retinal vasculitis remained in remission on maintenance of rituximab. Visual recovery was limited by the subretinal fibrosis (white arrow) and outer retinal damage.

4.3.3.3 *Treatments and Prognosis*

Managing the intraocular manifestations in patients with GPA primarily involves the use of glucocorticoids and cytotoxic medications to control the underlying systemic disease. Topical or intravitreal glucocorticoids are frequently employed as supplementary therapies to quickly achieve local disease control, especially for inflammation in the anterior segment or vitreous, as well as cystoid macular edema, which is a common complication from severe inflammation. Vision-threatening retinal vasculitis requires more intensive systemic immunosuppressive therapies (Figure 4.6). Moreover, aggressive panretinal photocoagulation has been proposed as an important component in managing retinal neovascularization, which is one of the problematic complications of retinal vasculitis.[57]

4.3.4 Infectious Masquerades in ANCA-Associated Vasculitis

Table 4.1 provides a summary of ophthalmologic manifestations in AAV. As emphasized in preceding sections, it is always critical to rule out infectious etiologies in any orbital or ocular diseases before initiating immunosuppressive therapies. Additionally, AAV patients on systemic immunosuppressants are susceptible to various infections, which can complicate the clinical picture by mimicking worsening inflammatory disease. For example, invasive fungal infection, such as mucormycosis and angioinvasive Aspergillus, can rapidly destroy nasosinus and orbital walls, simulating the clinical picture of progressing GPA with profound inflammation and necrosis in surrounding structures. Cytomegalovirus retinitis can present in immunocompromised patients as a hemorrhagic retinitis and vasculitis. It is important to remain vigilant for infectious masquerades when managing AAV with systemic immunosuppressants.

4.4 SUMMARY

Orbital disease is a common manifestation of GPA and can be vision threatening. Early diagnosis and aggressive treatment are essential for good outcomes. Conjunctivitis, episcleritis, and scleritis are common ocular manifestations and usually have good prognosis with treatment. Intraocular involvement remains rare but can be serious. Infectious masquerades are a concern in AAV patients on immunosuppressants.

Table 4.1 Summary of Common Ophthalmologic Manifestations in ANCA-Associated Vasculitis (AAV)

All patients should undergo an ocular examination including best corrected visual acuity, pupil examination, intraocular pressure, extraocular motility, slit lamp biomicroscopy, and dilated fundus examination.

Ancillary testing should be considered as indicated.

Disease	Symptoms	Findings/Testing	Treatment	Prognosis
Orbital complications	■ Decreased vision ■ Ocular/periorbital pain ■ Diplopia ■ Eye redness, eyelid/periorbital swelling ■ Tearing	■ Decreased color vision, relative afferent pupillary defect, ocular misalignment, extraocular motility restriction, proptosis, nasolacrimal duct obstruction ■ Orbital imaging (CT or MRI) ■ Orbital biopsy (if applicable)	■ Systemic immunosuppressants (glucocorticoids, methotrexate, mycophenolate mofetil, cyclophosphamide, rituximab) ■ Surgery (debulking, orbital decompression, dacryocystorhinostomy)	■ Can remain localized without systemic progression ■ Aggressive therapy leads to good outcomes, but local recurrence may occur
Conjunctivitis	■ Eye redness ■ Foreign body sensation ■ Blurred vision	■ Conjunctival hyperemia ■ Conjunctival ulceration, necrosis ■ Cicatricial changes: trichiasis, entropion, shortened fornix ■ Conjunctival biopsy (if applicable)	■ Address underlying disease ■ Topical glucocorticoids for mild disease	■ Recurrent conjunctivitis with atypical features and cicatricial conjunctivitis should raise the suspicion for GPA ■ Early treatment prevents cicatricial changes
Episcleritis	■ Eye redness, typically without severe pain or vision impairment	■ Injection of superficial episcleral vessels, mobile with cotton-tipped applicators ■ Blanches with 2.5% to 10% phenylephrine eye drop	■ Address underlying disease ■ Topical glucocorticoids as adjunctive therapy	■ Usually not self-limited in AAV, requires treatment
Scleritis	*Anterior scleritis:* ■ Intense scleral hyperemia with violet-bluish hue ■ Severe eye pain, tender to touch ■ Can be necrotizing *Posterior scleritis:* ■ No visible eye redness ■ Periocular dull, boring ache	*Anterior scleritis:* ■ Does not blanch with 2.5% to 10% phenylephrine eye drop ■ Inflamed scleral vessels immobile with cotton-tipped applicator *Posterior scleritis:* ■ Subtenon's fluid (T sign) on B-scan ultrasonography ■ May see thickened choroid, subretinal fluid and chorioretinal folds on OCT ■ Orbital MRI	■ Address underlying disease ■ Necrotizing scleritis warrants more aggressive immunosuppressants ■ Subconjunctival triamcinolone injection may be considered in non-necrotizing scleritis	■ Early diagnosis and treatment usually achieve good outcomes ■ Necrotizing scleritis is more severe and can lead to scarring or perforation rapidly

Table 4.1 (*Continued*) Summary of Common Ophthalmologic Manifestations in ANCA-Associated Vasculitis (AAV)

Disease	Symptoms	Findings/Testing	Treatment	Prognosis
Corneal involvement	■ Eye pain ■ Redness ■ Reduced vision ■ Corneal haze	■ May be associated with active scleritis as an adjacent corneal infiltrate ■ Interstitial keratitis ■ Peripheral ulcerative keratitis ■ Exposure keratopathy can develop as a secondary complication from orbital disease ■ Chronic cicatricial disease can result in conjunctivalization of the corneal epithelium	■ Address underlying disease ■ Topical glucocorticoids	■ Early treatment prevents complications like corneal scarring
Uveitis	■ Eye pain and redness ■ Photophobia ■ Blurred vision	■ Anterior chamber cell and flare ■ May have vitreous cell and haze	■ Address underlying disease ■ Systemic/topical/intravitreal glucocorticoids	■ Usually good, but depends on underlying cause and severity
Retinal and choroidal involvement	■ Decreased vision, scotoma	■ Fluorescein angiography for retinal vasculitis ■ Macular OCT ■ Optic nerve OCT	■ Address underlying disease ■ Intravitreal glucocorticoids ■ Can consider panretinal photocoagulation for retinal neovascularization	■ Variable, depends on early diagnosis and treatment

REFERENCES

1. Jennette JC, Falk RJ, Bacon PA, et al. 2012 revised international Chapel Hill conference nomenclature of vasculitides. *Arthritis Rheum.* 2013 Jan.;65(1):1–11. doi:10.1002/art.37715.
2. Redondo-Rodriguez R, Mena-Vazquez N, et al. Systematic review and metaanalysis of worldwide incidence and prevalence of antineutrophil cytoplasmic antibody (ANCA) associated vasculitis. *J Clin Med.* 2022 May 4;11(9). doi:10.3390/jcm11092573.
3. Jakes RW, Kwon N, Nordstrom B, et al. Burden of illness associated with eosinophilic granulomatosis with polyangiitis: a systematic literature review and meta-analysis. *Clin Rheumatol.* 2021 Dec.;40(12):4829–4836. doi:10.1007/s10067-021-05783-8.
4. Fujimoto S, Watts RA, Kobayashi S, et al. Comparison of the epidemiology of anti-neutrophil cytoplasmic antibody-associated vasculitis between Japan and the U.K. *Rheumatology (Oxford).* 2011 Oct.;50(10):1916–1920. doi:10.1093/rheumatology/ker205.
5. Lindberg H, Colliander C, Nise L, et al. Are farming and animal exposure risk factors for the development of granulomatosis with polyangiitis? Environmental risk factors revisited: a case-control study. *J Rheumatol.* 2021 June;48(6):894–897. doi:10.3899/jrheum.200210.
6. Aiyegbusi O, Frleta-Gilchrist M, Traynor JP, et al. ANCA-associated renal vasculitis is associated with rurality but not seasonality or deprivation in a complete national cohort study. *RMD Open.* Apr 2021;7(2). doi:10.1136/rmdopen-2020-001555.
7. Deshayes S, Dolladille C, Dumont A, et al. A worldwide pharmacoepidemiologic update on drug-induced antineutrophil cytoplasmic antibody-associated vasculitis in the era of targeted therapies. *Arthritis Rheumatol.* 2022 Jan.;74(1):134–139. doi:10.1002/art.41902.
8. Sreih AG, Cronin K, Shaw DG, et al. Diagnostic delays in vasculitis and factors associated with time to diagnosis. *Orphanet J Rare Dis.* 2021 Apr. 21;16(1):184. doi:10.1186/s13023-021-01794-5.

9. Hoffman GS, Specks U. Antineutrophil cytoplasmic antibodies. *Arthritis Rheum.* 1998 Sept.;41(9):1521–1537. doi:10.1002/1529-0131(199809)41:9<1521::AID-ART2>3.0.CO;2-A.
10. Guillevin L, Durand-Gasselin B, Cevallos R, et al. Microscopic polyangiitis: clinical and laboratory findings in eighty-five patients. *Arthritis Rheum.* 1999 Mar.;42(3):421–430. doi:10.1002/1529-0131(199904)42:3<421::AID-ANR5>3.0.CO;2-6.
11. Guillevin L, Cohen P, Gayraud M, et al. Churg-Strauss syndrome: clinical study and long-term follow-up of 96 patients. *Medicine (Baltimore).* 1999 Jan.;78(1):26–37. doi:10.1097/00005792-199901000-00003.
12. Ai S, Liu X, Chen G, et al. Characteristics and diagnostic challenge of antineutrophil cytoplasmic antibody positive infective endocarditis. *Am J Med.* 2022 Nov.;135(11):1371–1377. doi:10.1016/j.amjmed.2022.06.015.
13. McGrath MM, Isakova T, Rennke HG, et al. Contaminated cocaine and antineutrophil cytoplasmic antibody-associated disease. *Clin J Am Soc Nephrol.* 2011 Dec.;6(12):2799–2805. doi:10.2215/CJN.03440411.
14. Choi HK, Merkel PA, Walker AM, et al. Drug-associated antineutrophil cytoplasmic antibody-positive vasculitis: prevalence among patients with high titers of antimyeloperoxidase antibodies. *Arthritis Rheum.* 2000 Feb.;43(2):405–413. doi:10.1002/1529-0131(200002)43:2<405::AID-ANR22>3.0.CO;2-5.
15. Chung SA, Langford CA, Maz M, et al. 2021 American College of Rheumatology/Vasculitis Foundation Guideline for the management of antineutrophil cytoplasmic antibody-associated vasculitis. *Arthritis Care Res (Hoboken).* 2021 Aug.;73(8):1088–1105. doi:10.1002/acr.24634.
16. Stone JH, Merkel PA, Spiera R, et al. Rituximab versus cyclophosphamide for ANCA-associated vasculitis. *N Engl J Med.* 2010 Jul. 15;363(3):221–232. doi:10.1056/NEJMoa0909905.
17. Jones RB, Tervaert JW, Hauser T, et al. Rituximab versus cyclophosphamide in ANCA-associated renal vasculitis. *N Engl J Med.* 2010 Jul. 15;363(3):211–220. doi:10.1056/NEJMoa0909169.
18. Jayne DRW, Merkel PA, Schall TJ, et al. Avacopan for the treatment of ANCA-associated vasculitis. *N Engl J Med.* 2021 Feb. 18;384(7):599–609. doi:10.1056/NEJMoa2023386.
19. De Groot K, Rasmussen N, Bacon PA, et al. Randomized trial of cyclophosphamide versus methotrexate for induction of remission in early systemic antineutrophil cytoplasmic antibody-associated vasculitis. *Arthritis Rheum.* 2005 Aug.;52(8):2461–2469. doi:10.1002/art.21142.
20. Pagnoux C, Mahr A, Hamidou MA, et al. Azathioprine or methotrexate maintenance for ANCA-associated vasculitis. *N Engl J Med.* 2008 Dec. 25;359(26):2790–2803. doi:10.1056/NEJMoa0802311.
21. Guillevin L, Pagnoux C, Karras A, et al. Rituximab versus azathioprine for maintenance in ANCA-associated vasculitis. *N Engl J Med.* 2014 Nov. 6;371(19):1771–1780. doi:10.1056/NEJMoa1404231.
22. Hiemstra TF, Walsh M, Mahr A, et al. Mycophenolate mofetil vs azathioprine for remission maintenance in antineutrophil cytoplasmic antibody-associated vasculitis: a randomized controlled trial. *JAMA.* 2010 Dec. 1;304(21):2381–2388. doi:10.1001/jama.2010.1658.
23. Ribi C, Cohen P, Pagnoux C, et al. Treatment of Churg-Strauss syndrome without poor-prognosis factors: a multicenter, prospective, randomized, open-label study of seventy-two patients. *Arthritis Rheum.* 2008 Feb.;58(2):586–594. doi:10.1002/art.23198.
24. Cohen P, Pagnoux C, Mahr A, et al. Churg-Strauss syndrome with poor-prognosis factors: a prospective multicenter trial comparing glucocorticoids and six or twelve cyclophosphamide pulses in forty-eight patients. *Arthritis Rheum.* 2007 May 15;57(4):686–693. doi:10.1002/art.22679.
25. Springer JM, Kalot MA, Husainat NM, et al. Eosinophilic granulomatosis with polyangiitis: a systematic review and meta-analysis of test accuracy and benefits and harms of common treatments. *ACR Open Rheumatol.* 2021 Feb.;3(2):101–110. doi:10.1002/acr2.11194.
26. Wechsler ME, Akuthota P, Jayne D, et al. Mepolizumab or placebo for eosinophilic granulomatosis with polyangiitis. *N Engl J Med.* 2017 May 18;376(20):1921–1932. doi:10.1056/NEJMoa1702079.
27. Springer JM, Kalot MA, Husainat NM, et al. Granulomatosis with polyangiitis and microscopic polyangiitis: a systematic review and meta-analysis of benefits and harms of common treatments. *ACR Open Rheumatol.* 2021 Mar.;3(3):196–205. doi:10.1002/acr2.11230.
28. Ungprasert P, Crowson CS, Cartin-Ceba R, et al. Clinical characteristics of inflammatory ocular disease in anti-neutrophil cytoplasmic antibody associated vasculitis: a retrospective cohort study. *Rheumatology (Oxford).* 2017 Oct. 1;56(10):1763–1770. doi:10.1093/rheumatology/kex261.

29. Rothschild PR, Pagnoux C, Seror R, et al. Ophthalmologic manifestations of systemic necrotizing vasculitides at diagnosis: a retrospective study of 1286 patients and review of the literature. *Semin Arthritis Rheum.* 2013 Apr.;42(5):507–514. doi:10.1016/j.semarthrit.2012.08.003.

30. Junek ML, Zhao L, Garner S, et al. Ocular manifestations of ANCA-associated vasculitis. *Rheumatology (Oxford).* 2023 Jul. 5;62(7):2517–2524. doi:10.1093/rheumatology/keac663.

31. Bullen CL, Liesegang TJ, McDonald TJ, et al. Ocular complications of Wegener's granulomatosis. *Ophthalmology.* 1983 Mar.;90(3):279–290. doi:10.1016/s0161-6420(83)34574-7.

32. Haynes BF, Fishman ML, Fauci AS, et al. The ocular manifestations of Wegener's granulomatosis: fifteen years experience and review of the literature. *Am J Med.* 1977 Jul.;63(1):131–141. doi:10.1016/0002-9343(77)90125-5.

33. Hoffman GS, Kerr GS, Leavitt RY, et al. Wegener granulomatosis: an analysis of 158 patients. *Ann Intern Med.* 1992 Mar. 15;116(6):488–498. doi:10.7326/0003-4819-116-6-488.

34. Fauci AS, Haynes BF, Katz P, et al. Wegener's granulomatosis: prospective clinical and therapeutic experience with 85 patients for 21 years. *Ann Intern Med.* 1983 Jan.;98(1):76–85. doi:10.7326/0003-4819-98-1-76.

35. Pakrou N, Selva D, Leibovitch I. Wegener's granulomatosis: ophthalmic manifestations and management. *Semin Arthritis Rheum.* 2006 Apr.;35(5):284–292. doi:10.1016/j.semarthrit.2005.12.003.

36. Ismailova DS, Abramova JV, Novikov PI, et al. Clinical features of different orbital manifestations of granulomatosis with polyangiitis. *Graefes Arch Clin Exp Ophthalmol.* 2018 Sept.;256(9):1751–1756. doi:10.1007/s00417-018-4014-9.

37. Kubal AA, Perez VL. Ocular manifestations of ANCA-associated vasculitis. *Rheum Dis Clin North Am.* 2010 Aug.;36(3):573–586. doi:10.1016/j.rdc.2010.05.005.

38. Harman LE, Margo CE. Wegener's granulomatosis. *Surv Ophthalmol.* 1998 Mar.–Apr.;42(5):458–480. doi:10.1016/s0039-6257(97)00133-1.

39. Provenzale JM, Mukherji S, Allen NB, et al. Orbital involvement by Wegener's granulomatosis: imaging findings. *AJR Am J Roentgenol.* 1996 Apr.;166(4):929–934. doi:10.2214/ajr.166.4.8610576.

40. Holle JU, Voigt C, Both M, et al. Orbital masses in granulomatosis with polyangiitis are associated with a refractory course and a high burden of local damage. *Rheumatology (Oxford).* 2013 May;52(5):875–882. doi:10.1093/rheumatology/kes382.

41. Tan LT, Davagnanam I, Isa H, et al. Clinical and imaging features predictive of orbital granulomatosis with polyangiitis and the risk of systemic involvement. *Ophthalmology.* 2014 June;121(6):1304–1309. doi:10.1016/j.ophtha.2013.12.003.

42. Kwan AS, Rose GE. Lacrimal drainage surgery in Wegener's granulomatosis. *Br J Ophthalmol.* Mar. 2000;84(3):329–331. doi:10.1136/bjo.84.3.329.

43. Fechner FP, Faquin WC, Pilch BZ. Wegener's granulomatosis of the orbit: a clinicopathological study of 15 patients. *Laryngoscope.* 2002 Nov.;112(11):1945–1950. doi:10.1097/00005537-200211000-00007.

44. Tarabishy AB, Schulte M, Papaliodis GN, et al. Wegener's granulomatosis: clinical manifestations, differential diagnosis, and management of ocular and systemic disease. *Surv Ophthalmol.* 2010 Sept.–Oct.;55(5):429–444. doi:10.1016/j.survophthal.2009.12.003.

45. Jordan DR, Zafar A, Brownstein S, et al. Cicatricial conjunctival inflammation with trichiasis as the presenting feature of Wegener granulomatosis. *Ophthalmic Plast Reconstr Surg.* 2006 Jan.–Feb.;22(1):69–71. doi:10.1097/01.iop.0000196321.02011.c5.

46. Meier FM, Messmer EP, Bernauer W. Wegener's granulomatosis as a cause of cicatrising conjunctivitis. *Br J Ophthalmol.* 2001 May;85(5):628. doi:10.1136/bjo.85.5.625d.

47. Robinson MR, Lee SS, Sneller MC, et al. Tarsal-conjunctival disease associated with Wegener's granulomatosis. *Ophthalmology.* 2003 Sept.;110(9):1770–1780. doi:10.1016/S0161-6420(03)00616-X.

48. Kharel Sitaula R, Maskey HMS, et al. Scleritis as the harbinger of granulomatosis with polyangiitis. *Ann Med Surg (Lond).* 2022 Dec.;84:104908. doi:10.1016/j.amsu.2022.104908.

49. Sohn EH, Wang R, Read R, et al. Long-term, multicenter evaluation of subconjunctival injection of triamcinolone for non-necrotizing, noninfectious anterior scleritis. *Ophthalmology.* 2011 Oct.;118(10):1932–1937. doi:10.1016/j.ophtha.2011.02.043.

50. Charles SJ, Meyer PA, Watson PG. Diagnosis and management of systemic Wegener's granulomatosis presenting with anterior ocular inflammatory disease. *Br J Ophthalmol.* 1991 Apr.;75(4):201–207. doi:10.1136/bjo.75.4.201.

51. Messmer EM, Foster CS. Vasculitic peripheral ulcerative keratitis. *Surv Ophthalmol.* 1999 Mar.–Apr.;43(5):379–396. doi:10.1016/s0039-6257(98)00051-4.

52. Rosenbaum JT, Ku J, Ali A, et al. Patients with retinal vasculitis rarely suffer from systemic vasculitis. *Semin Arthritis Rheum.* 2012 June;41(6):859–865. doi:10.1016/j.semarthrit.2011.10.006.

53. Janknecht P, Mittelviefhaus H, Loffler KU. Sclerochoroidal granuloma in Wegener's granulomatosis simulating a uveal melanoma. *Retina.* 1995;15(2):150–153. doi:10.1097/00006982-199515020-00011.

54. Paul B, McElvanney AM, Agarwal S, et al. Two rare causes of posterior ischaemic optic neuropathy: eosinophilic fasciitis and Wegener's granulomatosis. *Br J Ophthalmol.* 2002 Sept.;86(9):1066–1068. doi:10.1136/bjo.86.9.1066-a.

55. Blaise P, Robe-Collignon N, Andris C, et al. Wegener's granulomatosis and posterior ischemic optic neuropathy: atypical associated conditions. *Eur J Intern Med.* 2007 Jul.;18(4):326–327. doi:10.1016/j.ejim.2006.11.013.

56. Kamei M, Yasuhara T, Tei M, et al. Vitreous hemorrhage from a ciliary granuloma associated with Wegener granulomatosis. *Am J Ophthalmol.* 2001 Dec.;132(6):924–926. doi:10.1016/s0002-9394(01)01149-7.

57. Levy-Clarke GA, Nussenblatt R. Retinal vasculitis. *Int Ophthalmol Clin.* 2005 Spring;45(2):99–113. doi:10.1097/01.iio.0000155905.95303.1d.

5 Ophthalmologic Disease in Giant Cell Arteritis, Takayasu Arteritis, and Other Systemic Non-ANCA Vasculitides

Christopher R. Rosenberg, Rebka Ephrem, Kimberly M. Winges, and Rennie L. Rhee

5.1 GIANT CELL ARTERITIS

5.1.1 Epidemiology

Giant cell arteritis (GCA) is predominantly a large-vessel vasculitis that primarily affects the branches of the external carotid artery, the ophthalmic artery, and the aorta and its major arterial branches. The most feared complication of GCA is acute vision loss, which can rapidly progress to blindness if left untreated. GCA was previously also known as temporal arteritis, granulomatous arteritis, cranial arteritis, and Horton's disease. GCA is the most common systemic vasculitis in people over 50 years old, with an estimated annual incidence in the United States of 19.8 per 100,000 people over the age of 50 years.[1] It has a female preponderance, affecting women 2 to 3 times as frequently as men.[1, 2] The prevalence of GCA is greater in people of Northern European descent, especially in those of Scandinavian descent, where the incidence has been reported as high as 33.6 per 100,000 people.[3]

Ophthalmic manifestations of GCA are often present and should be taken seriously. Studies have reported a wide range of frequency of visual symptoms in GCA, ranging from 6% to 70%.[4, 5] This variation may reflect the heterogeneity of studies, as studies performed at specialized, tertiary ophthalmologic referral centers tend to observe higher rates of ocular manifestations than the larger, population-based studies, perhaps due to selection and/or referral bias.[5] Moreover, older studies that were performed prior to widespread availability of glucocorticoid therapy report a greater incidence of ocular involvement, while recent population studies have reported a decrease in the incidence of visual complications in GCA, which is hypothesized to be in part due to prompt diagnosis and treatment of GCA in recent years.[6]

5.2 OCULAR MANIFESTATIONS

An inflammatory vasculitis, GCA may affect any part of the visual pathway, resulting in monocular or binocular sensory or motor deficits. These complications can be subtle or devastating. In this section, we will discuss related causes of transient and permanent vision loss, which are summarized in Table 5.1.

5.2.1 Transient Ophthalmic Symptoms

Amaurosis fugax (Latin for "transient blindness") represents transient occlusion in blood supply to the eye, resulting in transient (usually monocular) vision loss. In many cases, amaurosis fugax is the harbinger of permanent vision loss. One study reported up to 44% of patients with permanent vision loss experienced antecedent episodes of amaurosis fugax.[7] In GCA, these symptoms may be precipitated during maneuvers that either increase intraocular pressure, such as bending over, or reduce blood flow to the eye, such as orthostatic changes. Contrary to the pathophysiology of atherosclerotic carotid disease, which causes amaurosis by way of dislodged calcium emboli to retinal vessels, amaurosis in GCA typically occurs at the site of the optic nerve. The ophthalmic artery and its branches (e.g., central retinal artery, cilioretinal artery, posterior ciliary arteries) can suffer ischemia from stenosis and eventual blockage due to vascular inflammation of the ophthalmic artery (Figure 5.1). Amaurosis can be described as a "blurry, curtain over the vision," or "complete blackout" in one or both eyes. To clinically differentiate GCA-associated amaurosis from the more common dry eye, which may also result in transient blurriness, onset in GCA is acute, typically more severe "like an on/off switch," and does not change with blinking or artificial tear use. It may last several minutes and resolve as quickly as it came, or it may be shorter in duration and repeated in an accelerating pattern prior to permanent loss. In a patient at risk of GCA, the diagnosis should be investigated with laboratory testing and/or biopsy or imaging of the temporal artery. If the diagnosis is missed and high-dose glucocorticoids are not initiated, more than half of patients will experience permanent vision loss within an average of 8.5 days.[8]

Transient or permanent binocular diplopia may also occur secondary to ischemia of the cranial nerves or extraocular muscles. All patients complaining of diplopia should undergo a complete examination of extraocular movements and cranial nerve exam, including a cross-cover exam or prism testing to uncover a subtle ocular misalignment. Note that deficits may not map to a specific

DOI: 10.1201/9781003453710-5

Table 5.1 Ocular Manifestations in Giant Cell Arteritis

Ocular Diagnosis	Prevalence in GCA	Visual Symptoms	Distinguishing Ophthalmologic Exam Findings	Differential Diagnosis
Arteritic anterior ischemic optic neuropathy (A-AION)	6%	Acute, painless, severe vision loss (usually less than 20/200)	Chalky white edema of optic nerve head. Within weeks of the insult, edema resolves and optic nerve head develops prominent pallor. Often with a moderately enlarged cup:disc ratio and baring of the lamina cribrosa	Non-arteritic ischemic optic neuropathy. Other arteritic causes are extremely rare (polyarteritis nodosa, systemic lupus erythematosus, granulomatous polyangiitis, herpes zoster)
Arteritic posterior ischemic optic neuropathy (A-PION)	Very rare	Acute, painless, severe vision loss (usually less than 20/200)	Initially, normal-appearing optic nerve and retina but presents with profound clinical optic neuropathy and blindness. Confirm PION with fluorescein angiogram demonstrating absent/delayed choroidal arterial flow. Within weeks of the insult, edema resolves and optic nerve head develops prominent pallor	Surgical or non-surgical non-arteritic PION. Surgical PION is usually bilateral due to prone surgery with intraoperative blood loss and systemic hypotension
Central retinal artery occlusion (CRAO)	1.6%	Acute, severe, painless central vision loss, with far peripheral visual field sparing	Initially (< 1 day), normal-appearing exam. Within a day, demonstrates attenuation of the arterial arcades, macular whitening (representing edema), and a foveal "cherry red spot". With or without relative afferent pupillary defect, depending on extent of retinal injury	Embolism (from carotid atheromas, cardiac valves). Thrombosis (atherosclerotic, systemic autoimmune disease, hypercoagulable disease)
Branch retinal artery occlusion (BRAO)	Very rare	Acute, painless arcuate or altitudinal vision loss, often with central visual field sparing	Retinal whitening occurs along an arterial distribution (such as the upper or lower vascular arcade). With or without relative afferent pupillary defect, depending on extent of retinal injury	Embolism (from carotid atheromas, cardiac valves). Thrombosis (atherosclerotic, systemic autoimmune disease, hypercoagulable disease)
Cortical vision loss	< 1%	Binocular, homonymous visual field deficits	Confrontation visual fields with each eye covered, or formal visual field testing to localize the pathology of vision loss	Ischemic stroke, usually in the posterior cerebral artery territory affecting the occipital lobe

cranial nerve, and any extraocular muscle's function may be disrupted by transient ischemia. Binocular diplopia affects up to 6% of patients with ocular GCA.[9] Permanent ocular misalignment occurs with increased severity and duration of ischemia. While not as common, eye pain from ocular or orbital ischemia is endorsed by 8% of patients suffering vision loss and should be queried in the history of present illness.[9] Physical eye examination findings that may indicate chronic underlying ocular ischemia include mid-peripheral retinal hemorrhages or anterior chamber inflammation, often termed "cell and flare."

5.2.2 Causes of Permanent Visual Loss

5.2.2.1 *Anterior Ischemic Optic Neuropathy*

Feared complications of GCA relate to infarction of ocular or cortical structures. Often termed "the biggest medical emergency in ophthalmology," the most common cause of permanent vision loss is anterior ischemic optic neuropathy (referred to as "arteritic anterior ischemic optic neuropathy" or "AAION"). Usually presenting unilaterally but carrying a high risk of contralateral sequential involvement within the first week,[8, 10] AAION occurs in up to 6% of GCA patients and accounts for 85% of patients with permanent vision loss from GCA.[11] AAION results from infarction of the optic nerve head via occlusion of all posterior ciliary arteries due to complete stenosis of the ophthalmic artery (Figure 5.1). AAION manifests in the optic nerve head as chalky white edema due to diffuse, severe ischemia of the posterior ciliary artery vasculature (Figure 5.2). Vision loss is typically severe, with the majority of patients seeing worse than 20/200 and up to 21% of patients presenting with no light perception (NLP).[12] Within weeks of the insult, the edema typically resolves and the optic nerve head develops prominent pallor, often with a moderately enlarged cup:disc ratio and baring of the lamina cribrosa due to the severity of ophthalmic artery involvement (Figure 5.3).

Other key structures share the posterior ciliary artery blood supply, including the choroid and cilioretinal artery. The choroid nourishes the posterior retina, and the cilioretinal artery, which is present in 6% to 32% of the population, separately supplies the nasal macula.[13] Therefore, GCA patients suffering from AAION can present with solitary or simultaneous choroidal or cilioretinal artery occlusion, which may be seen on fundus examination or multimodal imaging (discussed in the next section).[14] Multifocal choroidal ischemia can result in widespread vision loss and eventual visible optic nerve atrophy on fundus examination, while selective cilioretinal artery occlusion causes injury to the nasal macula with or without involvement of the fovea.[14] Therefore, visual

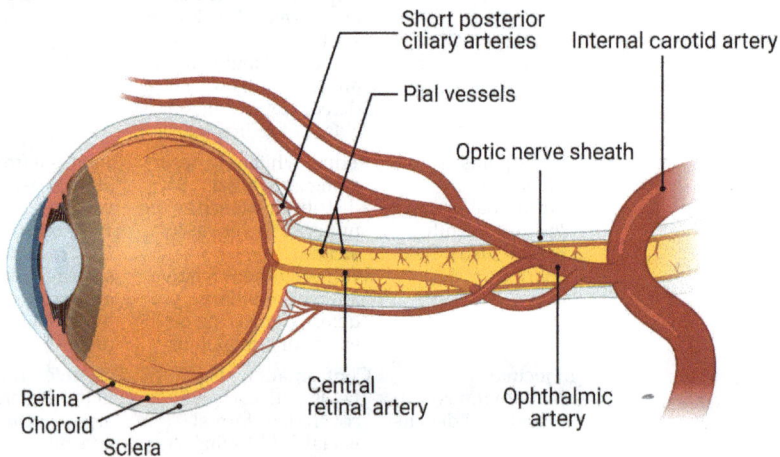

Figure 5.1 Vascular supply for the optic nerve and ocular globe. Nearly all the blood supply of the eye originates from the ophthalmic artery, a branch of the internal carotid artery. The central retinal artery supplies the inner retina (towards the vitreous cavity), while branches of the short posterior ciliary arteries supply the choroid and outer retina (towards the sclera). The optic nerve head is supplied by the short posterior ciliary arteries, and the body of the optic nerve is supplied by the pial vessels as branches from the central retinal artery. Any and all of these vessels can be affected by giant cell arteritis and result in the profound visual symptoms associated with the disease. (Created with BioRender.com.)

potential in cilioretinal artery occlusion is variable. Patients with simultaneous optic nerve, choroidal, or cilioretinal compromise should be strongly suspected of a vasculitic process such as GCA.

5.2.2.2 Posterior Ischemic Optic Neuropathy

The posterior optic nerve (behind the optic nerve head) may also be involved, resulting in arteritic posterior ischemic optic neuropathy (PION). PION is rarer than AAION and represents a total ophthalmic artery occlusion, which affects multiple arterial networks of the central retinal and pial arteries (Figure 5.1). As such, vision loss is severe, equal to, or worse than 20/200 in half of patients. However, given the posterior location of injury, there may be no discernible dilated fundus examination abnormalities at initial presentation.[15] Therefore, a complete review of systems, labs, and a careful examination for optic neuropathy (presence of a relative afferent pupillary defect [RAPD], poor visual field, and loss of visual acuity and color vision) is essential. Despite an initially normal-appearing optic nerve and retina, PION can be confirmed with a fluorescein angiogram that reveals an absence or severe delay of arterial flow to the choroid and retina. Like AAION, optic nerve pallor develops usually within the first month. If pallor does not occur or there is no initial RAPD in a unilateral case, the diagnosis of PION should be questioned. MRI enhancement on T1-weighted or diffusion-weighted imaging of the optic nerve and/or its sheath have been reported in arteritic optic neuropathies.[16–19]

5.2.2.3 Retinal Artery Occlusion

Central retinal artery occlusion (CRAO), particularly in patients without a cilioretinal artery, is a devastating event, resulting in severe central vision loss with relative peripheral visual field sparing. The majority of cases of CRAO seen in the eye clinic are from non-arteritic ischemic causes and are considered an acute embolic stroke until proven otherwise. However, GCA as a cause of CRAO must be considered in all individuals over 50 years old, especially if an intra-arterial Hollenhorst plaque is not visible on fundus exam. Regardless, physical exam may appear normal in the hyper-acute stage; however, within a day, it shows attenuation and "box-carring" of red blood cells within the arterial arcades, macular whitening, and a foveal "cherry red spot." The cherry-red spot occurs for several reasons. The fovea (central portion of the macula) is devoid of retinal ganglion cells or retinal nerve fiber layer and is therefore relatively thin compared to the rest of the macula. Additionally, the sub-foveal outer retina is supplied by a rich choriocapillaris due to the high metabolic demand of central photoreceptors. The foveal cherry-red spot occurs because the perifoveal inner retina develops edema and turns whiter than the central fovea, in which the choriocapillaris is well visualized. Thickening and hyper-reflectivity of the inner retina is seen in the acute stage of CRAO on optical coherence tomography (OCT). Once the macular edema resolves, the cherry-red spot fades, and diffuse inner retinal atrophy is easily seen on OCT.

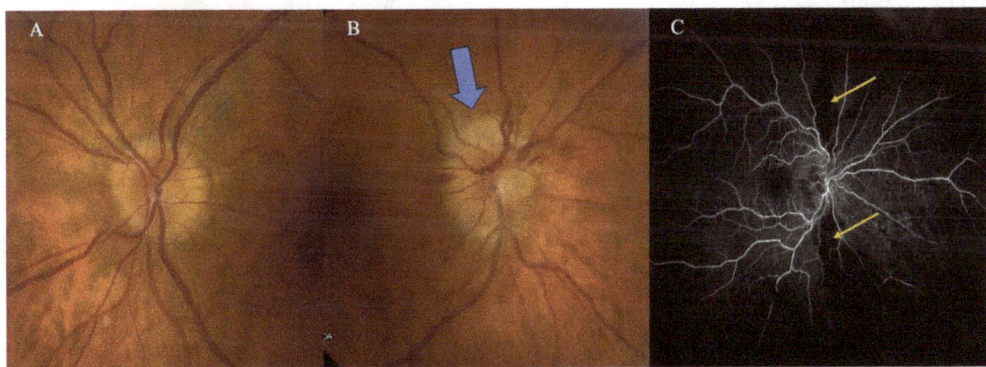

Figure 5.2 Ophthalmologic examination findings of ocular ischemia due to giant cell arteritis. (A) Fundus photo of a normal optic nerve. (B) Fundus photo of an optic nerve with acute arteritic anterior ischemic optic neuropathy with pallid optic disc edema (blue arrow). (C) Fluorescein angiogram showing patchy choroidal non-perfusion, most prominently emanating as wedges superiorly and inferiorly to the optic disc (yellow arrows). Note that the patient's eyelashes are obscuring the inferior fundus, which should not be confused with chorioretinal pathology. (Courtesy of Kimberly M. Winges, MD.)

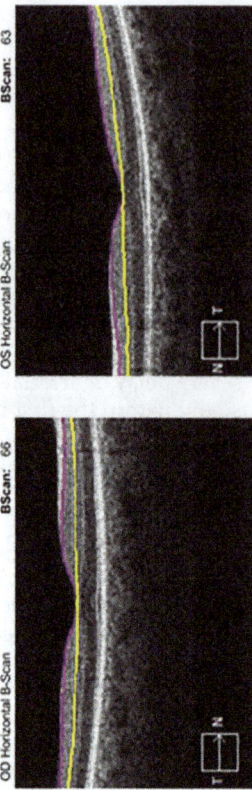
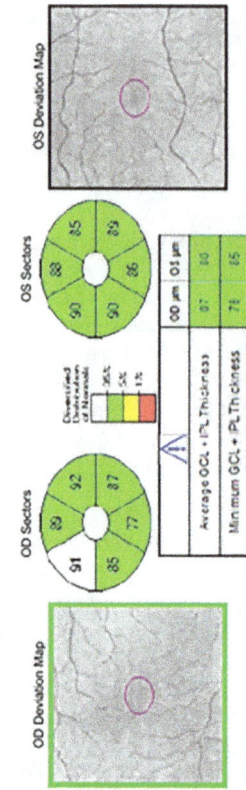
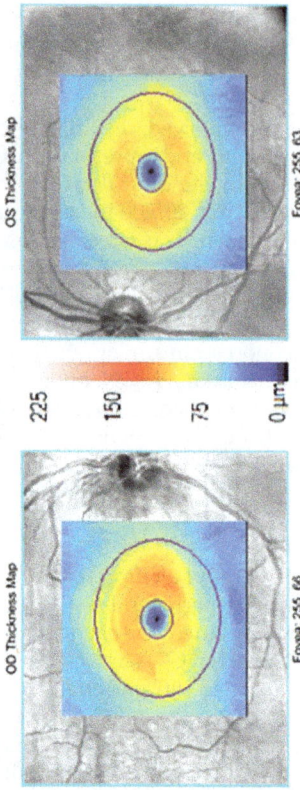

Ganglion Cell OU Analysis: Macular Cube 512x128

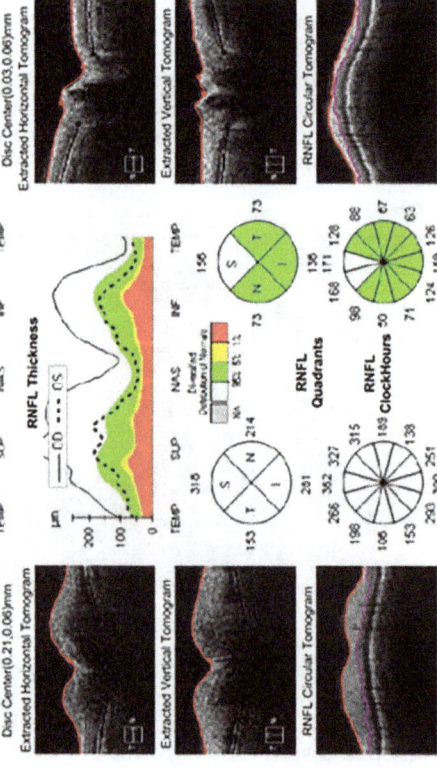
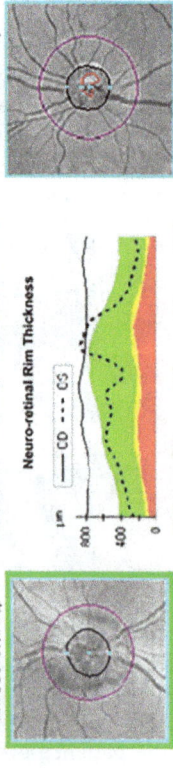
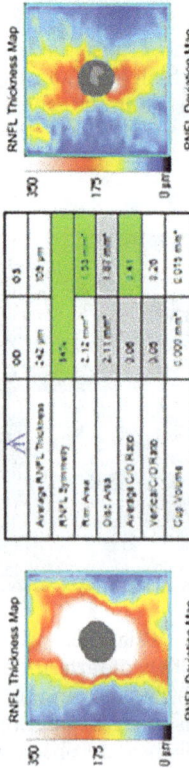

(A) ONH and RNFL OU Analysis: Optic Disc Cube 200x200

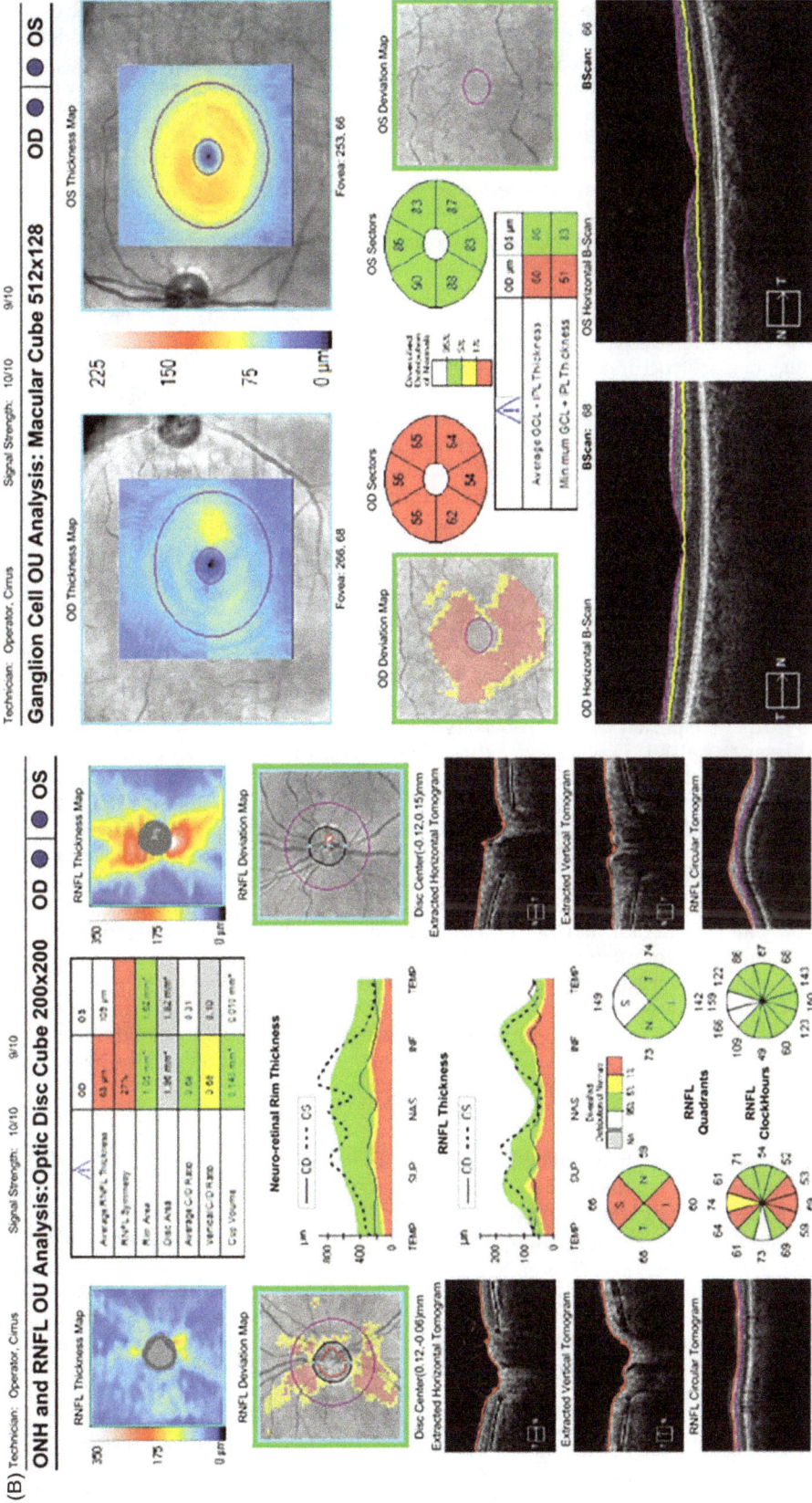

Figure 5.3 Optical coherence tomography of the retinal nerve fiber layer and macular ganglion cell layer in giant cell arteritis. (A) In the acute phase of arteritic anterior ischemic optic neuropathy of the right eye, there is global optic disc edema. (B) One year later, retinal nerve fiber layer and macular ganglion cell layer thinning is present in the same eye. The normal left eye is included for comparison (right side of panels). (Courtesy of Kimberly M. Winges, MD.)

While even rarer, GCA may also cause a branch retinal artery occlusion (BRAO).[5] In BRAO, retinal whitening occurs along an arterial distribution, such as the upper or lower vascular arcade. Central vision is typically not involved due to anastomoses between the superior and inferior arcades surrounding the fovea. A relative afferent pupillary defect with subsequent corresponding optic nerve atrophy may occur in either context, depending on the extent of retinal injury.

5.2.2.4 Cortical Vision Loss and Other Etiologies of Visual Disturbance

When GCA affects the vertebrobasilar arteries of the brain, ischemic stroke can occur and result in cortical vision loss. Cortical vision loss typically manifests as binocular, homonymous visual field deficits from the posterior cerebral arteries, which are branches of the vertebral arteries. Confusion may arise from patients erroneously pointing to one eye (i.e., left eye) when the hemifield loss is on that side (left visual field of both eyes), making confrontation visual fields with each eye covered (or formal visual field testing) an important exam tool to localize the pathology of vision loss. Cortical vision loss in GCA is relatively rare, reported to occur in less than 1% of cases.[5]

Lastly, other ocular structures may be complicated by GCA, including uveitis and posterior scleritis, although singular case reports leave a causal link unclear for the former.[15, 20-24] The pathophysiology of scleritis likely involves a vaso-occlusive component, but no examples of scleral histopathology have been reported to date. Physical exam features of posterior scleritis include pain described as "boring," painful eye movements, optic nerve head edema, subretinal fluid, and choroidal folds. The diagnosis is made with ultrasound, showing thickening of the posterior sclera, with or without the T sign, representing fluid in the subtenon space near the optic nerve's insertion on the globe (see Figure 3.3 in Chapter 3).

5.3 ANATOMIC PATHOLOGY AND PATHOPHYSIOLOGY

GCA is an immune-mediated vasculitis leading to systemic inflammatory manifestations and ischemia. While the pathophysiology of GCA is still poorly understood, significant insight has been gained. The architecture of the artery is an important aspect of the pathogenesis of GCA and may explain the predilection for certain vascular territories. The importance of the structure of the arterial wall is further supported by the propensity for GCA to affect arterial territories that have an adventitial layer and elastic lamina (e.g., extracranial arteries) while rarely involving vasculature which lacks these features (e.g., intracranial arteries).[25] The outer layer of the arterial wall, the adventitia, harbors dendritic cells, which are activated by an unknown stimulus. Upon activation, dendritic cells should normally migrate to lymph nodes. In GCA, however, the activated dendritic cells remain in situ and mature in the vessel wall, initiating an aberrant inflammatory process.[26] Dendritic cells produce a variety of pro-inflammatory cytokines and recruit CD4+ T cells to the arterial wall. CD4+ T cells differentiate into Th1 and Th17 cells, which produce cytokines such as interferon γ and interleukin 17 (IL-17) that modulate macrophage activation and functions.[27, 28] Macrophages produce pro-inflammatory cytokines such as tumor necrosis factor α, IL-1, and IL-6, contributing to systemic inflammation and destruction of the arterial wall.[29] Macrophages lead to formation of multinucleated giant cells and granulomatous inflammation. The arterial wall is further weakened by metalloproteases released by macrophages and vascular smooth muscle cells,[30] which contribute to intimal hyperplasia, luminal narrowing, and degradation of the internal elastic lamina, which are characteristic histopathologic features of GCA (Figure 5.4).

5.4 DIAGNOSTIC TESTING

Multiple tests are utilized for the diagnosis of GCA. Important imaging modalities include retinal fluorescein angiography (Figure 5.2), indocyanine green angiography to evaluate the choroidal circulation, temporal artery ultrasound (Figure 5.5), and extracranial vessel wall MRI to assess for contrast-enhancement of temporal and other cranial arteries (Figure 5.6). Elevated serologic tests signal systemic inflammation, including C-reactive protein (CRP), erythrocyte sedimentation rate (ESR), and platelet count (a surrogate marker of inflammation as an acute phase reactant), although they lack specificity for GCA. Other tests are used to stage GCA, such as CTA chest/abdomen/pelvis to evaluate for aortic and other large-vessel involvement, and cardiac (echocardiogram) and neck imaging to rule out other causes of acute vision loss (i.e., embolic stroke).

5.4.1 Systemic Diagnostic Tests

It is imperative to conduct an immediate initial investigation for cases of suspected GCA. This evaluation includes same-day laboratory testing, including ESR, CRP, and platelets. The sensitivity and specificity of ESR, CRP, and platelets are comparable, and they are elevated in most patients with GCA.[31, 32] While helpful if elevated, normal values do not rule out the diagnosis. If clinical suspicion is high despite normal values, a temporal artery biopsy should be pursued. Nomograms can be used to estimate a patient's likelihood of GCA to help guide clinical decision-making at presentation.[33, 34]

Temporal artery biopsy, the historical gold standard for GCA diagnosis, typically refers to biopsy of the superficial temporal artery or its branches. In a large meta-analysis of 32 studies, temporal artery biopsy showed an overall sensitivity of 77%, with wide variance by institution.[35] A vascular duplex probe may be used to locate the artery and trace its course before making the first incision. Care should be taken to avoid injuring the temporal branch of the facial nerve, which innervates the frontalis muscle responsible for elevating the eyebrow. The superficial temporal artery lies within the parietotemporal fascia-superficial musculoaponeurotic system (SMAS) layer, so dissection deep to this layer is recommended. Guidelines recommend a biopsy length no less than 1 cm and ideally greater than 2 cm in length to maximize diagnostic yield given the possibility of skip lesions.[36, 37]

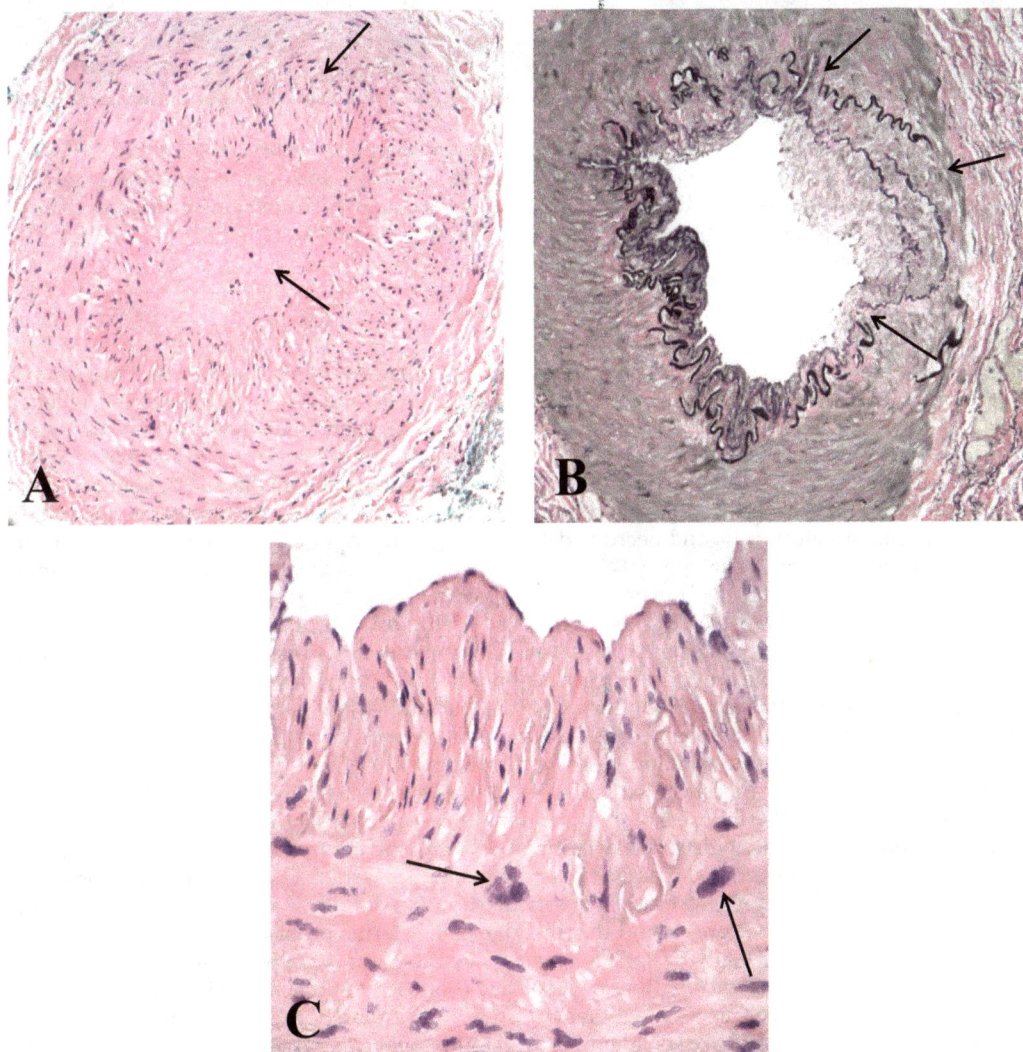

Figure 5.4 Histopathology of temporal artery in giant cell arteritis. (A) Hematoxylin and eosin stain of cross-section of temporal artery biopsy showed intimal hyperplasia with obliterated lumen (arrows) and lymphocytic infiltrate. (B) With elastin staining, large breaks in the internal elastic lamina are seen (arrows). (C) Higher magnification reveals presence of multinucleated giant cells (arrows). (Courtesy of Kimberly M. Winges, MD.)

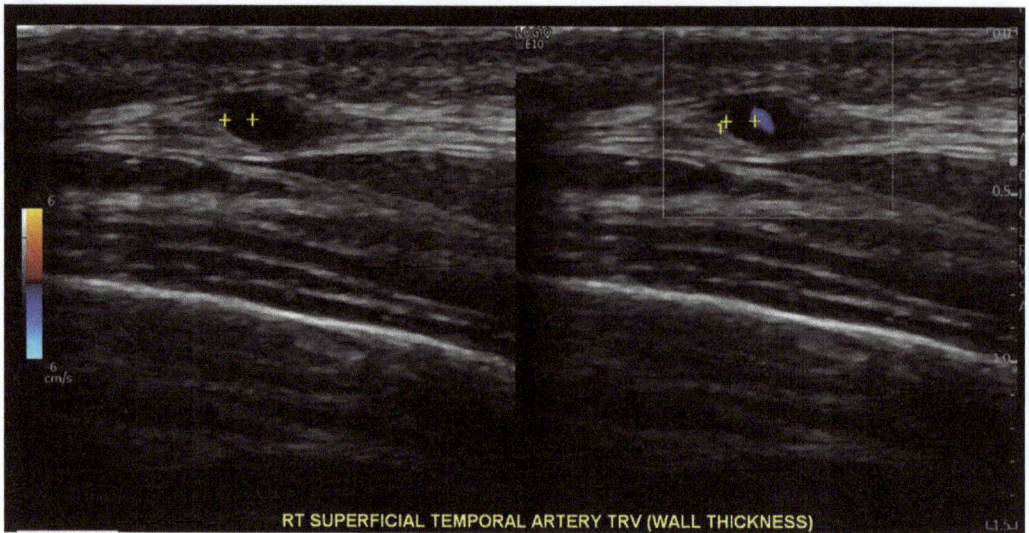

Figure 5.5 Halo sign on color Doppler ultrasound of temporal artery in giant cell arteritis. Ultrasound images of a superficial temporal artery in a patient with biopsy-positive giant cell arteritis. The "halo sign" is formed by the edematous vessel wall, which appears hypoechoic (black), through which vascular flow (blue) can be seen via Doppler. (Courtesy of Benjamin Osborne, MD and Mazin Elsarrag, MD.)

Aiming for a 3 cm target is recommended, as elasticity of the arterial wall will shrink the sample down significantly. The entire paraffin block should be sectioned and at least four levels evaluated.[38]

Biopsy should be obtained as soon as possible but no later than 14 days of starting high-dose corticosteroids. In the acute setting, histopathology shows a granulomatous infiltrate of histiocytes (CD68 stain) and multinucleated giant cells, seen most severely in the media and adventitia of the artery wall (Figure 5.4).[39] The intima is often thickened with fibrosis and may obliterate the lumen along with inflammatory cells and necrotic debris. An elastin stain may highlight large breaks in and subsequent scrolling of the internal elastic lamina, a finding that persists after acute inflammation heals. Late findings include transmural scarring with loss of the muscularis layer.

Color Doppler ultrasound may also be utilized by highly trained practitioners to evaluate for a hyperechoic "halo sign" around the lumen of superficial extracranial vessel walls, indicating localized vessel wall edema (Figure 5.5). A large meta-analysis of 23 studies showed a sensitivity and specificity of 67% and 95%, respectively, for GCA.[40] Recent studies have shown that ultrasound demonstrates non-inferior sensitivity compared to temporal artery biopsy for the diagnosis of GCA.[41, 42]

Novel techniques in high-resolution vessel wall MRI are also useful for diagnosis of GCA and have excellent sensitivity and specificity. MRI visualizes contrast enhancement of the superficial extracranial arterial walls (Figure 5.6).[43] This modality requires specialized scanners, MRI protocols, and trained neuroradiologists. It may be employed with greater frequency in the coming years.

Several groups have developed diagnostic prediction tools based on clinical manifestations with or without advanced imaging techniques, particularly ultrasound.[44–47] In one study, comparison of three clinical prediction scores found that the giant cell arteritis probability score (GCAPS, now referred to as the Southend GCAPS) had the greatest sensitivity for GCA, while the Bhavsar-Khalidi score had the greatest specificity.[48] Other groups have proposed approaches in incorporating high-resolution MRI into the diagnostic assessment of GCA.[49, 50] Ultimately, the most appropriate combination of diagnostic testing will depend on the availability of and expertise in these techniques at a given institution, and many centers may continue to rely on temporal artery biopsy.

5.4.2 Ocular Diagnostic Tests

In the context of acute visual loss, retinal angiography comprises the most useful ocular diagnostic imaging technique and includes both fluorescein angiography (FA) and indocyanine green angiography (ICGA). FA is the more commonly available modality and is generally used to document

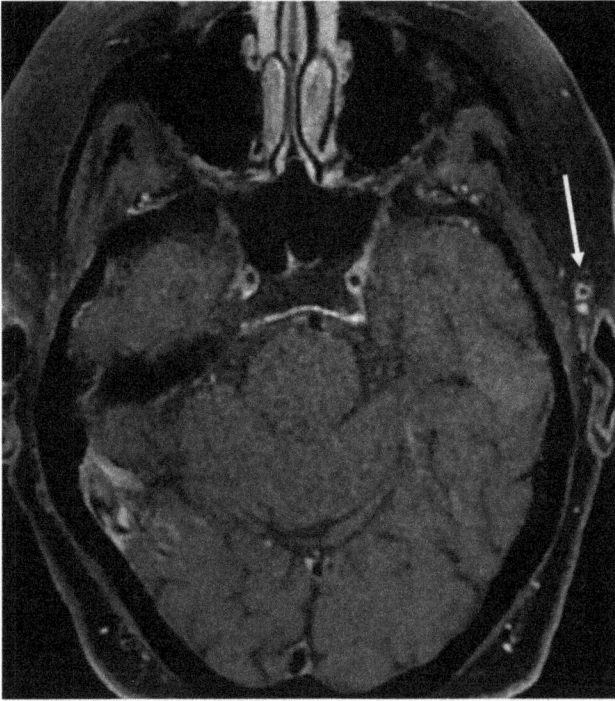

Figure 5.6 Vessel wall enhancement of superficial temporal artery on high-resolution MRI. Axial section of T1 post-contrast MRI in a patient with giant cell arteritis. Diffuse contrast enhancement of the vessel wall of the left superficial temporal artery is visualized (arrow). (Courtesy of Lulu Bursztyn, Msc, MD, FRCS.)

intraretinal leakage from the arteriole-to-venous circulation, but the first few seconds prior to the artery-to-venous phase perfuse the choroid itself. Patchy choroidal non-perfusion can be seen best in the first half of FA time, followed by attenuation of the retinal arterioles and leakage of the optic disc if there is arteritic anterior ischemic optic neuropathy (AAION). In FA, 80% of the fluorescent molecule, fluorescein sodium, is bound to protein.[51] Unbound fluorescein leaks through vessel walls if those walls are inflamed (such as in vasculitis) or have poor integrity (such as in neovascularization resulting from chronic ocular ischemia). In contrast, ICGA visualizes only the choroid itself, which lies deep to the retina and choriocapillaris. The fluorescent molecule in ICGA is indocyanine, which is bound to 99% of the serum protein molecule and therefore does not traverse the choriocapillaris into the retina, keeping the choroid visible. Sensitivity and specificity for GCA in FA are 88% and 69% and for ICGA are 76% and 81%, respectively.[52] FA is more commonly used, although indocyanine has lower rates of adverse events related to allergy and anaphylaxis. Other diagnostic considerations for patchy choroidal hypoperfusion include other inflammatory vasculitides or malignant hypertension. While non-arteritic anterior ischemic optic neuropathy (NAION) may be confused, at least clinically, with AAION, the pathophysiology of NAION is related to transient poor perfusion of the small posterior ciliary arterioles that supply the optic nerve head itself and therefore does not cause widespread choroidal hypoperfusion.

While not specific for GCA, optical coherence tomography (OCT) of the peripapillary retinal nerve fiber layer will show acute thickening in AAION, which reflects the acute ischemic edema seen on exam (Figure 5.3). Cotton wool spots – localized infarcts of the retinal nerve fiber layer (RNFL) – may also occur. The eventual atrophy and thinning of the RNFL on OCT can be useful in establishing a new baseline following resolution of optic disc edema, usually by 1 to 3 months after the event. OCT of the macula may also be helpful in characterizing disease status.[53] In instances of occlusive retinal vasculitis, such as in a central retinal artery occlusion (CRAO), the inner layers of the retina swell and become hyperreflective and thickened (Figure 5.3). If the superficial retinal capillary plexus is affected, acute thickening of the RNFL and GCL with eventual thinning and atrophy may occur. If the intermediate and deep capillary plexuses are affected, paracentral acute middle maculopathy (PAMM) lesions may occur, represented by focal hyperreflective bands within the inner nuclear layer.[54] Usually, the outer retina remains intact, including the retinal photoreceptors and retinal pigmented epithelium.

It is important to consider other etiologies when evaluating a patient with ischemic visual manifestations (e.g., amaurosis fugax, retinal artery occlusion). Given that patients with GCA are typically older than 50 years, on average in their 70s, many patients have other risk factors for cardiovascular disease and stroke. Therefore, emboli from internal carotid atherosclerosis or cardiac plaque or thrombus should be evaluated with CTA or MRA head and neck, as well as an echocardiogram and electrocardiogram to assess the quality of cardiac flow and rhythm. Contrast-enhanced head and neck imaging also may identify posterior circulation stroke in GCA. Systemic evaluation of GCA patients includes dedicated imaging of the aorta and epi-aortic vessels (i.e., carotid, subclavian, axillary arteries), either via CTA/MRA or fluorodeoxyglucose (FDG) positron emission tomography (PET).

5.5 DIAGNOSTIC DELAY AND NATURAL HISTORY

Non-ocular presentations of GCA include scalp tenderness, jaw claudication, headache, polymyalgia rheumatica, limb claudication, and general constitutional symptoms such as malaise and unintended weight loss.[55] Since these symptoms may be transient and/or nonspecific, patients are often diagnosed weeks or months after symptom onset. A retrospective analysis of 282 GCA patients showed that nearly 20% experienced permanent vision loss, preceded by non-ocular symptoms by a median of 21 days.[56] In several of these cases, patients presented to their primary care provider before the onset of vision loss, but they were misdiagnosed and treatment further delayed. Another study showed that vision loss was the presenting symptom in 16% of patients.[57] Fortunately, once the correct diagnosis is made, studies show that treatment is in fact initiated promptly, usually within 1 day. Rapid treatment is critical, as patients can expect to progress from transient visual symptoms to permanent loss within a mean of 8.5 days.[58] Prompt glucocorticoids improves visual acuity only slightly and only in 4% of patients.[59] Nevertheless, the main reason to treat vision loss from GCA immediately upon suspicion is to protect the remaining seeing eye from permanent irreversible blindness since 72% of sequential contralateral vision loss occurs within 1 week.[10]

Studies have sought to determine factors that predict duration of diagnostic delay and treatment. A large meta-analysis showed that patients with cranial symptoms (i.e., scalp tenderness, jaw claudication, headache) received an earlier diagnosis at 7.7 weeks compared to 17.6 weeks for patients with non-cranial presentations.[55] No study has shown a statistically significant difference in diagnosis between patients with and without vision loss, although this may be secondary to low sample size and statistical power.[57, 60, 61] Patients with vision symptoms have been diagnosed typically between 1.7 and 10.8 weeks after presentation. For GCA patients overall, the diagnosis is made on average 9 weeks after symptom onset.[55]

Recent initiatives or "fast-track" programs, similar to stroke protocols, have sought to expedite the diagnosis and treatment of suspected GCA. These programs work by creating a separate referral flow from general practitioners to rheumatologists and providing protected clinic time so that patients can be evaluated and treated urgently. A fast-track initiative in the United Kingdom lowered the incidence of vision loss from 37% to 9%.[62] Ophthalmologists and optometrists recognize GCA as an ophthalmic emergency; familiarity with and early recognition of the ocular symptoms, signs, and inflammatory labs is paramount to timely treatment for this preventable cause of irreversible blindness.

5.6 TREATMENT

5.6.1 Initial Glucocorticoid Therapy and Monitoring

The mainstay of treatment for GCA is high-dose glucocorticoid therapy. Early initiation of glucocorticoids is imperative to preventing permanent vision loss caused by GCA. Because visual morbidity can be prevented in the vast majority of GCA cases with treatment, early initiation of glucocorticoids at the first sign of visual symptoms in patients suspected of GCA is imperative and is the greatest predictor of visual recovery.[6, 63, 64] The recommended regimen of glucocorticoid therapy for patients with newly diagnosed ocular GCA is intravenous (IV) methylprednisolone daily for 1 to 3 days, followed by 60 to 80 mg/day oral prednisone. If IV pulse dosing cannot be rapidly initiated, then 1 mg/kg/day (up to 80 mg) of oral prednisone is recommended.[37, 65, 66] Studies comparing the efficacy of IV pulse dosing to high-dose oral dosing have been limited and have had conflicting results; however, one study has suggested that IV pulse dosing may be associated with greater improvement of visual acuity in biopsy-proven GCA patients with recent or impending visual loss.[67] Additionally, in recent years, national guidelines have provided conflicting recommendations on the role of tocilizumab as an adjunct to glucocorticoid therapy in newly diagnosed ocular GCA, in light of positive clinical trial data.[68] When used, tocilizumab is commonly administered subcutaneously at 162 mg weekly or at 6 mg/kg (up to) IV every 4 weeks.[69]

Glucocorticoid therapy is tapered clinically in a patient-dependent manner and with careful monitoring. A long-term approach to tapering is generally recommended, especially when glucocorticoids are used as monotherapy, as premature reduction of therapy can lead to flares of disease activity and progression of vision loss, even in the contralateral eye in patients with previously unilateral ocular GCA.[9] If glucocorticoids are being administered as monotherapy, then as long as symptoms have near-normalized, glucocorticoids can be gradually reduced over several months, typically 9 to 12 months or longer. If glucocorticoids are being administered in combination with tocilizumab, then glucocorticoids can be tapered more rapidly over 6 months, in accordance with the schedule used in the clinical trial of tocilizumab (GiACTA trial).[68] Notably in the GiACTA trial, none of the patients assigned to tocilizumab developed new permanent visual loss during follow-up; one patient on tocilizumab developed A-AION with disease flare, but vision loss resolved with glucocorticoid therapy.

Although relapse of systemic symptoms is common and occurs in between 34% and 75% of GCA patients,[70] the recurrence of ocular symptoms during relapse occurs very rarely and is estimated to be around 1.5% of GCA cases. Monitoring for disease activity through history, physical exam, and laboratory testing should be performed routinely throughout the clinical course. It is important to note that commonly used laboratory markers, ESR and CRP, are not reliable markers of disease activity and have further limited value in patients receiving tocilizumab as a result of IL-6 blockade.[71] While ESR and CRP should continue to be monitored, an isolated rise of ESR or CRP levels alone should not prompt escalation of glucocorticoid therapy without associated worsening of symptoms.

When relapse occurs, modification of therapy is warranted. In the rare occurrence of ocular relapse, escalating the glucocorticoid dose (via IV pulse dosing or high-dose oral prednisone, as described before) is recommended.[37, 65] For other types of relapse without visual symptoms, escalating to the last effective dose (or slightly greater) is appropriate.[37, 65, 66]

5.6.2 Non-Glucocorticoid Therapy Options for Giant Cell Arteritis

As a result of the long-term glucocorticoid regimen that is administered in GCA treatment, there is a high burden of toxicity associated with the therapy, such as glucocorticoid-induced osteoporosis and opportunistic infections secondary to immunosuppression.[72] Careful monitoring and potential prophylaxis for these conditions are paramount for GCA patients. Given the high burden of toxicity associated with glucocorticoid therapy, there is a need for steroid-sparing therapies that can be used adjunctively to reduce the cumulative steroid burden of extended treatment. Use of tocilizumab in GCA achieves sustained remission at 52 weeks and reduces cumulative prednisone exposure,[68, 73] although data on ophthalmologic manifestations is limited. Further investigation of long-term data on the safety of tocilizumab in the GCA population is needed. The limited safety data on the long-term use of tocilizumab in the older, comorbid population of GCA patients, as well as pragmatic concerns about its cost, has led to conflicting usage recommendations from various national guidelines, which are described in further detail in the next section. Another agent that has been tested in randomized trials is methotrexate, which has been shown to have, at best, a modest improvement in relapse rates and cumulative prednisone dose.[74] The efficacies of tocilizumab and methotrexate have not yet been compared, although studies are underway.

In the case of relapse while on tocilizumab, the addition of other immunosuppressives such as methotrexate may be considered.[37, 74] Abatacept may also be considered if patient is refractory to or cannot tolerate tocilizumab.[37] Several other agents, such as azathioprine, mycophenolate, cyclophosphamide, cyclosporin, dapsone, and leflunomide, have been suggested as potential adjuncts in GCA treatment; however, many of these have limited data to support their use.[75] In addition, there is conflicting evidence for the prophylactic use of aspirin to decrease the risk of cardiovascular and ischemic events in GCA patients,[76] resulting in conflicting recommendations from various national guidelines, as described in the next section. Clinical trials of other immunosuppressives are ongoing and may soon expand the armamentarium used to treat GCA.

Table 5.2 Society Guidelines for Management of GCA

	American College of Rheumatology/ Vasculitis Foundation (ACR/VF)	European Alliance of Associations for Rheumatology (EULAR)	British Society for Rheumatology (BSR)
Treatment of newly diagnosed GCA	Glucocorticoids + tocilizumab	Glucocorticoid monotherapy (unless disease is relapsing, refractory, or has a high risk of complications)	Either glucocorticoid monotherapy or in combination with tocilizumab (monotherapy may be more cost-effective)
Dosing of glucocorticoids in ocular GCA	Glucocorticoids should be administered as intravenous pulse dose, instead of oral		
Treatment of relapsing GCA	Tocilizumab should be added as an adjunctive agent if not already started, and methotrexate can be considered as an alternative to tocilizumab		
Aspirin as prophylaxis for cardiovascular and ischemic events	Start aspirin in newly diagnosed GCA patients with critical/flow-limiting involvement of vertebral/carotid arteries	Do not start aspirin in a prophylactic role for GCA-related stenoses, unless otherwise indicated for non-GCA pathology	
Fast-track pathways	Rapid multidisciplinary involvement though programs such as "fast-track" pathways have demonstrated better visual outcomes for patients with ocular GCA		

5.6.3 Guidelines for the Clinical Management of Giant Cell Arteritis

Multiple societies have published guidelines for the management of GCA, including the American College of Rheumatology/Vasculitis Foundation (ACR/VF),[37] the European Alliance of Associations for Rheumatology (EULAR),[65] and the British Society for Rheumatology (BSR).[66] Despite the conditional nature of many of the recommendations due to the low quantity and quality of available evidence, these societies agree across most recommendations with a few notable differences (Table 5.2).

For the initial treatment of newly diagnosed GCA, one such difference among the recommendations from these societies is present (Table 5.2). ACR/VF guidelines recommend the use of glucocorticoids in combination with tocilizumab for new GCA, while EULAR guidelines recommend the use of glucocorticoids alone unless disease is relapsing, refractory, or has a high risk of complications. BSR guidelines state that either glucocorticoid monotherapy or in combination with tocilizumab is acceptable and note that glucocorticoid monotherapy may be more cost-effective. However, the guidelines of all three societies agree that in the case of ocular GCA, irrespective of tocilizumab use, glucocorticoids should be administered as IV pulse dose instead of as oral prednisone, based on weak evidence from retrospective studies.[59, 67] BSR guidelines qualify this recommendation to clarify that treatment should not be delayed if IV pulse dose is not readily accessible.

For the treatment of relapsing GCA, the recommendations from all three societies are concordant: tocilizumab should be added as an adjunctive agent if not already started, and methotrexate can be considered as an alternative to tocilizumab (Table 5.2). For the use of aspirin as prophylaxis for cardiovascular and ischemic events, the societies' recommendations once again diverge: ACR/VF guidelines recommend starting aspirin in newly diagnosed GCA patients with critical or flow-limiting involvement of vertebral or carotid arteries, while EULAR and BSR guidelines do not recommend starting aspirin in a prophylactic role for GCA-related stenoses unless otherwise indicated. Finally, one overarching principle that was consistent across the guidelines of all societies was the need for rapid multidisciplinary involvement. Programs such as "fast-track" pathways have demonstrated better visual outcomes for patients with ocular GCA in particular,[62] thus demonstrating a non-pharmacologic method through which treatment can be improved for GCA patients at risk for blindness.

5.7 RARE OCULAR MANIFESTATIONS IN TAKAYASU ARTERITIS AND OTHER SYSTEMIC NON-ANCA VASCULITIDES

Ocular manifestations can also occur in another type of large-vessel vasculitis: Takayasu arteritis (TAK). Unlike GCA, TAK usually occurs in younger populations under the age of 40 years, with the highest reported prevalence in young, female, Asian populations, including Japan, where the prevalence is estimated at 40 per million.[77] In other parts of the world, the prevalence is much lower, such as in Kuwait at 7.8 per million.[78] The frequency of visual symptoms in TAK in case series ranges widely from 8% to 68%. Among these, the most common visual symptoms are decreased vision and amaurosis fugax, notably with a relatively well-preserved best-corrected visual acuity.[79]

The most common ocular complication of TAK is retinopathy. Hypertensive retinopathy, usually as a result of renal artery stenosis, was observed in 16% to 37% of TAK patients, and Takayasu retinopathy, which is instead caused by hypoperfusion as a result of carotid artery stenosis, has been observed in 14% to 33% of TAK patients.[80] In addition to retinopathy, another rarer complication of TAK includes uveitis, but this is seen in children much more commonly than in adults.[81] Like in GCA, the mainstay of treatment for TAK is systemic glucocorticoids; however, given the chronic nature of TAK, a glucocorticoid-sparing agent, such as tumor necrosis factor-alpha inhibitors, tocilizumab, methotrexate, mycophenolate, or leflunomide, is also recommended as an adjunctive therapy to reduce the cumulative glucocorticoid burden.[37, 65]

In addition, there have been rare reports of ocular manifestations in the vasculitides affecting small and/or medium vessels, many of which are more similar in clinical presentation to ANCA-associated vasculitis. Among the small-vessel vasculitides, there have been reports of episcleritis, uveitis, and keratitis in IgA vasculitis, albeit exceedingly rare.[82, 83] In cryoglobulinemic vasculitis, corneal deposits have been observed as well as various types of retinopathy.[84, 85] In hypocomplementemic urticarial vasculitis syndrome, conjunctivitis, episcleritis, and uveitis are known to occur.[86] Of the vasculitides that affect medium-sized vessels, polyarteritis nodosa (PAN) has ocular involvement in 10% to 20% of cases[87] with wide-ranging manifestations such as episcleritis, scleritis, and keratitis, and ischemic optic neuropathy.[88] Identification of the ocular manifestations of these vasculitides is critical to providing organ-saving treatment.

5.8 SUMMARY

Ophthalmologic complications are a major concern in GCA, which is a systemic large-vessel vasculitis. Patients over the age of 50 years with abrupt, severe vision loss in one or both eyes or other GCA-associated visual symptoms should seek medical attention immediately to promptly initiate therapy. Comprehensive ophthalmologic evaluation, laboratory, imaging, and/or temporal artery biopsy are needed to diagnose GCA. High-dose glucocorticoids and possibly other systemic immunosuppressives are effective treatments of GCA. Ocular manifestations are less common but can occur in Takayasu arteritis and other systemic non-ANCA vasculitides.

REFERENCES

1. Chandran AK, Udayakumar PD, Crowson CS, et al. The incidence of giant cell arteritis in Olmsted County, Minnesota, over a 60-year period 1950–2009. *Scand J Rheumatol.* 2015;44(3):215–218.
2. Salvarani C, Gabriel SE, O'Fallon WM, et al. The incidence of giant cell arteritis in Olmsted County, Minnesota: apparent fluctuations in a cyclic pattern. *Ann Intern Med.* 1995;123(3): 192–194.
3. Noltorp S, Svensson B. High incidence of polymyalgia rheumatica and giant cell arteritis in a Swedish community. *Clin Exp Rheumatol.* 1991;9(4):351–355.
4. Skanchy DF, Vickers A, Prospero Ponce CM, et al. Ocular manifestations of giant cell arteritis. *Expert Rev Ophthalmol.* 2019;14(1):23–32.
5. Vodopivec I, Rizzo JF, III. Ophthalmic manifestations of giant cell arteritis. *Rheumatology (Oxford, England).* 2018;57(Suppl 2):ii63–ii72.
6. Soriano A, Muratore F, Pipitone N, et al. Visual loss and other cranial ischaemic complications in giant cell arteritis. *Nat Rev Rheumatol.* 2017;13(8):476–484.
7. Salvarani C, Cantini F, Boiardi L, et al. Polymyalgia rheumatica and giant-cell arteritis. *N Engl J Med.* 2002;347(4):261–271.
8. Kawasaki A, Purvin V. Giant cell arteritis: an updated review. *Acta Ophthalmol.* 2009;87(1):13–32.

9. Hayreh SS, Podhajsky PA, Zimmerman B. Ocular manifestations of giant cell arteritis. *Am J Ophthalmol*. 1998;125(4):509–520.

10. Jonasson F, Cullen JF, Elton RA. Temporal arteritis: a 14-year epidemiological, clinical and prognostic study. *Scott Med J*. 1979;24(2):111–117.

11. Chen JJ, Leavitt JA, Fang C, et al. Evaluating the Incidence of arteritic ischemic optic neuropathy and other causes of vision loss from giant cell arteritis. *Ophthalmology*. 2016;123(9):1999–2003.

12. Liu GT, Glaser JS, Schatz NJ, et al. Visual morbidity in giant cell arteritis: clinical characteristics and prognosis for vision. *Ophthalmology*. 1994;101(11):1779–1785.

13. Michalinos A, Zogana S, Kotsiomitis E, et al. Anatomy of the ophthalmic artery: a review concerning its modern surgical and clinical applications. *Anat Res Int*. 2015;2015:591961.

14. Hayreh SS. Giant cell arteritis: its ophthalmic manifestations. *Indian J Ophthalmol*. 2021; 69(2):227–235.

15. Hayreh SS. Posterior ischaemic optic neuropathy: clinical features, pathogenesis, and management. *Eye (London)*. 2004;18(11):1188–1206.

16. Danyel LA, Miszczuk M, Pietrock C, et al. Utility of standard diffusion-weighted magnetic resonance imaging for the identification of ischemic optic neuropathy in giant cell arteritis. *Sci Rep*. 2022;12(1):16553.

17. Rhee RL, Rebello R, Tamhankar MA, et al. Combined orbital and cranial vessel wall magnetic resonance imaging for the assessment of disease activity in giant cell arteritis. *ACR Open Rheumatol*. 2024;6(4):189–200. doi:10.1002/acr2.11649. Epub 2024 Jan 24.

18. Guggenberger KV, Vogt ML, Song JW, et al. Intraorbital findings in giant cell arteritis on black blood MRI. *Eur Radiol*. 2023;33(4):2529–2535.

19. Mohammed-Brahim N, Clavel G, Charbonneau F, et al. Three Tesla 3D high-resolution vessel wall MRI of the orbit may differentiate arteritic from nonarteritic anterior ischemic optic neuropathy. *Invest Radiol*. 2019;54(11):712–718.

20. Bandini F, Benedetti L, Ceppa P, et al. Uveitis as a presenting sign of giant cell arteritis. *J Neuroophthalmol*. 2005;25(3):247–248.

21. Rajesh CV, Cole M. Panuveitis as a presenting feature of giant cell arteritis. *Br J Ophthalmol*. 2000;84(3):340.

22. Nguyen NV, Karkhur S, Yuksel M, et al. Posterior uveitis associated with large vessel giant cell arteritis. *Ocul Immunol Inflamm*. 2022;30(7–8):2019–2022.

23. Zulfiqar AA. Giant cell arteritis and scleritis: a rare association. *Caspian J Intern Med*. 2022;13(3):642–645.

24. Erdogan M, Sayin N, Yildiz Ekinci D, et al. Bilateral posterior scleritis associated with giant cell arteritis: a case report. *Ocul Immunol Inflamm*. 2018;26(8):1244–1247.

25. Penet T, Lambert M, Baillet C, et al. Giant cell arteritis-related cerebrovascular ischemic events: a French retrospective study of 271 patients, systematic review of the literature and meta-analysis. *Arthritis Res Ther*. 2023;25(1):116.

26. Krupa WM, Dewan M, Jeon MS, et al. Trapping of misdirected dendritic cells in the granulomatous lesions of giant cell arteritis. *Am J Pathol*. 2002;161(5):1815–1823.

27. Weyand CM, Hicok KC, Hunder GG, et al. Tissue cytokine patterns in patients with polymyalgia rheumatica and giant cell arteritis. *Ann Intern Med*. 1994;121(7):484–491.

28. Deng J, Younge BR, Olshen RA, et al. Th17 and Th1 T-cell responses in giant cell arteritis. *Circulation*. 2010;121(7):906–915.

29. Weyand CM, Wagner AD, Bjornsson J, et al. Correlation of the topographical arrangement and the functional pattern of tissue-infiltrating macrophages in giant cell arteritis. *J Clin Invest*. 1996;98(7):1642–1649.

30. Rodriguez-Pla A, Bosch-Gil JA, Rossello-Urgell J, et al. Metalloproteinase-2 and -9 in giant cell arteritis: involvement in vascular remodeling. *Circulation*. 2005;112(2):264–269.

31. Gonzalez-Gay MA, Lopez-Diaz MJ, Barros S, et al. Giant cell arteritis: laboratory tests at the time of diagnosis in a series of 240 patients. *Medicine (Baltimore)*. 2005;84(5):277–290.

32. Chan FLY, Lester S, Whittle SL, et al. The utility of ESR, CRP and platelets in the diagnosis of GCA. *BMC Rheumatol*. 2019;3:14.

33. Ing EB, Miller NR, Nguyen A, et al. Neural network and logistic regression diagnostic prediction models for giant cell arteritis: development and validation. *Clin Ophthalmol*. 2019;13:421–430.

34. Selby LD, Park-Egan BAM, Winges KM. Temporal artery biopsy in the workup of giant cell arteritis: diagnostic considerations in a veterans administration cohort. *J Neuroophthalmol*. 2020;40(4):450–456.

35. Rubenstein E, Maldini C, Gonzalez-Chiappe S, et al. Sensitivity of temporal artery biopsy in the diagnosis of giant cell arteritis: a systematic literature review and meta-analysis. *Rheumatology (Oxford, England)*. 2020;59(5):1011–1020.

36. McMurran AE, Boom SJ. Temporal artery biopsies: do they make the cut? *Scott Med J*. 2015;60(1):9–12.

37. Maz M, Chung SA, Abril A, et al. 2021 American College of Rheumatology/Vasculitis Foundation Guideline for the Management of giant cell arteritis and Takayasu arteritis. *Arthritis Rheumatol (Hoboken, NJ)*. 2021;73(8):1349–1365.

38. Stone JR, Basso C, Baandrup UT, et al. Recommendations for processing cardiovascular surgical pathology specimens: a consensus statement from the standards and definitions committee of the Society for Cardiovascular Pathology and the Association for European Cardiovascular Pathology. *Cardiovasc Pathol*. 2012;21(1):2–16.

39. Wang AL, Raven ML, Surapaneni K, et al. Studies on the histopathology of temporal arteritis. *Ocul Oncol Pathol*. 2017;3(1):60–65.

40. Sebastian A, Coath F, Innes S, et al. Role of the halo sign in the assessment of giant cell arteritis: a systematic review and meta-analysis. *Rheumatol Adv Pract*. 2021;5(3):rkab059.

41. Hansen MS, Terslev L, Jensen MR, et al. Comparison of temporal artery ultrasound versus biopsy in the diagnosis of giant cell arteritis. *Eye (London)*. 2023;37(2):344–349.

42. Luqmani R, Lee E, Singh S, et al. The role of ultrasound compared to biopsy of temporal arteries in the diagnosis and treatment of giant cell arteritis (TABUL): a diagnostic accuracy and cost-effectiveness study. *Health Technol Assess*. 2016;20(90):1–238.

43. Zhang KJ, Li MX, Zhang P, et al. Validity of high resolution magnetic resonance imaging in detecting giant cell arteritis: a meta-analysis. *Eur Radiol*. 2022;32(5):3541–3552.

44. Laskou F, Coath F, Mackie SL, et al. A probability score to aid the diagnosis of suspected giant cell arteritis. *Clin Exp Rheumatol*. 2019;37((2) Suppl 117):104–108.

45. Czihal M, Lottspeich C, Bernau C, et al. A diagnostic algorithm based on a simple clinical prediction rule for the diagnosis of cranial giant cell arteritis. *J Clin Med*. 2021;10(6).

46. Sebastian A, van der Geest KSM, Tomelleri A, et al. Development of a diagnostic prediction model for giant cell arteritis by sequential application of Southend giant cell arteritis probability score and ultrasonography: a prospective multicentre study. *Lancet Rheumatol*. 2024;6(5):e291–e299.

47. Ing EB, Lahaie Luna G, Toren A, et al. Multivariable prediction model for suspected giant cell arteritis: development and validation. *Clin Ophthalmol*. 2017;11:2031–2042.

48. Sargi C, Ducharme-Benard S, Benard V, et al. Assessment and comparison of probability scores to predict giant cell arteritis. *Clin Rheumatol*. 2024;43(1):357–365.

49. Junek M, Hu A, Garner S, et al. Contextualizing temporal arterial magnetic resonance angiography in the diagnosis of giant cell arteritis: a retrospective cohort study. *Rheumatology*. 2021;60(9):4229–4237. doi:10.1093/rheumatology/keaa916.

50. Lecler A, Hage R, Charbonneau F, et al. Validation of a multimodal algorithm for diagnosing giant cell arteritis with imaging. *Diagn Interv Imaging*. 2022;103(2):103–110.

51. O'Goshi K, Serup J. Safety of sodium fluorescein for in vivo study of skin. *Skin Res Technol*. 2006;12(3):155–161.

52. Dentel A, Clavel G, Savatovsky J, et al. Use of retinal angiography and MRI in the diagnosis of giant cell arteritis with early ophthalmic manifestations. *J Neuroophthalmol*. 2022;42(2):218–225.

53. Casella AMB, Mansour AM, Ec S, et al. Choroidal ischemia as one cardinal sign in giant cell arteritis. *Int J Retina Vitreous*. 2022;8(1):69.

54. Yu S, Pang CE, Gong Y, et al. The spectrum of superficial and deep capillary ischemia in retinal artery occlusion. *Am J Ophthalmol*. 2015;159(1):53–63.e1–e2.

55. Prior JA, Ranjbar H, Belcher J, et al. Diagnostic delay for giant cell arteritis – a systematic review and meta-analysis. *BMC Med*. 2017;15(1):120.

56. Hemmig AK, Aschwanden M, Seiler S, et al. Long delay from symptom onset to first consultation contributes to permanent vision loss in patients with giant cell arteritis: a cohort study. *RMD Open*. 2023;9(1).

57. Ezeonyeji AN, Borg FA, Dasgupta B. Delays in recognition and management of giant cell arteritis: results from a retrospective audit. *Clin Rheumatol*. 2011;30(2):259–262.

58. Gordon LK, Levin LA. Visual loss in giant cell arteritis. *JAMA*. 1998;280(4):385–386.

59. Hayreh SS, Zimmerman B, Kardon RH. Visual improvement with corticosteroid therapy in giant cell arteritis: report of a large study and review of literature. *Acta Ophthalmol Scand*. 2002;80(4):355–367.

60. Gonzalez-Gay MA, Garcia-Porrua C, Llorca J, et al. Visual manifestations of giant cell arteritis: trends and clinical spectrum in 161 patients. *Medicine (Baltimore)*. 2000;79(5):283–292.

61. Schmidt D, Vaith P, Hetzel A. Prevention of serious ophthalmic and cerebral complications in temporal arteritis? *Clin Exp Rheumatol*. 2000;18((4) Suppl 20):S61–S63.

62. Patil P, Williams M, Maw WW, et al. Fast track pathway reduces sight loss in giant cell arteritis: results of a longitudinal observational cohort study. *Clin Exp Rheumatol*. 2015;33((2) Suppl 89):S103–S106.

63. Cid MC, Merkel PA. Chapter 43 – giant cell arteritis. In: Creager MA, Beckman JA, Loscalzo J, eds, *Vascular medicine: a companion to Braunwald's heart disease*, 2nd edn. Philadelphia: W.B. Saunders, 2013:525–532.

64. Gonzalez-Gay MA, Blanco R, Rodriguez-Valverde V, et al. Permanent visual loss and cerebrovascular accidents in giant cell arteritis: predictors and response to treatment. *Arthritis Rheum*. 1998;41(8):1497–1504.

65. Hellmich B, Agueda A, Monti S, et al. 2018 update of the EULAR recommendations for the management of large vessel vasculitis. *Ann Rheum Dis*. 2020;79(1):19–30.

66. Mackie SL, Dejaco C, Appenzeller S, et al. British Society for Rheumatology guideline on diagnosis and treatment of giant cell arteritis: executive summary. *Rheumatology*. 2020;59(3):487–494.

67. Chan CC, Paine M, O'Day J. Steroid management in giant cell arteritis. *Br J Ophthalmol*. 2001;85(9):1061–1064.

68. Stone JH, Tuckwell K, Dimonaco S, et al. Trial of tocilizumab in giant-cell arteritis. *N Engl J Med*. 2017;377(4):317–328.

69. Schirmer M, Muratore F, Salvarani C. Tocilizumab for the treatment of giant cell arteritis. *Expert Rev Clin Immunol*. 2018;14(5):339–349.

70. Muratore F, Boiardi L, Restuccia G, et al. Relapses and long-term remission in large vessel giant cell arteritis in Northern Italy: characteristics and predictors in a long-term follow-up study. *Semin Arthritis Rheum*. 2020;50(4):549–558.

71. van der Geest KSM, Sandovici M, Brouwer E, et al. Diagnostic accuracy of symptoms, physical signs, and laboratory tests for giant cell arteritis: a systematic review and meta-analysis. *JAMA Intern Med*. 2020;180(10):1295–1304.

72. Harris E, Tiganescu A, Tubeuf S, et al. The prediction and monitoring of toxicity associated with long-term systemic glucocorticoid therapy. *Curr Rheumatol Rep*. 2015;17(6):513.

73. Stone JH, Han J, Aringer M, et al. Long-term effect of tocilizumab in patients with giant cell arteritis: open-label extension phase of the giant cell arteritis actemra (GiACTA) trial. *Lancet Rheumatol*. 2021;3(5):e328–e336.

74. Mahr AD, Jover JA, Spiera RF, et al. Adjunctive methotrexate for treatment of giant cell arteritis: an individual patient data meta-analysis. *Arthritis Rheum*. 2007;56(8):2789–2797.

75. Dejaco C, Brouwer E, Mason JC, et al. Giant cell arteritis and polymyalgia rheumatica: current challenges and opportunities. *Nat Rev Rheumatol*. 2017;13(10):578–592.

76. Qureshi A, Halilu F, Serafi SW, et al. Evidence-based role of aspirin in giant cell arteritis: a literature review. *J Community Hosp Intern Med Perspect*. 2022;12(5):11–16.

77. Toshihiko N. Current status of large and small vessel vasculitis in Japan. *Int J Cardiol*. 1996;(Suppl 54):S91–S98.

78. el-Reshaid K, Varro J, al-Duwairi Q, et al. Takayasu's arteritis in Kuwait. *J Trop Med Hyg*. 1995;98(5):299–305.

79. Peter J, David S, Danda D, et al. Ocular manifestations of Takayasu arteritis: a cross-sectional study. *Retina (Philadelphia, PA)*. 2011;31(6):1170–1178.

80. Chun YS, Park SJ, Park IK, Lee J. The clinical and ocular manifestations of Takayasu arteritis. *Retina (Philadelphia, PA)*. 2001;21(2):132–140.

81. Szydelko-Pasko U, Przezdziecka-Dolyk J, Nowak L, et al. Ocular manifestations of Takayasu's arteritis: a case-based systematic review and meta-analysis. *J Clin Med*. 2023;12(11).

82. Lorentz WB, Jr., Weaver RG. Eye involvement in anaphylactoid purpura. *Am J Dis Child*. 1980;134(5):524–525.

83. Yamabe H, Ozawa K, Fukushi K, et al. IgA nephropathy and Henoch-Schonlein purpura nephritis with anterior uveitis. *Nephron*. 1988;50(4):368–370.

84. Kremer I, Wright P, Merin S, et al. Corneal subepithelial monoclonal kappa IgG deposits in essential cryoglobulinaemia. *Br J Ophthalmol*. 1989;73(8):669–673.

85. Myers JP, Di Bisceglie AM, Mann ES. Cryoglobulinemia associated with Purtscher-like retinopathy. *Am J Ophthalmol*. 2001;131(6):802–804.

86. Jara LJ, Navarro C, Medina G, et al. Hypocomplementemic urticarial vasculitis syndrome. *Curr Rheumatol Rep.* 2009;11(6):410–415.
87. Vingopoulos F, Karagiotis T, Palioura S. Bilateral interstitial keratitis, erythema nodosum and atrial fibrillation as presenting signs of polyarteritis nodosa. *Am J Ophthalmol Case Rep.* 2020;18:100619.
88. Vazquez-Romo KA, Rodriguez-Hernandez A, Paczka JA, et al. Optic neuropathy secondary to polyarteritis nodosa, case report, and diagnostic challenges. *Front Neurol.* 2017;8:490.

6 Ophthalmologic Diseases in the Spondyloarthritides

Cassidy Pinion, George Mount, and Grace A. Levy-Clarke

The spondyloarthritides (SpA) encompass a large group of rheumatic inflammatory disorders with similar clinical features and genetic predisposition (Table 6.1). The SpA group of disorders can be considered in two sub-groups: axial SpA and peripheral SpA. The typical presenting symptoms include chronic lower back pain deemed inflammatory, with an insidious onset. The lower back disorder can present as morning stiffness, which improves with exercise, not rest.[1] The most common extra-articular manifestation among this group is acute anterior uveitis (AAU), occurring in up to one-third of patients.[2] The patient population showing the highest incidence of anterior uveitis of all the spondyloarthropathies are the patients with ankylosing spondylitis (AS). AS patients with uveitis appear to have a more significant delay in diagnosis and a trend toward higher AS disease activity scores as compared to AS patients without uveitis.[3] Some studies report that the patient population affected by AS-associated AAU is predominantly male, while other studies report no differences based on gender.[4]

Worldwide, 60% to 90% of the axial SpA population carry the HLA-B27 haplotype; it is a highly heritable disorder.[5] An estimated 50% to 75% of AAU patients with an underlying SpA are also HLA-B27 haplotype positive.[6] As the prevalence of HLA-B27 positivity varies between the different spondyloarthropathies, the occurrence of uveitis also differs. Diseases that have a high association with HLA-B27 report a much higher incidence of uveitis. Uveitis occurs in approximately 40% of patients with ankylosing spondylitis, the spondyloarthropathy most associated with the carriage of HLA-B27.[7] Spondyloarthropathies less frequently associated with HLA-B27, such as psoriatic arthritis and enteropathic arthritis, are also less commonly associated with uveitis, 10% to 20% and 2% to 5%, respectively.[8, 9]

Three main hypotheses regarding HLA-B27 and the development of AS are commonly cited in the literature. The first hypothesis, coined the "arthritogenic peptide theory," proposes the presentation of exogenous peptides to CD8 lymphocytes, resulting in an inflammatory response to cross-reactive antigens. The second hypothesis proposes an intracellular misfolding of the HLA-B27 molecule, resulting in inflammatory cytokine release. The final hypothesis proposes that the free heavy chain of the HLA-B27 molecule may stimulate the innate and adaptive immune system, leading to the release of pro-inflammatory mediators.[5]

Gut bacteria share microbial-derived metabolites like vitamin K and are critical to the immune system. Therefore, changes in the gut microbiota can ultimately alter immune function.[10] Research into the involvement of the gut microbiome in the spondyloarthritides has been increasingly important. It is reported that HLA-B27 affects transgenic rats' gut microbiota and predisposes them to AS and possibly AAU. Many theories exist regarding the pivotal role of homeostasis between the immune system and the microbiota.[11] These concepts also support the postulate that dysbiosis plays a role in the risk gene HLA-B27 and its association with the development of SpA and AAU.[12, 13]

6.1 CLINICAL FEATURES: Presenting Symptoms and Signs

In 2021, the Standardization of Uveitis Nomenclature (SUN) Working Group published classification criteria for HLA-B27-associated spondyloarthritis anterior uveitis, using machine learning, coupled with case selection-based informatics, followed by consensus technique-based case selection. Three key uveitic diagnostic features were identified: acute/recurrent in onset and duration, unilateral/alternating in laterality, and anterior in anatomical location.[14]

AAU is defined as inflammation limited to the anterior chamber, which is sudden in onset with a limited duration, typically 3 months or less. AAU is also known as iritis, iridocyclitis, or anterior cyclitis.[15, 16] The most prominent feature is an acute onset of eye pain, often described as a deep, varying intensity of discomfort localized in and around the afflicted eye. The pain typically will be preceded by a prodromal stage, and patients will report a foreign body sensation within the eye, which exacerbates overall discomfort. Along with pain, patients will present with redness (ciliary injection) and photophobia. Due to the inflammation of the anterior chamber, blurry or hazy vision may also be a presenting symptom. Decreased visual acuity could also result from inflammatory cells in the anterior vitreous (intermediate uveitis) with associated cystoid macular edema. Spondyloarthritis-associated AAU is usually recurrent, with one to four limited episodes occurring in a year. SUN defines recurrent as repeated episodes of uveitis separated by periods of inactivity without treatment of at least 3 months.[17]

DOI: 10.1201/9781003453710-6

Table 6.1 Clinical Features and Ocular Findings in the Spondyloarthropathies

		Clinical Findings	Ocular Findings	HLA-B27	Age	Sex
Axial SpA	Ankylosing Spondylitis	Spondylitis, sacroiliitis	Acute anterior uveitis	90%	15–40	M > F
	Non-Radiographic Axial Spondyloarthritis[2]	Inflammation of spine as seen with MRI	Acute anterior uveitis	80%	< 45	M = F
Peripheral SpA	Reactive Arthritis	Arthritis, urethritis, mucocutaneous lesions	Acute anterior uveitis, conjunctivitis	60%	15–40	M > F
	Psoriatic Arthritis	Inflammation of small joints, psoriasis, dactylitis	Chronic uveitis	< 15%	30–55	F > M
	Enteropathic Arthritis[5]	Inflammatory back/joint pain; Inflammation of bowel: Crohn's disease, ulcerative colitis and undifferentiated colitis	Chronic uveitis	< 10%	15–40	F > M
	Juvenile Spondyloarthritis[6, 7]	SpA symptoms beginning in childhood, enthesitis, spinal arthritis	Acute anterior uveitis	45%	3–16	F > M
	Undifferentiated Spondyloarthritis[8]	Combination of disease features suggestive of spondyloarthritis	Uveitis	20–25%	< 45	F > M

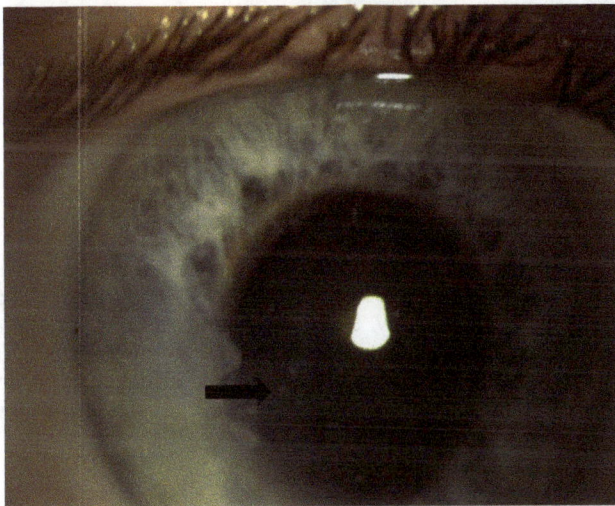

Figure 6.1 Keratic precipitates (black arrow, GLC, WVU).

Clinical signs involving the anterior segment include anterior chamber cell and flare, endothelial keratic precipitates (typically non-granulomatous) (Figure 6.1), posterior synechiae (Figure 6.2), and normal or low intraocular pressure. The reduced intraocular pressure (hypotony) in the affected eye compared to the contralateral eye is an essential clinical sign in developing the differential diagnosis. This hypotony is due to inflammation of the ciliary body, resulting in hyposecretion.[18] In severe cases, hypopyon (Figure 6.3) and anterior chamber fibrin may be present in the anterior chamber.

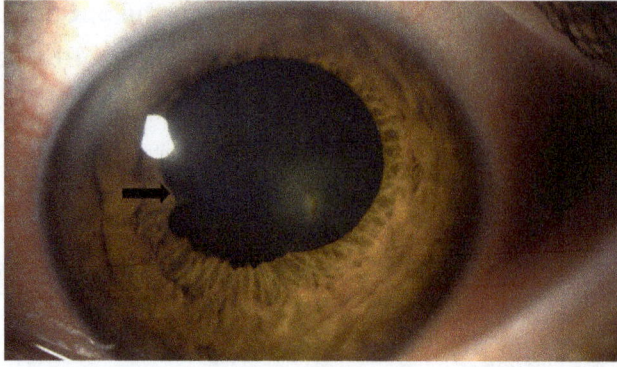

Figure 6.2 Posterior synechiae. Abnormal adhesions between the iris and underlying structures (black arrow) (GLC, WVU).

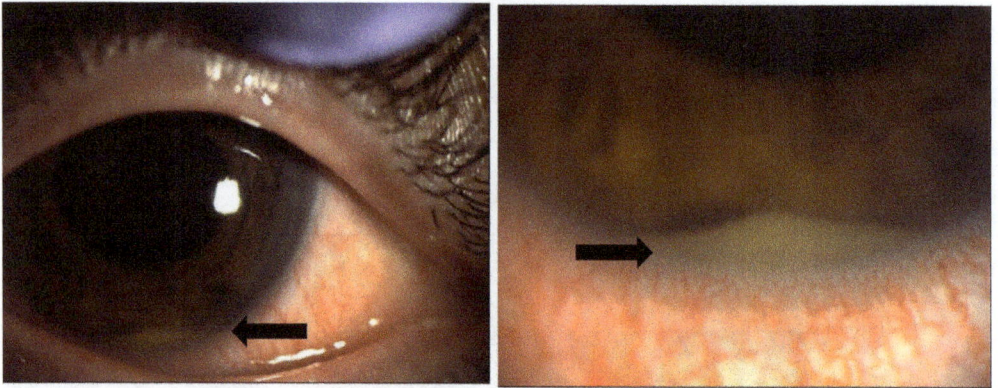

Figure 6.3 Hypopyon. Accumulation of white blood cells as a layer in the anterior chamber (black arrows) (GLC, WVU).

6.2 UVEITIS ASSOCIATED WITH OTHER FORMS OF SpA

The patient's underlying SpA often dictates the clinical presentation of associated uveitis. Uveitis in reactive arthritis, like ankylosing spondylitis, generally presents with the typical phenotype for HLA-B27-associated uveitis.[19] Alternatively, uveitis in patients with psoriatic arthritis or enteropathic arthritis is more likely to present with less typical manifestations. These include bilateral involvement, insidious rather than acute onset, chronic rather than recurrent duration, and increased involvement of the intermediate segment. Moreover, patients with these conditions may demonstrate other forms of ocular inflammation, such as scleritis.[20, 21]

6.3 DIFFERENTIAL DIAGNOSIS (TABLE 6.2)[22–26]

The differential diagnosis includes infectious and noninfectious etiologies for anterior uveitis. Infectious etiologies must be considered in the differential and excluded through a careful clinical examination and laboratory evaluation, as treatment of such entities requires antimicrobial therapy and avoidance of potential worsening if immunotherapy is utilized. The classic pattern and phenotype of HLA-B27-associated anterior uveitis often allows for differentiation from other etiologies of anterior uveitis, which may present with other clinical features (e.g., elevated intraocular pressure, transillumination defects, and stellate keratic precipitates in herpetic anterior uveitis).

6.4 CLINICAL EXAMINATION

A comprehensive examination includes examination of the ocular adnexal structures, pupillary and extraocular motility examination, slit lamp biomicroscopy of the anterior segment, measurement of

Table 6.2 Differential Diagnosis of Acute Anterior Uveitis

Inflammatory	<ul><li>HLA-B27-Associated</li><li>Sarcoidosis</li><li>Tubulo-Interstitial Nephritis and Uveitis (TINU)</li><li>Behçet's Disease</li><li>Inflammatory Bowel Disease</li><li>Psoriatic Arthritis</li></ul>
Infectious	<ul><li>Tuberculosis</li><li>Viral (HSV, VZV, CMV, Rubella)</li><li>Syphilis</li><li>Toxoplasmosis</li></ul>
Medication-Induced	<ul><li>Bisphosphonates</li><li>Anti-Tumor Necrosis Factor</li><li>Sulfonamides</li><li>Cancer Immunotherapy</li></ul>
Masquerade or Malignancies	<ul><li>Lymphoma/Leukemia</li><li>Retinoblastoma</li><li>Intraocular Foreign Body</li></ul>
Idiopathic or Undifferentiated Syndromes	<ul><li>Posner–Schlossman Syndrome</li><li>Glaucomatocyclitic Crisis</li><li>Post-Traumatic</li><li>Post-Infectious</li><li>Post-Vaccination</li></ul>

the intraocular pressure, gonioscopy, and a dilated fundus examination to evaluate the vitreous and the structures of the posterior segment. In addition to the clinical examination, diagnostic imaging studies are performed as appropriate: slit lamp photography to document anterior segment findings; fundus photography to document posterior segment findings; optical coherence tomography (OCT), which provides high-resolution, cross-sectional images of the retina; fluorescein angiography (FA), an imaging study used to evaluate the integrity of the retinal vasculature, the extent of retinal edema, and to evaluate for any associated retinal vasculitis; color vision testing to assess optic nerve function; automated perimetry to assess optic nerve function; indocyanine green angiography to assess choroidal and retinal vasculature; and B-scan ultrasonography to assess the posterior pole if the view is obscured.

A thorough history of present illness (HPI), a comprehensive review of systems (ROS), and a comprehensive clinical examination are critical in developing an accurate differential diagnosis. The key features of the HPI and ROS should include but not be limited to the following:

- Onset, duration, laterality, course, precipitating and alleviating factors, associated clinical symptoms, ocular surgery or injury

- Demographic features to include age, gender, ethnicity, race, and occupation

- Social history, travel history, socio-economic history

- Pertinent positives and negatives by organ systems

The clinical examination should document pertinent positive and negative findings. Those patients presenting with classic features of HLA-B27-associated uveitis should be queried on the presence of typical symptoms seen in the seronegative spondyloarthropathies. These would include back pain, focusing on inflammatory components such as improvement with activity, exacerbation with rest, insidious onset and persistence, and association with morning stiffness. Additionally, asking about the presence of a rash, particularly those consistent with psoriatic plaques or nail changes of psoriasis, should be part of the ROS. Gastrointestinal symptoms may also serve as a clue for underlying inflammatory bowel disease.

Laboratory and imaging evaluations would include those utilized to exclude the common etiologies of uveitis, including testing for syphilis, angiotensin-converting enzyme testing, and chest imaging with a chest X-ray. If unknown, screening for HLA-B27 status should be undertaken in those patients presenting with acute anterior uveitis exhibiting the classic phenotype of HLA-B27-associated uveitis. Additional lab considerations would include urinary testing for beta-2-microglobulin, especially in those patients fitting the typical demographic for tubulointerstitial uveitis (TINU) and those with less classic presentation of HLA-B27-associated anterior uveitis, such as bilateral presentations.[27]

6.5 TREATMENT

The priority in treating SpA-associated uveitis is controlling inflammation to resolve symptoms and prevent further complications. Choosing a specific treatment strategy is often based on the severity, recurrence pattern, and underlying SpA. The treatment options can be divided into local or systemic modalities.

Local: Initial treatment involves the use of local corticosteroids and mydriatics.

Topical

Corticosteroids: Corticosteroids are the drug of choice when treating anterior uveitis. They act by modifying and decreasing the inflammatory response in the eye. Topical drops are effective with manageable side effects. The severity of anterior uveitis determines the potency and severity of the chosen topical steroid, with prednisolone acetate and difluprednate used most.[28]

Cycloplegics: These agents serve three purposes in the treatment of anterior uveitis: relieve pain by immobilizing the iris, prevent adhesion of the iris to the anterior lens, which can lead to posterior synechiae, iris bombe, and may precipitate elevated intraocular pressure (IOP), and to stabilize the blood–aqueous barrier to help prevent further protein leakage.[22]

Regional

Sub-Tenon: Depending on the severity, recurrence rates, or posterior pole complications, periocular corticosteroid injections are utilized.

Intravitreal: Intraocular corticosteroids may be administered through intravitreal injection for severe anterior uveitis with associated intermediate uveitis and retinal edema or intraoperatively/perioperatively in high-risk anterior uveitis patients undergoing intraocular surgery.

Systemic: Though most cases of HLA-B27-associated anterior uveitis are managed with topical therapy, more severe episodes, those involving the posterior segment or those complicated by macular edema, may require systemic immunotherapy (IMT).[22] Additionally, patients with frequent episodes of uveitis or those who experience adverse effects from topical or local corticosteroids may also require steroid-sparing systemic IMT. Systemic therapies include oral or intravenous corticosteroids and non-steroidal immunotherapies such as antimetabolites or biologic DMARDs.

Corticosteroids: Prednisone is the primary oral corticosteroid used in patients with severe and visually impactful inflammation. Intravenous corticosteroids, utilizing agents such as methylprednisolone, are rarely required. Of note, systemic corticosteroids are not typically efficacious in managing axial spondyloarthritis and do not form part of the recommended treatment for patients with axial SpA.

Traditional Immunotherapies: A stepwise approach is often utilized for patients requiring steroid-sparing agents, starting with conventional DMARDs. Sulfasalazine, an agent occasionally used in the management of the articular features of peripheral SpA, may be employed to reduce the frequency and severity of uveitis in patients with SpA.[29, 30] The choice of steroid-sparing agents in HLA-B27-associated uveitis often depends on the subset and severity of the patient's associated SpA when present. For example, antimetabolite DMARDs such as methotrexate or mycophenolate, though potentially efficacious for a patient's uveitis, are not typically effective for axial spondyloarthritis.[31, 32] However, such DMARDs are often employed for the management of other B27-associated spondyloarthropathies, such as psoriatic arthritis or enteropathic arthritis.[33] Therefore, coordination of care between ophthalmology and rheumatology is critical in selecting systemic IMT that will most likely be effective for both the ocular and articular or systemic features of a patient with HLA-B27-associated disease.

Biologic DMARDs

Anti-Tumor Necrosis Factor (TNF): Biologic agents may be employed in patients who require systemic IMT and fail to respond or tolerate traditional DMARDs. Additionally, as noted, patients with concomitant axial spondyloarthritis may require biologic therapy, given the lack of efficacy of traditional DMARDs in managing inflammatory back disease. Anti-TNF agents are the first line of biologic treatment for axial SpA patients who have failed a non-steroid anti-inflammatory (NSAID) trial.[34] Though there are currently five available anti-TNF medications, adalimumab has the most robust data for its use in uveitis. Currently, it is the only biologic with FDA approval for the management of noninfectious intermediate, posterior, or panuveitis.[35] As HLA-B27-associated uveitis is most often anterior, the use of adalimumab for ocular inflammation alone presents challenges in light of this indication. However, adalimumab also carries indications for treating several systemic HLA-B27-associated diseases, including ankylosing spondylitis, psoriatic arthritis, and inflammatory bowel disease.[34] The patient may meet an indication for their systemic disease while often receiving benefits from use for their concomitant ocular inflammation. Infliximab, a chimeric monoclonal antibody against TNF, administered as an infusion, also carries indications for the aforementioned systemic conditions and demonstrates benefit in ocular inflammation in patients with these conditions.[36-38] Two additional anti-TNF agents, certolizumab and golimumab, have more limited data supporting their use in B27-associated ocular inflammation. The final commercially available anti-TNF medication, etanercept, is typically avoided in the management of ocular inflammation, given mixed or poor results.[39-41]

Interleukin (IL) Inhibitors: Interleukins 17 and 23 are implicated in the pathogenesis of spondyloarthritis.[42] Additionally, patients with HLA-B27-associated anterior uveitis demonstrate elevated levels of IL-17 T cells, suggesting a role for inhibiting these pathways in managing uveitis.[43] Secukinumab, a monoclonal antibody against IL-17, carries an indication for the management of several seronegative arthropathies.[34, 44] There are variable data for the use of secukinumab in the management of uveitis.[45, 46] Similarly, there is limited evidence for treating uveitis with ustekinumab, a monoclonal antibody that inhibits the IL-12/23 pathway, which is approved for the treatment of psoriatic arthritis.[47]

Janus Kinase (JAK) Inhibitors: Inhibition of the JAK pathway is utilized in treating several systemic rheumatic diseases, including psoriatic arthritis and ankylosing spondylitis.[34, 48] Tofacitinib, baracitinib, and upadacitinib are commercially available JAK inhibitors. Early investigations examining the use of tofacitinib in the treatment of uveitis are primarily limited to small case series.[49, 50]

6.5.1 Special Treatment Considerations

Use of topical corticosteroids should be limited or avoided in the event of intraocular pressure elevations. Retinal edema or other structural complications may be managed with adjunctive intraocular or periocular corticosteroid injections, which can help deliver medication directly to the site of inflammation. If corticosteroids are contraindicated or the patient experiences side effects, alternative medications such as immunomodulatory drugs may be considered. Early collaboration with a rheumatologist should be considered for patients with systemic or ocular disease who would benefit from systemic immunotherapy.

6.5.2 Monitoring Response

The SUN criteria recommend a two-step increase or decrease in anterior chamber cell count (reviewed in Chapter 2) as the best method to determine whether uveitis is improving or worsening. Improvement of inflammation is defined as a two-step decrease or the uveitis being deemed "inactive." Worsening of inflammation is defined as a two-step increase in inflammation or an increase to the maximum grade of 4+.[16] Remission of uveitis is defined as an inactive disease for 3 months or more after termination of all treatments for eye disease. Educational brochures should be provided to patients, and the importance of compliance should be likewise discussed with written instructions on medication dosing and frequency.

6.6 COMPLICATIONS AND SEQUELAE

Anterior Segment: A primary concern in AAU of the spondyloarthropathies is the risk of frequent recurrence or persistent inflammation, increasing the likelihood of structural complications.

> **Posterior Synechiae:** Posterior synechiae is a common finding in anterior uveitis. It results in the adhesion of the iris to the lens capsule. These synechiae restrict the movement of the pupil and can cause the pupil to remain fixed. The most concerning risk is that adhesion can obstruct fluid drainage from the eye. This complication may lead to chronic or acute glaucoma.

> **Cataract:** Cataract is a common complication of uveitis and results from prolonged inflammation in the anterior segment and the use of corticosteroids in treating inflammation.

Ocular Hypertension, Glaucoma

> **Steroid Responder:** Steroid-induced glaucoma can occur with the use of any form of steroid administration. The elevated IOP is primarily due to the increase of resistance in the outflow mechanisms of the trabecular meshwork. The term "steroid responder" is applied to a clinically significant increase in intraocular pressure compared to baseline after topical or regional corticosteroid treatment.[51]

> **Extensive Posterior Synechiae, Compromised Angle:** Secondary glaucoma poses a significant risk in cases of AAU associated with the mechanism as previously described.

Posterior Segment

> **Cystoid Macular Edema:** Uveitis is a risk factor for developing cystoid macular edema and is the most frequent cause of visual deterioration in uveitis patients.[52]

> **Epiretinal Membrane (ERM):** Defined as a pre-retinal proliferation of fibroblastic cells associated with the deposition of extracellular matrix.[53] Studies have shown that ERM formation is present in 40% to 50% of patients with uveitis. Epiretinal membrane development can lead to compromised visual acuity, metamorphopsia, macropsia, or micropsia.[53]

6.7 SUMMARY

A collaborative approach between ophthalmologists and rheumatologists is essential for effectively diagnosing and managing HLA-B27-associated uveitis. Understanding the clinical features of uveitis associated with spondyloarthropathies is necessary for this collaboration to be successful. Ophthalmologists can identify red flags through careful history taking, uncovering potential underlying spondyloarthropathies. This valuable information empowers rheumatologists to confirm or rule out systemic disease, ultimately leading to a more comprehensive diagnosis and tailored treatment plan for the patient's uveitis, optimal treatment outcomes, and improved visual prognosis.

REFERENCES

1. Poddubnyy D. Classification vs diagnostic criteria: the challenge of diagnosing axial spondyloarthritis. *Rheumatology (Oxford)*. 2020;59(Suppl4):iv6–iv17.
2. Rademacher J, Poddubnyy D, Pleyer U. Uveitis in spondyloarthritis. *Ther Adv Musculoskelet Dis*. 2020;2. doi:10.1177/1759720X20951733.
3. Lee SC, Yang CH, Tsai YC, et al. The effect of uveitis and undiagnosed spondyloarthritis: a systematic review and meta-analysis. *Sci Rep*. 2023;13(1):14779.
4. Rusman T, van Vollenhoven RF, van der Horst-Bruinsma IE. Gender differences in axial spondyloarthritis: women are not so lucky. *Curr Rheumatol Rep*. 2018;20(6):35.
5. Braun J, Sieper J. Fifty years after the discovery of the association of HLA B27 with ankylosing spondylitis. *RMD Open*. 2023;9(3).
6. Kopplin LJ, Mount G, Suhler EB, Review for disease of the year: epidemiology of HLA-B27 associated ocular disorders. *Ocul Immunol Inflamm*. 2016; 24(4):470–475.
7. Martin TM, Smith JR, Rosenbaum JT. Anterior uveitis: current concepts of pathogenesis and interactions with the spondyloarthropathies. *Curr Opin Rheumatol*. 2002;14(4):337–341.
8. Salek SS, Pradeep A, Guly C, et al. Uveitis and juvenile psoriatic arthritis or psoriasis. *Am J Ophthalmol*. 2018;185:68–74.

9. Rosenbaum JT. Uveitis in spondyloarthritis including psoriatic arthritis, ankylosing spondylitis, and inflammatory bowel disease. *Clin Rheumatol*. 2015;34(6):999–1002.

10. Gholami H, Chmiel JA, Burton JP, et al. The role of microbiota-derived vitamins in immune homeostasis and enhancing cancer immunotherapy. *Cancers (Basel)*. 2023;15(4).

11. Belkaid Y, Harrison OJ. Homeostatic immunity and the microbiota. *Immunity*. 2017;46(4):562–576.

12. Rosenbaum JT, Asquith M. The microbiome and HLA-B27-associated acute anterior uveitis. *Nat Rev Rheumatol*. 2018;14(12):704–713.

13. Peluso R, Di Minno MN, Iervolino S, et al. Enteropathic spondyloarthritis: from diagnosis to treatment. *Clin Dev Immunol*. 2013;2013:631408.

14. Standardization of Uveitis Nomenclature (SUN) Working Group. Classification criteria for spondyloarthritis/HLA-B27-associated anterior uveitis. *Am J Ophthalmol*. 2021;228:117–125.

15. Whitcup SM, Sen HN. *Whitcup and Nussenblatt's uveitis: fundamentals and clinical practice*. Elsevier Health Sciences, 2021 Mar. 31.

16. Jabs DA, Nussenblatt RB, Rosenbaum JT. Standardization of uveitis nomenclature for reporting clinical data: results of the first international workshop. *Am J Ophthalmol*. 2005;140(3):509–516.

17. Standardization of Uveitis Nomenclature (SUN) Working Group. Development of classification criteria for the uveitides. *Am J Ophthalmol*. 2021;228:96–105.

18. Toris CB, Gregerson DS, Pederson JE. Uveoscleral outflow using different-sized fluorescent tracers in normal and inflamed eyes. *Exp Eye Res*. 1987;45(4):525–532.

19. D'Ambrosio EM, La Cava M, Tortorella P. Clinical features and complications of the HLA-B27-associated acute anterior uveitis: a metanalysis. *Semin Ophthalmol*. 2017;32(6):689–701.

20. Lyons JL, Rosenbaum JT. Uveitis associated with inflammatory bowel disease compared with uveitis associated with spondyloarthropathy. *Arch Ophthalmol*. 1997;115(1):61–64.

21. Paiva ES, Macaluso DC, Edwards A, et al. Characterisation of uveitis in patients with psoriatic arthritis. *Ann Rheum Dis*. 2000;59(1):67–70.

22. Agrawal RV, Murthy S, Sangwan V, et al. Current approach in diagnosis and management of anterior uveitis. *Indian J Ophthalmol*. 2010;58(1):11–19.

23. Iqbal KM, Hay MW, Emami-Naeini P. Medication-induced uveitis: an update. *J Ophthalmic Vis Res*. 2021;16(1):84–92.

24. Babu K, Konana VK, Ganesh SK, et al. Viral anterior uveitis. *Indian J Ophthalmol*. 2020;68(9):1764–1773.

25. Aboul Naga SH, Hassan LM, El Zanaty RT, et al. Behçet uveitis: current practice and future perspectives. *Front Med (Lausanne)*. 2022;9:968345.

26. Mahendradas P, Shetty R, Malathi J, et al. Chikungunya virus iridocyclitis in Fuchs' heterochromic iridocyclitis. *Indian J Ophthalmol*. 2010;58(6):545–547.

27. McKay KM, Lim LL, Van Gelder RN. Rational laboratory testing in uveitis: a Bayesian analysis. *Surv Ophthalmol*. 2021;66(5):802–825.

28. Rosenbaum JT. The eye in spondyloarthritis (☆). *Semin Arthritis Rheum*. 2019;49(3s):S29–S31.

29. Benitez-Del-Castillo JM, Garcia-Sanchez J, Iradier T, et al. Sulfasalazine in the prevention of anterior uveitis associated with ankylosing spondylitis. *Eye (London)*. 2000;14(Part 3A):340–343.

30. Muñoz-Fernández S, Hidalgo V, Fernández-Melón J, et al. Sulfasalazine reduces the number of flares of acute anterior uveitis over a one-year period. *J Rheumatol*. 2003;30(6):1277–1279.

31. Gangaputra S, Newcomb CW, Liesegang TL, et al. Methotrexate for ocular inflammatory diseases. *Ophthalmology*. 2009;116(11):2188–2198.e1.

32. Daniel E, Thorne JE, Newcomb CW, et al. Mycophenolate mofetil for ocular inflammation. *Am J Ophthalmol*. 2010;149(3): 423–432.e1–e2.

33. Gossec L, Baraliakos X, Kerschbaumer A, et al. EULAR recommendations for the management of psoriatic arthritis with pharmacological therapies: 2019 update. *Ann Rheum Dis*. 2020;79(6):700–712.

34. Ward MM, Deodhar A, Gensler LS, et al. 2019 update of the American College of Rheumatology/ Spondylitis Association of America/Spondyloarthritis research and treatment network recommendations for the treatment of ankylosing spondylitis and nonradiographic axial spondyloarthritis. *Arthritis Care Res (Hoboken)*. 2019;71(10):1285–1299.

35. Jaffe GJ, Dick AD, Brézin AP, et al. Adalimumab in patients with active noninfectious uveitis. *N Engl J Med*. 2016;375(10):932–943.

36. Suhler EB, Smith JR, Giles TR, et al. Infliximab therapy for refractory uveitis: 2-year results of a prospective trial. *Arch Ophthalmol*. 2009;127(6):819–822.

37. Braun J, Baraliakos X, Listing J, et al. Decreased incidence of anterior uveitis in patients with ankylosing spondylitis treated with the anti-tumor necrosis factor agents infliximab and etanercept. *Arthritis Rheum*. 2005;52(8):2447–2451.

38. Kim M, Won JY, Choi SY, et al. Anti-TNFα treatment for HLA-B27-positive ankylosing spondylitis-related uveitis. *Am J Ophthalmol*. 2016;170:32–40.

39. Calvo-Río V, Blanco R, Santos-Gómez M, et al. Golimumab in refractory uveitis related to spondyloarthritis: multicenter study of 15 patients. *Semin Arthritis Rheum*. 2016;46(1):95–101.

40. Rudwaleit M, Rosenbaum JT, Landewé R, et al. Observed incidence of uveitis following certolizumab pegol treatment in patients with axial spondyloarthritis. *Arthritis Care Res (Hoboken)*. 2016;68(6):838–844.

41. Levy-Clarke G, Jabs DA, Read RW, et al. Expert panel recommendations for the use of anti-tumor necrosis factor biologic agents in patients with ocular inflammatory disorders. *Ophthalmology*. 2014;121(3):785–796.e3.

42. Paine A, Ritchlin CT. Targeting the interleukin-23/17 axis in axial spondyloarthritis. *Curr Opin Rheumatol*. 2016;28(4):359–367.

43. Guedes MC, Borrego LM, Proença RD. Roles of interleukin-17 in uveitis. *Indian J Ophthalmol*. 2016;64(9):628–634.

44. Blair HA. Secukinumab: a review in ankylosing spondylitis. *Drugs*. 2019;79(4):433–443.

45. Dick AD, Tugal-Tutkun I, Foster S, et al. Secukinumab in the treatment of noninfectious uveitis: results of three randomized, controlled clinical trials. *Ophthalmology*. 2013;120(4):777–787.

46. Letko E, Yeh S, Foster CS, et al., Efficacy and safety of intravenous secukinumab in noninfectious uveitis requiring steroid-sparing immunosuppressive therapy. *Ophthalmology*. 2015;122(5):939–948.

47. Mugheddu C, Atzori L, Del Piano M, et al. Successful ustekinumab treatment of noninfectious uveitis and concomitant severe psoriatic arthritis and plaque psoriasis. *Dermatol Ther*. 2017;30(5).

48. Klavdianou K, Papagoras C, Baraliakos X. JAK inhibitors for the treatment of axial spondyloarthritis. *Mediterr J Rheumatol*. 2023;34(2):129–138.

49. Paley MA, Karacal H, Rao PK, et al. Tofacitinib for refractory uveitis and scleritis. *Am J Ophthalmol Case Rep*. 2019;13:53–55.

50. Wang Y, Wan Z, Jin R, et al. Tofacitinib for extraintestinal manifestations of inflammatory bowel disease: a literature review. *Int Immunopharmacol*. 2022;105:108517.

51. Feroze KB, Zeppieri M, Khazaeni L. Steroid-induced glaucoma. In: *StatPearls*. Treasure Island, FL: StatPearls Publishing LLC, 2024. Copyright © 2024.

52. Massa H, Pipis SY, Adewoyin T, et al. Macular edema associated with non-infectious uveitis: pathophysiology, etiology, prevalence, impact and management challenges. *Clin Ophthalmol*. 2019;13:1761–1777.

53. Yap A, Lu LM, Sims JL, et al. Epiretinal membrane in uveitis: rate, visual prognosis, complications and surgical outcomes. *Clin Exp Ophthalmol*. 2023;52.

7 Ophthalmic Disease in Sarcoidosis

Timothy M. Janetos, Taylor L. Koenig, Rula A. Hajj-Ali, and Debra A. Goldstein

7.1 EPIDEMIOLOGY

7.1.1 Systemic Sarcoidosis

The epidemiology of sarcoidosis is significantly affected by geography and patient ethnicity. Incidence and prevalence vary widely based on geographical region. An analysis of the worldwide distribution of sarcoidosis found that fewer than 1% of patients with sarcoidosis live in the Southern Hemisphere.[2] The Nordic region countries have the highest incidence rates; 11.4 and 11.5 persons per 1000 in Finland and Sweden, respectively. Sarcoidosis is much less common in Asia, with incidence rates of only 0.48 per 100,000 in South Korea and 1 per 100,000 in Japan.[3]

In the United States (US), there are differences in the incidence and prevalence rates among racial ethnicities. Sarcoidosis is more than twice as common in Black patients as White patients, and Hispanic and Asian patients living in the United States have even lower disease rates.[2, 4] This disparity in the prevalence of sarcoidosis across varying ethnicities and regions suggest that genetics as well as environmental factors influence disease rates.[2]

Globally, sarcoidosis is more common in women than men; the specific gender breakdown varies based on ethnicity and geographic location.[2, 3] In the US, women comprise at least 60% of the sarcoidosis population. Sarcoidosis has been reported in patients of all ages but most commonly presents between 25 and 40 years of age. Women tend to be diagnosed at an older age than men, and there is a second incidence peak in women greater than age 50.[3, 5, 6]

There is also variation in the clinical phenotype of sarcoidosis across regions and ethnicities, both globally and in the US. In Northern countries, particularly in Europe, thoracic disease is more severe, and ocular involvement is the most common extra-thoracic systemic feature; this is compared to Southern European countries, where patients have milder thoracic disease, and cutaneous involvement is the main extra-thoracic systemic feature. Sarcoidosis patients in the Northwest US have mostly extra-thoracic systemic manifestations, while patients in the US South and Midwest more commonly have thoracic disease.[2] In the US, Black patients have more severe thoracic disease and extra-thoracic involvement compared to White patients lending towards an overall higher rate of hospitalization and mortality for US Black patients.[2, 7]

7.1.2 Ocular Sarcoidosis

The prevalence of ocular involvement in patients with sarcoidosis again varies by study population, geography, and ethnic group. In the US, among a population-based cohort, only 7% of sarcoidosis patients ever developed ocular disease during follow-up.[8] A Veteran Health Administration population-based study showed a similar rate of ocular involvement.[9] This is a low estimate among most US studies, with some showing a rate of up to 50% of ocular involvement in patients with sarcoidosis.[10] Differences may partially be due to lack of a definite diagnosis in many series. Furthermore, cohort studies among referral centers may have higher rates of severe disease with ocular involvement and not be representative of total population prevalence. Regardless, this places estimates of ocular involvement among patients with sarcoidosis anywhere from 7% to 50%. Despite the potentially high prevalence, routine screening for eye involvement of patients with systemic sarcoidosis who do not have ocular symptoms has been shown to have a low yield.[11]

In the US, ocular involvement is more frequent, symptomatic, and aggressive in Black patients compared with White.[12] Black patients tend to have an earlier disease onset, present with more aggressive anterior inflammation, and have a positive family history.[9, 12–14] Furthermore, the type and presentation of uveitis may vary among race. Anterior uveitis is consistently the most common form of ocular inflammation reported among all patients.[8, 9, 12, 15] However, the rate of posterior uveitis has been shown in several studies to be higher among White patients than Black patients.[16, 17] White patients overall may have higher rates of chorioretinal lesions and cystoid macular edema.[16, 18–20]

Differences in sex also exist. Women consistently have higher overall rates of chronic ocular inflammation and present with inflammation later compared with men.[8, 9, 21–23] Specifically, White women greater than 50 years old have higher rates of cystoid macular edema and multifocal choroiditis, and several studies show ultimate worse visual acuity outcomes compared to younger male patients.[16, 17, 22, 24] This suggests a potential hormonal component that may influence ocular disease course.

DOI: 10.1201/9781003453710-7

79

Across the globe, prevalence of ocular sarcoidosis appears to vary greatly. A Korean cohort showed a rate of 21% of ocular sarcoidosis among patients with sarcoidosis, whereas a Japanese study showed a prevalence of 50% with sarcoidosis being the leading cause of uveitis in Japan.[25, 26] Among Turkish patients with biopsy-proven sarcoidosis, only 12.9% had ocular involvement.[23] In a Northern Ireland population-based study, ocular sarcoidosis prevalence was estimated as 4.5 cases per 100,000.[27]

7.2 PATHOGENESIS OF SARCOIDOSIS

7.2.1 ACCESS Study

A Case Control Etiologic Study of Sarcoidosis (ACCESS) was a National Institutes of Health large prospective study of newly diagnosed sarcoidosis patients from 10 clinical centers within the United States.[28] Greater than 700 biopsy-proven cases of sarcoidosis and control subjects were included. The goal of the study was to identify etiologic causes of sarcoidosis – including genetic, environmental, infectious, or immune-related triggers of the disease. Etiologic causes were explored using detailed questionnaires for environmental, occupational, and genetic causes, while serum laboratory testing was used for potential infectious causes. In addition to confirming that certain ethnic groups within the US have higher rates of sarcoidosis, a genetic link was confirmed with an increased risk of developing sarcoidosis among siblings and parents of subjects with sarcoidosis, which was present in all ethnic groups.[29] A portion of research participants had HLA testing, with a significantly higher proportion of patients with sarcoidosis having HLA-DRB1 alleles compared to controls.

The ACCESS study additionally examined various environmental and occupational exposures via detailed questionnaires. Although a large number of associations were significant (e.g., occupations involving interaction with birds, automobile manufacturing, radiation exposure, insecticide use, mold exposure), most odds ratios were low or had wide confidence intervals, and the clinical relevance behind such associations is unknown. Furthermore, patient questionnaires were extensive, which, given the large sample size, may have identified clinically irrelevant associations. There was no one large association that might explain an environmental trigger, suggesting that a multifactorial cause is likely. Last, serum testing including cultures and PCR testing did not reveal any differences between patients and controls of potential infectious triggers; however, it is debatable whether this methodology would identify any causes given the low utility of routine cultures and PCR testing.[30]

7.2.2 Proposed Pathogenesis

The pathophysiology of sarcoidosis is incompletely understood; however, advancements in genetic and immunology research have led to improved comprehension of disease mechanisms. The pathogenic mechanisms of granuloma formation are the defining features of sarcoidosis and cause the end-organ damage associated with the disease.[31]

Granuloma formation is initiated by a trigger in a genetically susceptible host. The seasonal variation of sarcoidosis with clustering of new diagnoses in the months of June and July and latitude-dependent epidemiology supports environmental and transmissible infectious agents as potential disease triggers.[32] In the ACCESS study, sarcoidosis after exposure to insecticide at work was associated with the HLA-DRB1*1101 and HLA-DRB*1501 alleles.[33] Exposure to molds, mildews, and dusty odors is also positively associated with sarcoidosis.[33, 34] Additionally, other environmental factors, such as silica, talc, man-made fibers, and other inhalational workplace exposures, have been observed in sarcoidosis cohorts.[32] After the 9/11 World Trade Center disaster, an increased rate of sarcoidosis was noted among populations exposed to the disaster, including firefighters and first responders.[35, 36] Skin tattoos can also trigger granuloma formation with both cutaneous disease at the tattoo site and systemic manifestations.[37]

Infectious triggers of sarcoidosis, such as *Mycobacterium* and *Propionibacterium*, have also been postulated given these microbiotas' propensity to form granulomas in animal hosts.[38] Studies have demonstrated culture growth of *Cutibacterium acnes* in lymph node tissue in patients with sarcoidosis. A meta-analysis found that mycobacteria genetic material was detected in body tissues and fluid, including lymph nodes, lacrimal glands, lung tissue, and bronchial fluid, in 26% of sarcoidosis patients – a rate 10 to 20 times greater than healthy controls.[39] Furthermore, mycobacterium proteins have been shown to induce granulomatous inflammation in patients with sarcoidosis.[40] However, data on the role of mycobacteria in the pathogenesis of sarcoidosis has overall been inconclusive.[32, 41]

Vimentin, a cytoskeletal cell filament protein, may also be involved in the pathogenesis of sarcoidosis.[42] Vimentin plays a key role in the cellular interactions of the immune system and is the predominant cytoskeleton protein within sarcoid granulomas.[42, 43] Vimentin has been demonstrated to stimulate the immune response in patients with sarcoidosis. Peripheral blood mononuclear cells (PBMCs) isolated from patients with sarcoidosis incubated with vimentin ex vivo produced significantly increased levels of inflammatory cytokines compared to PBMCs from healthy controls.[44] Furthermore, vimentin can undergo post-translational modifications including citrullination, which disrupts the electrical charge of the filaments, leading to change in the cytoskeletal structure and function.[42] Autoantibodies to mutated citrullinated vimentin (anti-MCV) have been detected at higher rates in sarcoidosis patients than healthy controls, and it has therefore emerged as a possible antigenic target in sarcoidosis.[45]

After a genetically susceptible host is exposed to an antigenic trigger for sarcoidosis, a cascade of immunologic events leads to granuloma formation. The antigenic trigger activates macrophages that use toll-like receptor signaling of HLA molecules to further activate the immune system in a T cell dominant response.[31, 34] The macrophage response in sarcoidosis can be polarized to an M1, pro-inflammatory, macrophage or M2, anti-inflammatory/anti-fibrotic, macrophage response.[46]

M1 macrophages initiate the T cell response characterized by CD4 positive T cells (helper T cells), which differentiate into specific helper T cell subtypes; differentiation is dictated by the unique cytokine environment. The T helper 1 (Th1) subtype produces pro-inflammatory cytokines including interferon (IFN)-γ and interleukin 12 (IL-12).[46] Analysis of bronchoalveolar lavage (BAL) fluid of sarcoidosis patients shows elevated levels of both these cytokines as well as M1 macrophages compared to control patients.[47, 48] These pro-inflammatory cytokines amplify the immune response, driving more inflammatory cells to the site, and lead to granuloma formation.[34, 49]

Alternative to this conventional pro-inflammatory M1 and Th1 response, M2 macrophages and a resulting T helper 2 (Th2) response can also be seen in sarcoidosis patients. M2 macrophages have been isolated in sarcoid granulomas and drive a Th2 response.[50] The Th2 cells produce IL-10, an anti-inflammatory cytokine that has been found in the BAL fluid of sarcoidosis patients. IL-10 down-regulates the M1/Th1 pro-inflammatory response.[51] In addition to tempering this inflammatory response, Th2 cells also secrete pro-fibrotic cytokines, such as IL-4, IL-13, and transforming growth factor-β1.[46] A shift toward a Th2 response, therefore, may be associated with downstream fibrosis and poorer outcomes. Biomarkers of a Th2 response have been associated with greater and more advanced sarcoid organ involvement.[52]

7.2.3 HLA Associations and GWAS Studies

Sarcoidosis is a highly genetic disorder – siblings of sarcoidosis patients are 5 times more likely to develop sarcoidosis compared to patients without a family history of the disease.[53] There has been significant investigation into genes that contribute to this risk. The ACCESS study findings of HLA-DRB1 allele associations with sarcoidosis has been reproduced across several genome-wide associated studies.[54, 55]

Genome-wide studies have also found genetic markers for specific sarcoidosis phenotypes. For example, Lofgren's syndrome, an acute presentation of sarcoidosis, is associated with the HLA-DRB1*03 allele.[56] HLA-DRB1*0401 is a marker for sarcoid ocular involvement in White and Black patients.[57]

Non-HLA genes have also been investigated in genome-wide studies. The BTNL2 gene on chromosome 6, which is suspected to suppress T cell activation, was first linked to sarcoidosis after a genome analysis of German families with sarcoidosis; further studies have found similar associations in White and Black patients within the US.[58] Another chromosome 6 variant, the RAB23 gene, which encodes a negative regulator of the sonic hedgehog signaling pathway, has also been identified as a genetic risk factor of sarcoidosis.[59]

7.2.4 Familial Juvenile Systemic Granulomatosis (Blau Syndrome)

In contrast to sarcoidosis, which is likely due to a complex interaction of genetic and environmental factors, familial juvenile systemic granulomatosis (also known as Blau syndrome) is an autosomal dominant monogenic granulomatous disease.[60] The disease was initially thought of as early-onset sarcoidosis due to the granulomatous nature of systemic inflammation, but it is now recognized as a distinct autoinflammatory process caused by a mutation in the NOD2/CARD15 gene. The disease presents in early childhood, typically before the age of 5. The ocular inflammation shares many characteristics with ocular sarcoidosis but is usually very resistant to conventional treatments.[61] The disease has the classic triad of uveitis, arthritis, and a diffuse rash, but other organ systems can be involved.[62, 63] Notably, however, pulmonary involvement is rare.

The NOD2/CARD15 protein acts within macrophages and dendritic cells to recognize bacterial cell wall components and functions to activate an inflammatory cascade in response.[64] Therefore, it is involved in activation of the innate immune response. There are multiple known mutations of NOD2/CARD15, with the R334W and R334Q mutations being the most common and potentially having more severe ocular inflammation.[65] NOD2-mediated mouse models of inflammation have demonstrated downstream production of interleukin-1-beta (IL-1β), leading to IL-1 antagonists as a potential therapeutic agent for patients with Blau syndrome.[66] However, the little evidence available has had mixed success with these agents.[67, 68] Blau syndrome, although distinct from sarcoidosis, demonstrates that genetic factors can play a role in the development of granulomatous sarcoid-like inflammation.

7.3 DIAGNOSIS OF OCULAR SARCOIDOSIS

The diagnosis of ocular sarcoidosis remains difficult, and there is no one laboratory or imaging finding that is very sensitive and specific. Rather, it is multiple studies in conjugation with clinical examination and ultimately biopsy demonstrating noncaseating granulomas that makes the diagnosis. The International Workshop on Ocular Sarcoidosis (IWOS) proposed criteria for the diagnosis – first in 2009 and then updated in 2017 (Table 7.1) after validation studies questioned the sensitivity of some of the original criteria.[69, 70] In particular, liver function testing, which was included in the original criteria, appears to have very little relevance in diagnosis and was removed from the updated criteria.[71] The criteria categorizes patients with ocular sarcoidosis into "definite," "presumed," and "probable" based on biopsy results, systemic investigations, and ocular findings. None of the intraocular clinical findings of ocular sarcoidosis are particularly sensitive.[70]

The Standardization of Uveitis Nomenclature (SUN) Working Group proposed a simpler set of criteria for the diagnosis of ocular sarcoidosis. In essence, the SUN criteria require findings of uveitis with either tissue biopsy of noncaseating granulomas or bilateral hilar adenopathy on chest imaging. Syphilis and tuberculosis infection must be excluded.

Laboratory and imaging studies that may support the diagnosis include elevated serum angiotensin-converting enzyme (ACE), elevated serum lysozyme, elevated serum soluble IL-2 receptor (sIL-2R), elevated CD4/CD8 T cell ratio (> 3.5) in bronchoalveolar lavage, abnormal gallium-67 scintigraphy or 18F-fluorodeoxyglucose positron emission tomography, lymphopenia, or chest imaging

Table 7.1 IWOS Revised Criteria for the Diagnosis of Ocular Sarcoidosis[71]

Criteria	Description
I. Exclusion Criteria	Other causes of granulomatous uveitis must be ruled out.
II. Intraocular Clinical Signs	1. Mutton-fat keratic precipitates and/or iris nodules (Koeppe/Busacca). 2. Trabecular meshwork nodules and/or tent-shaped peripheral anterior synechia. 3. Snowballs/string-of-pearls vitreous opacities. 4. Multiple chorioretinal peripheral lesions (active and atrophic). 5. Nodular and/or segmental periphlebitis (± candle wax drippings) and/or macroaneurysm in an inflamed eye. 6. Optic disc nodule(s)/granuloma(s) and/or solitary choroidal nodule. 7. Bilaterality (assessed by ophthalmological examination including ocular imaging showing subclinical inflammation).
III. Systemic Investigation Results	1. Bilateral hilar lymphadenopathy (BHL) by chest X-ray and/or CT scan. 2. Negative tuberculin test or interferon-gamma-releasing assays. 3. Elevated serum ACE. 4. Elevated serum lysozyme. 5. Elevated CD4/CD8 ratio (> 3.5) in bronchoalveolar lavage fluid. 6. Abnormal accumulation of gallium-67 scintigraphy or 18F-fluorodeoxyglucose PET imaging. 7. Lymphopenia. 8. Parenchymal lung changes consistent with sarcoidosis, as determined by pulmonologists or radiologists.
IV. Diagnostic Criteria	*Definite OS:* Diagnosis supported by biopsy with compatible uveitis. *Presumed OS:* Diagnosis not supported by biopsy, but BHL present with two intraocular signs. *Probable OS:* Diagnosis not supported by biopsy and BHL absent, but three intraocular signs and two systemic investigations selected from two to eight are present.

with bilateral hilar lymphadenopathy or parenchymal lung changes. Bilateral hilar adenopathy is the only relatively sensitive finding, with chest computed tomography being more sensitive than chest X-ray.[14, 24, 70]

Serum ACE and lysozyme levels have quite variable reported sensitivity and specificity depending on the study, but in general, both are more specific than sensitive.[14, 72] The ACE level is uninterpretable if the patient is on an ACE inhibitor. Lysozyme can be elevated in other infectious diseases such as tuberculosis or syphilis. Lymphopenia may have a relatively higher sensitivity and specificity than ACE or lysozyme, especially when used in combination with serum ACE levels.[73] Elevated sIL-2R has been shown to have a higher sensitivity than serum ACE levels but a comparable specificity.[74, 75] sIL-2R was also found to be elevated, however, in patients with HLA-B27-associated uveitis and varicella-zoster virus-associated uveitis.[74]

Chest imaging, and in particular chest CT, more frequently identifies patients with sarcoidosis than any serum biomarker.[14] Patients with negative chest X-rays and subsequently positive chest CTs, in at least two studies, have been generally White women greater than 50 years of age.[14, 24] 18F-fluorodeoxyglucose positron emission tomography (18F-FDG PET) can be used to identify areas of hypermetabolic foci that may represent disease activity and a target for biopsy. It, therefore, may be useful in identifying patients without pulmonary involvement on presentation; in one study of patients with sarcoid uveitis and a normal CT chest, 30% had abnormal findings on 18F-FDG PET.[76]

Bronchoalveolar lavage (BAL) demonstrating lymphocytosis with an elevated CD4/CD8 ratio can have a high diagnostic value, even in cases with normal chest imaging.[77, 78] Elevated CD4/CD8 in vitreous and aqueous samples has also been shown to be a sensitive and specific biomarker for sarcoidosis, but its invasive nature limits its use.[79, 80]

Ultimately, the gold standard for diagnosis is biopsy demonstrating noncaseating epithelioid giant cell granulomas, with negative staining for mycobacteria. Tissue biopsy can be of any organ with involvement. In the eye, blind conjunctival biopsy is likely of low yield, but when directed at conjunctival granulomas seen on examination, the yield may be up to 63% in obtaining a diagnosis; this method is minimally invasive compared to targeting other organs such as the lungs.[81] Minor salivary gland biopsy has a relatively low diagnostic value in cases of ocular sarcoidosis.[82] Ultimately, biopsy of any site should be guided by clinical findings (e.g., skin lesions, conjunctival granulomas) or imaging suggestive of disease activity rather than blind biopsy.

7.4 SYSTEMIC MANIFESTATIONS OF SARCOIDOSIS

Sarcoidosis can cause granulomatous inflammation in nearly every organ in the body. Systemic manifestations are variable and depend on the organ involved. Multiorgan involvement is common as well, with 30% of patients having at least two organs affected at initial presentation.[83]

Constitutional – Constitutional symptoms are common in sarcoidosis. Fatigue is the most frequent constitutional symptom affecting 50% to 70% of patients; weight loss, night sweats, loss of appetite, and fever may also be seen. The fever is generally low grade and should prompt an evaluation for infectious microorganisms in a patient presenting with radiographic or pathologic evidence of granulomatous inflammation.[84]

Pulmonary – Pulmonary involvement is the most common systemic manifestation, affecting 70% to 90% of sarcoidosis patients.[34] Bilateral perihilar lymphadenopathy, including mediastinal lymphadenopathy, and parenchymal infiltrates and nodules are typical.[34, 84, 85] Pulmonary infiltrates are classically reticulonodular but can also present as alveolar or lobar infiltrates.[85] Less frequently, patients can have fibrocystic pulmonary disease, bronchiectasis, pleural effusions, and pulmonary fibrosis.[34, 84] Pulmonary involvement can lead to obstructive and restrictive lung disease as well.[34]

Cutaneous – Cutaneous involvement is seen in up to 30% of patients with sarcoidosis and can be the initial sign of sarcoidosis in up to 67% of patients.[86] Like involvement of other organs, cutaneous manifestations are variable. Cutaneous sarcoidosis is often termed "the Great Mimicker" because the cutaneous manifestations of sarcoidosis can overlap with other dermatologic conditions.[84] Erythema nodosum (EN), presenting as painful nodules on the lower legs, is the most common cutaneous manifestation and is associated with acute forms of sarcoidosis.[87] Other than EN, cutaneous sarcoidosis is generally painless. Patients may present with cutaneous or subcutaneous nodules, erythematous macules, plaques, or papules.[84, 88] Lupus pernio is a distinctive cutaneous manifestation and causes violaceous indurated lesions on the face.[87, 88] It is more common in Black and female patients. Other skin lesions include atrophic lesions that may share features with morphea and can present as necrobiosis lipoidica-like or lipodermatosclerosis-like lesions. Other manifestations include ulcerative lesions, angiolupoid, psoriasiform verrucous, and disseminated lichenoid sarcoidosis.[89]

Hematologic – Hematologic involvement is seen in 20% to 30% of sarcoidosis patients.[34] Extra-thoracic peripheral lymphadenopathy is the most common hematologic manifestation, occurring in 10% to 20% of patients.[34] Less frequently, patients can have bone marrow and splenic involvement, seen in approximately 4% and 7% of sarcoidosis patients, respectively.[83] Splenic involvement is often asymptomatic but is associated with the development of cytopenias secondary to splenic sequestration. Bone marrow involvement can result in cytopenias through granulomatous infiltration and replacement of the bone marrow. Cytopenias not secondary to bone marrow infiltration, such as autoimmune hemolytic anemia, are rarer.[90] Patients with sarcoidosis also have an increased risk of developing lymphoproliferative disorders, such as lymphoma.[91]

Cardiac – Symptomatic cardiac sarcoidosis occurs in 5% to 10% of patients; however, autopsy studies show cardiac granulomas in 20% to 30% of sarcoidosis patients.[87] Cardiac manifestations in sarcoidosis are most often asymptomatic yet are associated with the highest mortality.[84, 87] Conduction abnormalities and arrhythmias are the most common cardiac manifestations, with atrioventricular block accounting for almost half of cardiac involvement. Cardiomyopathy and heart failure, valvular abnormalities, and pericardial disease are less common.[31, 34, 84, 87, 92] There is a significant risk for sudden cardiac death in cardiac sarcoidosis patients due to fatal arrythmias and conduction blocks. These electrophysiologic abnormalities account for 25% to 65% of deaths caused by cardiac sarcoidosis.[31, 34, 92] Coronary artery disease can rarely develop in sarcoidosis presenting as unstable angina or myocardial infarction.[93] Cardiac involvement in sarcoidosis should be distinguished from atherosclerotic heart disease, as both can coexist, and it may be challenging to differentiate between these entities.

ENT – Otolaryngologic involvement is seen in 10% to 15% of patients with sarcoidosis. Patients can present with nonspecific symptoms such as nasal congestion, bleeding, and crusting secondary to chronic sinusitis or hoarseness and stridor due to laryngeal or tracheal obstruction from a granulomatous mass.[31, 34, 84, 94] Auricular involvement is uncommon but can present as hearing loss and tinnitus from middle ear involvement.[94] Glandular enlargement of the head and neck, such as the parotid and lacrimal glands, can also occur.[34, 84]

Musculoskeletal – Musculoskeletal clinical manifestations occur in up to 25% of sarcoidosis patients.[31] Acute inflammatory arthritis can occur as part of Lofgren's syndrome and most commonly affects the bilateral ankles. Chronic inflammatory arthritis is uncommon, occurring in fewer than 5% of patients, and is associated with diffuse organ involvement, specifically lupus pernio, lung involvement, and chronic uveitis.[95] Patients can present with joint pain and swelling as well as dactylitis. Radiographic findings of cystic and lytic bone lesions with sclerotic margins may be seen in these patients and can also be asymptomatic.[34, 84, 95] Tenosynovitis without arthritis can occur in sarcoidosis and mainly affects the Achilles or flexor tendons of the wrists and fingers.[95] Clinical myopathy is exceedingly rare, but granulomatous involvement of muscle has been found in up to 80% of patients with sarcoidosis.[87, 95]

Neurologic – Neurosarcoidosis is rare and only present in up to 5% of cases.[83] Patients may present with a variety of neurologic symptoms depending on the site of neurologic involvement. The most common neurologic manifestation is cranial nerve dysfunction; facial nerve palsy may develop in 25% to 50% of patients with neurosarcoidosis.[87, 96] Symptomatic meningeal disease is seen in up to 20% of neurosarcoidosis patients, although rates of subclinical disease are likely much higher.[97] Meningeal involvement presents as aseptic meningitis but can rarely present as a mass lesion; both can result in hydrocephalus and symptoms of elevated intracranial pressure.[96] From a central nervous system perspective, the brain parenchyma and spinal cord can also be affected.[87, 96] In the brain parenchyma, patients can develop granulomatous infiltration of the pituitary and hypothalamus, resulting in pituitary insufficiency and mass effect.[98] Peripheral nerve involvement presenting as mononeuropathy, mononeuritis multiplex, and generalized polyneuropathy is less common than central nervous system involvement.[84, 96]

Gastrointestinal/Hepatic – Hepatic sarcoidosis occurs in up to one-third of patients and most frequently manifests as asymptomatic elevation in liver function tests – alkaline phosphatase is more reliably elevated in these patients than alanine transaminase or aspartate transferase.[84, 99] Liver granulomas can occur although need to be evaluated for other etiologies, specifically infectious causes, prior to attributing these to systemic sarcoidosis.[87, 99] Outside of the liver, gastrointestinal involvement is very rare. Pancreatitis, gastrointestinal dysmotility, and peritoneal involvement are all possible manifestations.[34, 99] Gastric and esophageal ulceration can be seen and appear similar to peptic ulcer disease on endoscopy.[100] Small intestinal involvement can rarely mimic Crohn's disease.[101]

Endocrine – Endocrine involvement is an uncommon clinical manifestation of sarcoidosis, occurring in fewer than 10% of patients.[34] The most common endocrine manifestation in sarcoidosis is hypercalcemia. The percentage of sarcoidosis patients with hypercalcemia varies across studies although was found to be approximately 6% in the largest available cohort.[102] Hypercalcemia is caused by production of 1, 25 dihydroxyvitamin D3 from granulomas via the overactive alpha-1-hydroxylase enzyme.[34, 87] Other endocrine manifestations include granulomatous involvement of the pituitary, which can cause hypopituitarism.[34]

Renal – Significant renal disease is very uncommon in sarcoidosis, affecting 0.5% to 2% of patients.[31] Interstitial nephritis or membranous glomerulonephritis can occur from granulomatous inflammation but is rare.[87, 103] Patients can also develop nephrocalcinosis secondary to hypercalciuria, which can result in renal insufficiency secondary to obstructive uropathy.[31, 34, 87, 103]

7.4.1 Ocular Manifestations of Sarcoidosis

Ocular sarcoidosis may involve any part of the eye or orbit, causing disease manifestations that range from ocular surface disease to intraocular inflammation or orbital and optic nerve lesions. Orbital and adnexal lesions may be present in up to 30% of patients with ocular sarcoidosis.[79, 104] Orbital inflammation can mimic thyroid eye disease or orbital cellulitis. Lacrimal gland involvement is relatively common and can result in keratoconjunctivitis sicca or, less commonly, proptosis or diplopia due to lacrimal gland enlargement. Other non-intraocular manifestations that have been reported include dacryoadenitis, eyelid granulomas, acquired nasolacrimal duct obstruction, and lesions of the posterior optic nerve.[79, 105, 106]

Uveitis typically presents as a bilateral, granulomatous, chronic inflammation. Many of the below discussed findings are included in the IWOS clinical criteria. Uveitis type varies among cohort studies but is most frequently reported to be anterior uveitis or panuveitis.[105] Anterior uveitis is most frequently granulomatous; however, non-granulomatous disease is also reported (Figure 7.1). Of note, granulomatous disease is referring to clinical findings, not histopathological, and includes mutton-fat keratic precipitates and iris nodules. Other frequent findings in sarcoid anterior uveitis include tent-like peripheral anterior synechiae, posterior synechiae, and trabecular meshwork nodules. Anterior uveitis can be associated with increased intraocular pressure due to acute inflammation or chronic complications of the disease (e.g., peripheral anterior synechiae of the angle).[107]

Primary intermediate uveitis is less frequent but not uncommon.[72, 105] Retinal vasculitis, snowballs in a "string of pearls" formation, cystoid macular edema, and epiretinal membrane are all frequent complications of sarcoid intermediate uveitis. All patients with intermediate uveitis require fluorescein angiography to identify subclinical retinal vasculitis. Ciliary body granulomas have also been reported as a manifestation of ocular sarcoidosis, with one case series reporting both diffuse and discrete nodular masses of the ciliary body associated with intraocular inflammation; treatment outcomes were not reported.[108]

Posterior and panuveitis can be characterized by multifocal choroiditis, isolated choroidal or optic nerve granulomas, or retinal granulomas. Multifocal retinal or choroidal granulomas are a common presentation of posterior uveitis; granulomas may resolve, leaving atrophic scars throughout the midperiphery and periphery (Figure 7.2).[72, 109] Retinal vasculitis, cystoid macular edema, and epiretinal membrane formation are common complications of sarcoid posterior and panuveitis. Retinal vasculitis in sarcoidosis is typically a periphlebitis. The vasculitis can be occlusive in nature, causing branch retinal vein occlusions, and may be complicated by retinal ischemia and neovascularization (Figure 7.3).[72] Isolated choroidal granulomas have also been described in sarcoidosis and may present without any associated anterior chamber, vitreous, or retinal inflammation.[110] In these cases, choroidal granulomas may be mistaken for malignancy – distinguishing features include a vermiform or "worm-like" appearance to the lesion.

The differential diagnosis of these ocular findings is often broad, as sarcoidosis can present in many fashions; however, tuberculosis is one infectious cause that may have considerable overlap. Indeed, some have even proposed that tuberculosis and sarcoidosis are on a disease spectrum with a shared infectious trigger.[111] Both are diseases characterized by granulomatous inflammation, often

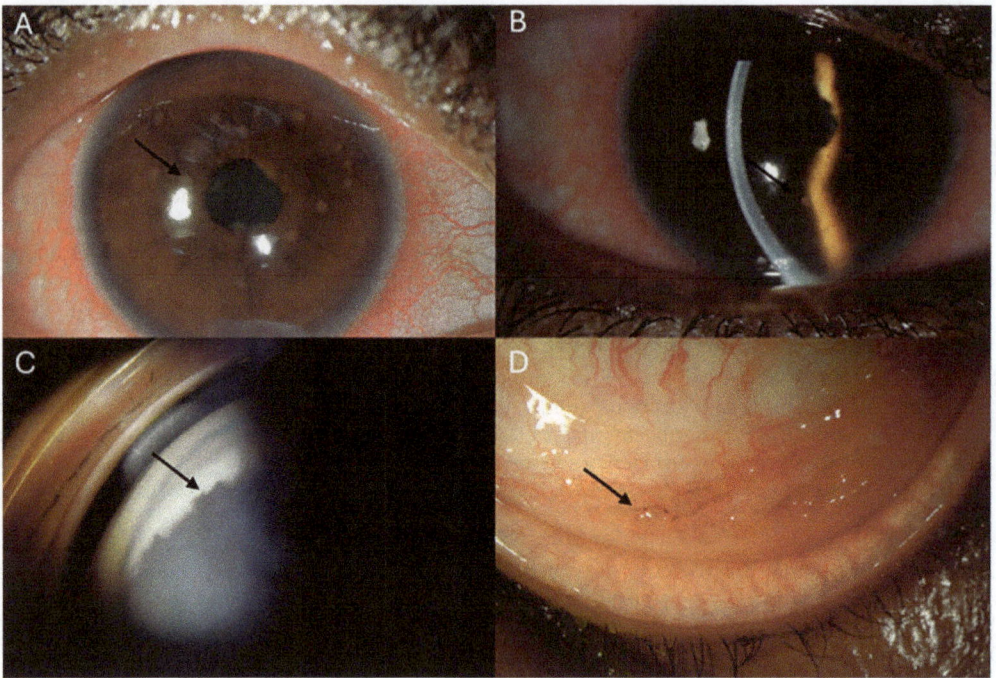

Figure 7.1 Anterior segment inflammation in sarcoidosis. Iris with granulomatous nodules (A). Granulomatous "mutton-fat" keratic precipitates on the corneal endothelium (B). "Tent-shaped" peripheral anterior synechiae on gonioscopy (C). String of conjunctival granulomas in the fornix (D).

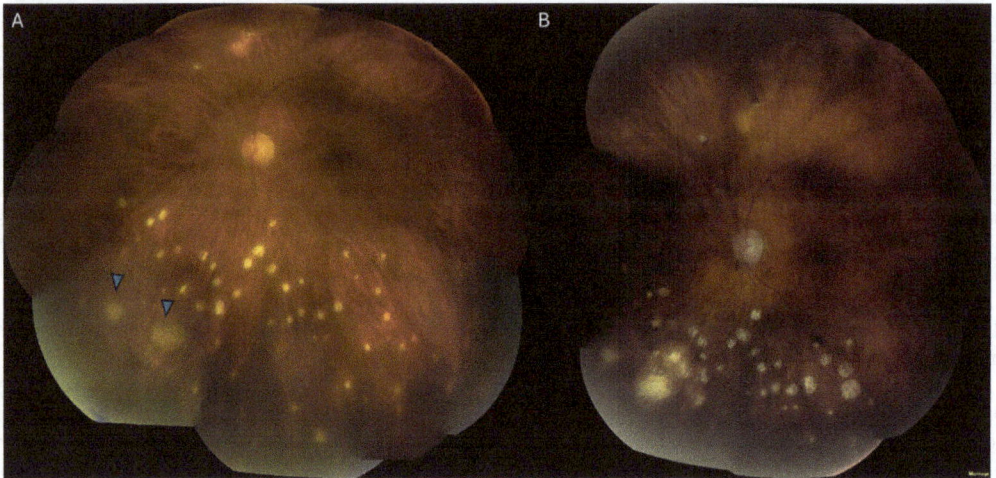

Figure 7.2 Multifocal retinal granulomas in sarcoidosis. Areas of chorioretinal scarring from prior inflammatory granulomas with two large active retinal granulomas inferonasal to the optic nerve (A; blue arrowheads). Post-treatment several years later showing resolution of granulomas with residual chorioretinal scarring (B).

with choroidal and pulmonary involvement. In cases of uveitis with a positive interferon gamma release assay (IGRA) suggesting exposure to or infection with tuberculosis, it can frequently be difficult to exclude tuberculosis as an infectious cause of ocular inflammation.

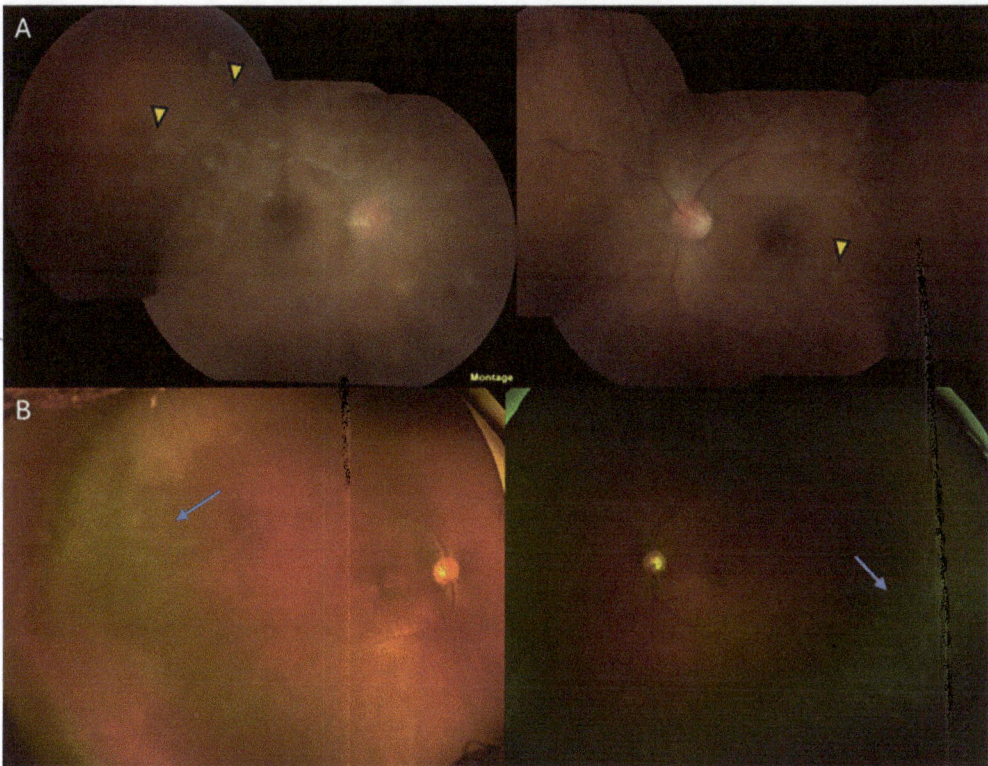

Figure 7.3 Vitritis and retinal vasculitis in a patient with sarcoid uveitis. (A) Dense vitreous cell obscuring the view of the posterior pole and optic nerve in the right eye (left upper panel) with clumps of inflammatory cells (yellow arrowheads). The left eye (right upper panel) has fewer vitreous cells, allowing better visualization of the optic nerve and posterior pole. (B) Retinal vasculitis affecting the large veins is highlighted by a perivascular white infiltrate, or sheathing, surrounding the venous system (blue arrows).

7.4.2 Imaging in Ocular Sarcoidosis

Fluorescein angiography (FA), indocyanine green angiography (ICGA), optical coherence tomography (OCT), and fundus autofluorescence (FAF) are the most frequently employed and useful imaging modalities for both diagnosing and monitoring treatment response in patients with ocular sarcoidosis.[112] FA can identify subclinical retinal vasculitis, cystoid macular edema, macroaneurysms, areas of occlusions, ischemia, and neovascularization of the retina or optic disc – all of which are complications of sarcoidosis inflammation.[71] FA is often repeated to monitor response to treatment. ICGA can highlight choroidal granulomas as hypofluorescent scattered areas in the early to mid-phases of angiography.[113] However, this is a nonspecific finding and can be seen in a number of inflammatory and infectious diseases involving the choroid. In particular, tuberculosis is a major infectious etiology in which choroidal granulomas can have a similar appearance on ICGA.

OCT with enhanced depth imaging is an invaluable tool to visualize the vitreo-retinal interface, retina, and choroid in detail. OCT can identify and quantitatively monitor cystoid macular edema. Pre-retinal or intra-retinal sarcoid granulomas can be identified by hyper-reflective foci within or on the retina that can resolve with treatment (Figure 7.4).[114] Sarcoidosis choroidal granulomas are hyporeflective focal enlargements within the choroid with well-defined margins and can have overlying structural changes within the retina.[115] OCT-angiography uses repeated b-scans to identify erythrocyte movement and therefore map blood flow and vasculature. Similar to ICGA, choroidal granulomas may be identified as dark areas with displacement of surrounding vasculature on OCTA.[112] FAF may highlight choroidal granulomas as mixed areas of hypo- and hyperautofluoresence.

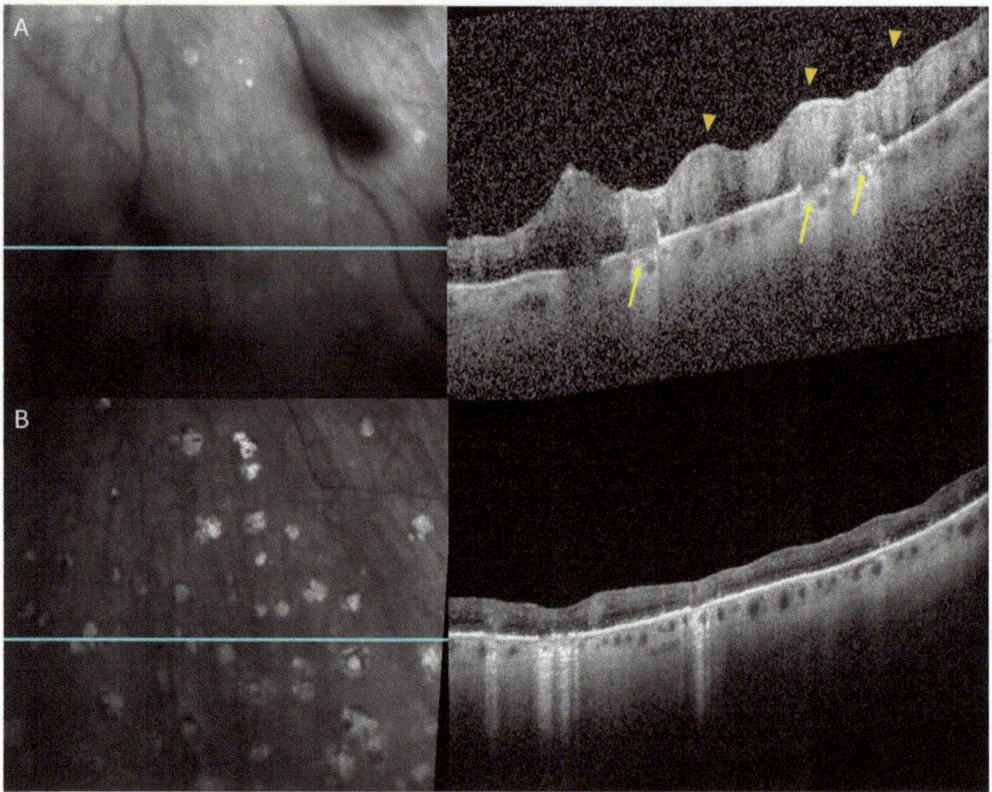

Figure 7.4 OCT imaging of retinal granulomas in sarcoidosis. (A) Active retinal granulomas captured by OCT as hyperreflective foci within all layers of the retina (yellow arrowheads) as well as granulomas in the outer retina causing retinal pigment epithelium disruption (yellow arrows). (B) Post-treatment showing resolution of the hyperreflective foci.

7.5 MANAGEMENT AND TREATMENT OF OCULAR SARCOIDOSIS

In 2019, IWOS developed a set of recommendations from experts around the world for the treatment and management of ocular sarcoidosis.[116] Ocular sarcoidosis is most often a bilateral, chronic uveitis, and therefore, treatment should be aimed at initial quiescence with short-term corticosteroids followed by long-term control with corticosteroid-sparing agents. Chronic disease can be identified by disease that relapses when attempting to taper corticosteroid therapy or by findings of chronic inflammation on presentation such as band keratopathy and epiretinal membrane formation. It is important to work with other specialists (e.g., pulmonologists, rheumatologists) when treating if multiple organs are involved.

7.5.1 Local Ocular Therapy

Local ocular therapy includes topical, periocular, or intravitreal corticosteroids. It is most often used to treat disease flares or in conjunction with systemic immunomodulatory therapy (IMT) to treat breakthrough disease but is typically not considered as long-term therapy. The exception to this is long-term fluocinolone implants, which are sometimes used to treat chronic disease. Side effects of chronic corticosteroids in any form include development of glaucoma and cataract. In cases of anterior uveitis, topical corticosteroids are most frequently used and include prednisolone acetate 1% or difluprednate 0.05%. Difluprednate is a more potent steroid that may treat cystoid macular edema as well as anterior uveitis, but it is associated with a higher rate of cataract and elevated intraocular pressure than prednisolone.

Intermediate uveitis, if manifested solely by vitreous cells, may be observed if there are no structural complications such as retinoschisis, cystoid macular edema, or retinal vasculitis. IWOS experts agree that diffuse vitreous opacities, snowballs, active snowbanks, and macular edema require treatment.[116] First-line local therapy includes periocular (e.g., subtenon triamcinolone acetonide 40 mg/mL) or intravitreal therapy (e.g., dexamethasone 0.7 mg implant or triamcinolone acetonide 40 mg/mL).

Active posterior findings, including choroidal and retinal granulomas, optic disc granulomas, retinal vasculitis, and cystoid macular edema, should be treated.[116] First-line local treatment may include the mentioned periocular or intravitreal corticosteroids. If disease is bilateral and/or severe, a short course of systemic prednisone may be administered. Local treatments for ischemic complications may include anti-vascular endothelial growth factor agents or retinal laser treatment to areas of retinal ischemia, but these are typically only considered after quiescence of the inflammatory disease, as neovascularization may be induced by inflammation rather than ischemia.

7.5.2 Systemic Therapy

Systemic corticosteroids are the first-line treatment for severe ocular disease at dosages of 0.5 to 1 mg/kg of prednisone followed by slow taper over months. This may be used in conjunction with topical or periocular/intravitreal corticosteroids.[116] However, corticosteroid monotherapy is not effective to control disease in the long term due to systemic side effects of corticosteroids, which include insulin resistance, hypertension, osteoporosis, weight gain, and mood changes. Patients who relapse when corticosteroids are tapered, are unable to achieve remission with corticosteroid monotherapy, or have organ-threatening involvement on presentation require the addition of corticosteroid-sparing immunosuppressive medication.[117]

There are multiple non-glucocorticoid treatment options for the treatment of ocular sarcoidosis. Methotrexate, a folate antimetabolite that impairs DNA synthesis, is an effective first-line steroid-sparing agent.[118] It has been shown to treat thoracic manifestations and improves pulmonary function tests and radiologic findings.[119, 120] It is also effective for improving skin lesions, central nervous system manifestations, and other systemic organ involvement including ocular involvement.[119, 120] Other antimetabolites include mycophenolate, leflunomide, and azathioprine, all of which have been used in the treatment of chronic uveitis.[121]

Tumor necrosis factor-alpha (TNF-α) inhibitors have emerged as the cornerstone of sarcoidosis treatment in the biologic era, including for ocular manifestations. Both infliximab and adalimumab have shown efficacy for the treatment of thoracic and extra-thoracic manifestations of systemic sarcoidosis.[122–126] Adalimumab is the only systemic treatment approved by the Food and Drug Administration for the treatment of noninfectious intermediate, posterior, or panuveitis. Approval was based on two large randomized controlled trials, VISUAL I and VISUAL II, demonstrating decreased uveitis flares, visual loss, and corticosteroid use in patients on adalimumab versus placebo.[127, 128] These clinical trials included patients with sarcoid uveitis. However, not all TNFα inhibitors have demonstrated benefit in treating sarcoidosis. The TNF-α inhibitor etanercept has shown no benefit in the treatment of uveitis.[129] Golimumab can be effective for uveitis but is associated with treatment failure in pulmonary manifestation of sarcoidosis.[130, 131] Other biologics are under investigation. Studies of rituximab, a B cell depleting agent, have demonstrated mixed results, although it may be effective in the treatment of refractory disease.[117, 132] Both IL-6 inhibitors and JAK inhibitors also have some limited evidence for use in refractory cases of ocular sarcoidosis, but they are often only employed after failure of TNF-alpha inhibitors.[133]

7.6 NATURAL HISTORY AND PROGNOSIS

7.6.1 Ocular Sarcoidosis

With appropriate treatment, ocular sarcoidosis can have an excellent prognosis with preserved visual acuity. As discussed, the disease is most frequently manifest by chronic inflammation. Interestingly, the severity of ocular disease may be independent from and have a different course from pulmonary or other systemic disease. The number of pulmonary relapses was inversely related with ocular disease activity in one study, and several other studies have shown little correlation between pulmonary disease activity and ocular manifestations.[12, 23, 104]

Complications of chronic uveitis most commonly include glaucoma, cataract, cystoid macular edema, and epiretinal membrane formation. Cystoid macular edema is the most frequent cause of visual deterioration, particularly among older White women.[1] Overall, the visual prognosis is relatively good, with most studies indicating only a small minority of patients with severe vision loss (e.g., vision less than 20/200).[134–137] Factors associated with a worse prognosis include Black race, female sex, posterior segment involvement, and cystoid macular edema.[72]

7.6.2 Systemic Sarcoidosis

Patients with systemic manifestations of sarcoidosis have an overall favorable prognosis. Fifty to 70% of patients achieve remission within 2 to 3 years – and a portion of these patients, such as patients with Lofgren's syndrome, will have spontaneous remission without receiving immunosuppressive treatment.[31, 34, 138] In the ACCESS study, 80% of patients with pulmonary sarcoidosis had improved or stable pulmonary function testing, chest radiographs, and dyspnea scores after 2 years of treatment.[139] Systemic manifestations of EN, acute arthritis, and mediastinal and hilar lymphadenopathy portend a favorable prognosis.[138, 140] Additionally, it is uncommon for patients to develop new organ involvement that was not present at the time of their initial diagnosis. In the 2 years following the initial diagnosis, less than a quarter of patients will develop new organ involvement. The development of new systemic involvement is more common in Black than White patients and in those with extra-thoracic disease at diagnosis.[139]

After achieving remission, whether this is spontaneous or secondary to treatment, sarcoidosis patients can relapse with recurrence of active disease. Relapse rates vary among cohorts from 16% to 74% depending on how remission was achieved and treatment course.[141] Relapse rates are higher for patients requiring treatment to achieve remission compared to patients with spontaneous remission without treatment; relapse rates are also higher in Black patients and those with musculoskeletal and hepatic involvement.[142]

Patients with sarcoidosis frequently develop a chronic disease course requiring long-term treatment. The proportion of patients developing chronic sarcoidosis, including ocular involvement requiring long-term immunosuppression, varies across studies from 28% to 79% depending on the length of follow-up.[138, 143] Risk factors for developing chronic disease include severe pulmonary involvement with fibrosis, hepatosplenic involvement, lupus pernio, sinopulmonary manifestations, neurosarcoidosis, cardiac sarcoidosis, nephrocalcinosis, and multi-organ involvement.[34, 138, 140, 143, 144]

Mortality rates of sarcoidosis are low and are estimated at around 5% at 5 years from diagnosis and up to 9% 10 years out from diagnosis.[31, 138] Increased mortality is associated with severe thoracic disease complicated by pulmonary fibrosis and pulmonary hypertension.[144] There are racial influences on mortality rates as well, with Black patients having higher mortality rates than White patients in the United States.[31, 144]

7.7 SUMMARY

As a multisystem inflammatory disorder, sarcoidosis can be a challenging disease to diagnose and treat. The clinical presentation, evaluation, and management of sarcoidosis can be complex due to the disease's multiorgan involvement and requires coordination and communication among multiple subspecialists. The interdisciplinary care of subspecialists, specifically rheumatologists, pulmonologists, and ophthalmologists, is critical for the timely and appropriate diagnosis and treatment of sarcoidosis patients with ocular disease involvement.

REFERENCES

1. Jones N, Mochizuki M. Sarcoidosis: epidemiology and clinical features. *Ocul Immunol Inflamm.* 2010;18(2):72–79. doi:10.3109/09273941003710598.
2. Brito-Zerón P, Kostov B, Superville D, et al. Geoepidemiological big data approach to sarcoidosis: geographical and ethnic determinants. *Clin Exp Rheumatol.* 2019;37(6):1052–1064.
3. Arkema EV, Cozier YC. Sarcoidosis epidemiology: recent estimates of incidence, prevalence and risk factors. *Curr Opin Pulm Med.* 2020;26(5):527–534. doi:10.1097/MCP.0000000000000715.
4. Baughman RP, Field S, Costabel U, et al. Sarcoidosis in America: analysis based on health care use. *Ann Am Thorac Soc.* 2016;13(8):1244–1252. doi:10.1513/AnnalsATS.201511-760OC.
5. Costabel U, Hunninghake GW, On Behalf of the Sarcoidosis Statement Committee. ATS/ERS/WASOG statement on sarcoidosis. *Eur Respir J.* 1999;14(4):735. doi:10.1034/j.1399-3003.1999.14d02.x.
6. Ungprasert P, Crowson CS, Matteson EL. Influence of gender on epidemiology and clinical manifestations of sarcoidosis: a population-based retrospective cohort study 1976–2013. *Lung.* 2017;195(1):87–91. doi:10.1007/s00408-016-9952-6.
7. Hena KM. Sarcoidosis epidemiology: race matters. *Front Immunol.* 2020;11:537382. doi:10.3389/fimmu.2020.537382.
8. Ungprasert P, Tooley AA, Crowson CS, et al. Clinical characteristics of ocular sarcoidosis: a population-based study 1976–2013. *Ocul Immunol Inflamm.* 2019;27(3):389–395. doi:10.1080/09273948.2017.1386791.
9. Birnbaum AD, French DD, Mirsaeidi M, et al. Sarcoidosis in the national veteran population. *Ophthalmology.* 2015;122(5):934–938. doi:10.1016/j.ophtha.2015.01.003.

10. Jamilloux Y, Kodjikian L, Broussolle C, et al. Sarcoidosis and uveitis. *Autoimmun Rev.* 2014;13(8):840–849. doi:10.1016/j.autrev.2014.04.001.

11. Lee J, Zaguia F, Minkus C, et al. The role of screening for asymptomatic ocular inflammation in sarcoidosis. *Ocul Immunol Inflamm.* 2022;30(7–8):1936–1939. doi:10.1080/09273948.2021.1976216.

12. Evans M, Sharma O, LaBree L, et al. Differences in clinical findings between Caucasians and African Americans with biopsy-proven sarcoidosis. *Ophthalmology.* 2007;114(2):325–333.e1. doi:10.1016/j.ophtha.2006.05.074.

13. Judson MA, Boan AD, Lackland DT. The clinical course of sarcoidosis: presentation, diagnosis, and treatment in a large white and black cohort in the United States. *Sarcoidosis Vasc Diffuse Lung Dis Off J WASOG.* 2012;29(2):119–127.

14. Birnbaum AD, Oh F, Chakrabarti A, et al. Clinical features and diagnostic evaluation of biopsy-proven ocular sarcoidosis. *Arch Ophthalmol.* 2011;129(4):409. doi:10.1001/archophthalmol.2011.52.

15. Heiligenhaus A, Wefelmeyer D, Wefelmeyer E, et al. The eye as a common site for the early clinical manifestation of sarcoidosis. *Ophthalmic Res.* 2011;46(1):9–12. doi:10.1159/000321947.

16. Khalatbari D, Stinnett S, McCallum RM, et al. Demographic-related variations in posterior segment ocular sarcoidosis. *Ophthalmology.* 2004;111(2):357–362. doi:10.1016/S0161-6420(03)00793-0.

17. Rothova A, Alberts C, Glasius E, et al. Risk factors for ocular sarcoidosis. *Doc Ophthalmol.* 1989;72(3–4):287–296. doi:10.1007/BF00153496.

18. Thorne JE, Brucker AJ. Choroidal white lesions as an early manifestation of sarcoidosis. *Retina.* 2000;20(1):8–14. doi:10.1097/00006982-200001000-00002.

19. Hershey JM, Pulido JS, Folberg R, et al. Non-caseating conjunctival granulomas in patients with multifocal choroiditis and panuveitis. *Ophthalmology.* 1994;101(3):596–601. doi:10.1016/S0161-6420(94)31296-6.

20. Lardenoye CWTA, Van Der Lelij A, De Loos WS, et al. Peripheral multifocal chorioretinitis. *Ophthalmology.* 1997;104(11):1820–1826. doi:10.1016/S0161-6420(97)30021-9.

21. Nagata K, Maruyama K, Sugita S, et al. Age differences in sarcoidosis patients with posterior ocular lesions. *Ocul Immunol Inflamm.* 2014;22(4):257–262. doi:10.3109/09273948.2013.855796.

22. Lee SY, Lee HG, Kim DS, et al. Ocular Sarcoidosis in a Korean population. *J Korean Med Sci.* 2009;24(3):413. doi:10.3346/jkms.2009.24.3.413.

23. Atmaca LS, Atmaca-Sönmez P, İdil A, et al. Ocular involvement in sarcoidosis. *Ocul Immunol Inflamm.* 2009;17(2):91–94. doi:10.1080/09273940802596526.

24. Febvay C, Kodjikian L, Maucort-Boulch D, et al. Clinical features and diagnostic evaluation of 83 biopsy-proven sarcoid uveitis cases. *Br J Ophthalmol.* 2015;99(10):1372–1376. doi:10.1136/bjophthalmol-2014-306353.

25. Ohguro N, Sonoda KH, Takeuchi M, et al. The 2009 prospective multi-center epidemiologic survey of uveitis in Japan. *Jpn J Ophthalmol.* 2012;56(5):432–435. doi:10.1007/s10384-012-0158-z.

26. Matsuo T, Fujiwara N, Nakata Y. First presenting signs or symptoms of sarcoidosis in a Japanese population. *Jpn J Ophthalmol.* 2005;49(2):149–152. doi:10.1007/s10384-004-0154-z.

27. Reid G, Williams M, Compton M, et al. Ocular sarcoidosis prevalence and clinical features in the Northern Ireland population. *Eye.* 2022;36(10):1918–1923. doi:10.1038/s41433-021-01770-0.

28. Rossman MD, Kreider ME. State of the art: lesson learned from ACCESS (a case controlled etiologic study of sarcoidosis). *Proc Am Thorac Soc.* 2007;4(5):453–456. doi:10.1513/pats.200607-138MS.

29. Rybicki BA, Iannuzzi MC, Frederick MM, et al. Familial aggregation of sarcoidosis: a case-control etiologic study of sarcoidosis (ACCESS). *Am J Respir Crit Care Med.* 2001;164(11):2085–2091. doi:10.1164/ajrccm.164.11.2106001.

30. Brown ST, Brett I, Almenoff PL, et al. Recovery of cell wall-deficient organisms from blood does not distinguish between patients with sarcoidosis and control subjects. *Chest.* 2003;123(2):413–417. doi:10.1378/chest.123.2.413.

31. Firestein GS. *Firestein & Kelley's textbook of rheumatology,* volume 2, 11th edn. Elsevier, 2021.

32. Müller-Quernheim J, Prasse A, Zissel G. Pathogenesis of sarcoidosis. *Presse Medicale Paris Fr 1983.* 2012;41(6 Pt 2):e275–e287. doi:10.1016/j.lpm.2012.03.018.

33. Rossman MD, Thompson B, Frederick M, et al. HLA and environmental interactions in sarcoidosis. *Sarcoidosis Vasc Diffuse Lung Dis Off J WASOG.* 2008;25(2):125–132.

34. Stone J. *Current diagnosis & treatment: rheumatology,* 4th edn. McGraw Hill, 2021.

35. Jordan HT, Stellman SD, Prezant D, et al. Sarcoidosis diagnosed after Sept. 11, 2001, among adults exposed to the world trade center disaster. *J Occup Environ Med.* 2011;53(9):966–974. doi:10.1097/JOM.0b013e31822a3596.

36. Hena KM, Yip J, Jaber N, et al. Clinical course of sarcoidosis in World Trade Center-exposed firefighters. *Chest*. 2018;153(1):114–123. doi:10.1016/j.chest.2017.10.014.

37. Kluger N. Tattoo-associated uveitis with or without systemic sarcoidosis: a comparative review of the literature. *J Eur Acad Dermatol Venereol JEADV*. 2018;32(11):1852–1861. doi:10.1111/jdv.15070.

38. Saidha S, Sotirchos ES, Eckstein C. Etiology of sarcoidosis: does infection play a role? *Yale J Biol Med*. 2012;85(1):133–141.

39. Gupta D, Agarwal R, Aggarwal AN, et al. Molecular evidence for the role of mycobacteria in sarcoidosis: a meta-analysis. *Eur Respir J*. 2007;30(3):508–516. doi:10.1183/09031936.00002607.

40. Song Z, Marzilli L, Greenlee BM, et al. Mycobacterial catalase-peroxidase is a tissue antigen and target of the adaptive immune response in systemic sarcoidosis. *J Exp Med*. 2005;201(5):755–767. doi:10.1084/jem.20040429.

41. Judson MA. Environmental risk factors for sarcoidosis. *Front Immunol*. 2020;11:1340. doi:10.3389/fimmu.2020.01340.

42. Musaelyan A, Lapin S, Nazarov V, et al. Vimentin as antigenic target in autoimmunity: a comprehensive review. *Autoimmun Rev*. 2018;17(9):926–934. doi:10.1016/j.autrev.2018.04.004.

43. Cain H, Kraus B. Immunofluorescence microscopic demonstration of vimentin filaments in asteroid bodies of sarcoidosis: a comparison with electron microscopic findings. *Virchows Arch B Cell Pathol Incl Mol Pathol*. 1983;42(1):213–226. doi:10.1007/BF02890384.

44. Eberhardt C, Thillai M, Parker R, et al. Proteomic analysis of Kveim reagent identifies targets of cellular immunity in sarcoidosis. Dieli F, ed. *PLoS One*. 2017;12(1):e0170285. doi:10.1371/journal.pone.0170285.

45. Starshinova A, Malkova A, Zinchenko U, et al. Detection of anti-vimentin antibodies in patients with sarcoidosis. *Diagn Basel Switz*. 2022;12(8):1939. doi:10.3390/diagnostics12081939.

46. Zhou ER, Arce S. Key players and biomarkers of the adaptive immune system in the pathogenesis of sarcoidosis. *Int J Mol Sci*. 2020;21(19):7398. doi:10.3390/ijms21197398.

47. Wojtan P, Mierzejewski M, Osińska I, et al. Macrophage polarization in interstitial lung diseases. *Cent-Eur J Immunol*. 2016;41(2):159–164. doi:10.5114/ceji.2016.60990.

48. Moller DR, Forman JD, Liu MC, et al. Enhanced expression of IL-12 associated with Th1 cytokine profiles in active pulmonary sarcoidosis. *J Immunol Baltim Md 1950*. 1996;156(12):4952–4960.

49. Moller DR. Treatment of sarcoidosis – from a basic science point of view. *J Intern Med*. 2003;253(1):31–40. doi:10.1046/j.1365-2796.2003.01075.x.

50. Shamaei M, Mortaz E, Pourabdollah M, et al. Evidence for M2 macrophages in granulomas from pulmonary sarcoidosis: a new aspect of macrophage heterogeneity. *Hum Immunol*. 2018;79(1):63–69. doi:10.1016/j.humimm.2017.10.009.

51. Oltmanns U, Schmidt B, Hoernig S, et al. Increased spontaneous interleukin-10 release from alveolar macrophages in active pulmonary sarcoidosis. *Exp Lung Res*. 2003;29(5):315–328. doi:10.1080/01902140303786.

52. Nguyen CTH, Kambe N, Ueda-Hayakawa I, et al. TARC expression in the circulation and cutaneous granulomas correlates with disease severity and indicates Th2-mediated progression in patients with sarcoidosis. *Allergol Int Off J Jpn Soc Allergol*. 2018;67(4):487–495. doi:10.1016/j.alit.2018.02.011.

53. Rybicki BA, Iannuzzi MC, Frederick MM, et al. Familial aggregation of sarcoidosis: a case-control etiologic study of sarcoidosis (ACCESS). *Am J Respir Crit Care Med*. 2001;164(11):2085–2091. doi:10.1164/ajrccm.164.11.2106001.

54. Fischer A, Grunewald J, Spagnolo P, et al. Genetics of sarcoidosis. *Semin Respir Crit Care Med*. 2014;35(3):296–306. doi:10.1055/s-0034-1376860.

55. Liao SY, Jacobson S, Hamzeh NY, et al. Genome-wide association study identifies multiple HLA loci for sarcoidosis susceptibility. *Hum Mol Genet*. 2023;32(16):2669–2678. doi:10.1093/hmg/ddad067.

56. Grunewald J, Spagnolo P, Wahlström J, et al. Immunogenetics of disease-causing inflammation in sarcoidosis. *Clin Rev Allergy Immunol*. 2015;49(1):19–35. doi:10.1007/s12016-015-8477-8.

57. Rossman MD, Thompson B, Frederick M, et al. HLA-DRB1*1101: a significant risk factor for sarcoidosis in blacks and whites. *Am J Hum Genet*. 2003;73(4):720–735. doi:10.1086/378097.

58. Iannuzzi MC. Advances in the genetics of sarcoidosis. *Proc Am Thorac Soc*. 2007;4(5):457–460. doi:10.1513/pats.200606-136MS.

59. Hofmann S, Fischer A, Till A, et al. A genome-wide association study reveals evidence of association with sarcoidosis at 6p12.1. *Eur Respir J*. 2011;38(5):1127–1135. doi:10.1183/09031936.00001711.

60. Pillai P, Sobrin L. Blau syndrome-associated uveitis and the *NOD2* gene. *Semin Ophthalmol.* 2013;28(5–6):327–332. doi:10.3109/08820538.2013.825285.
61. Latkany PA, Jabs DA, Smith JR, et al. Multifocal choroiditis in patients with familial juvenile systemic granulomatosis. *Am J Ophthalmol.* 2002;134(6):897–904. doi:10.1016/S0002-9394(02)01709-9.
62. Saini SK, Rose CD. Liver involvement in familial granulomatous arthritis (Blau syndrome). *J Rheumatol.* 1996;23(2):396–399.
63. Ting SS, Ziegler J, Fischer E. Familial granulomatous arthritis (Blau syndrome) with granulomatous renal lesions. *J Pediatr.* 1998;133(3):450–452. doi:10.1016/S0022-3476(98)70286-0.
64. Ogura Y, Inohara N, Benito A, et al. Nod2, a Nod1/Apaf-1 family member that is restricted to monocytes and activates NF-κB. *J Biol Chem.* 2001;276(7):4812–4818. doi:10.1074/jbc.M008072200.
65. Okafuji I, Nishikomori R, Kanazawa N, et al. Role of the NOD2 genotype in the clinical phenotype of Blau syndrome and early-onset sarcoidosis. *Arthritis Rheum.* 2009;60(1):242–250. doi:10.1002/art.24134.
66. Rosenzweig HL, Martin TM, Planck SR, et al. Activation of NOD2 in vivo induces IL-1β production in the eye via caspase-1 but results in ocular inflammation independently of IL-1 signaling. *J Leukoc Biol.* 2008;84(2):529–536. doi:10.1189/jlb.0108015.
67. Simonini G, Xu Z, Caputo R, et al. Clinical and transcriptional response to the long-acting interleukin-1 blocker canakinumab in Blau syndrome–related uveitis. *Arthritis Rheum.* 2013;65(2):513–518. doi:10.1002/art.37776.
68. Martin TM, Zhang Z, Kurz P, et al. The *NOD2* defect in Blau syndrome does not result in excess interleukin-1 activity. *Arthritis Rheum.* 2009;60(2):611–618. doi:10.1002/art.24222.
69. Takase H, Shimizu K, Yamada Y, et al. Validation of international criteria for the diagnosis of ocular sarcoidosis proposed by the first international workshop on ocular sarcoidosis. *Jpn J Ophthalmol.* 2010;54(6):529–536. doi:10.1007/s10384-010-0873-2.
70. Acharya NR, Browne EN, Rao N, et al. Distinguishing features of ocular sarcoidosis in an international cohort of uveitis patients. *Ophthalmology.* 2018;125(1):119–126. doi:10.1016/j.ophtha.2017.07.006.
71. Mochizuki M, Smith JR, Takase H, et al. Revised criteria of international workshop on ocular sarcoidosis (IWOS) for the diagnosis of ocular sarcoidosis. *Br J Ophthalmol.* 2019;103(10):1418–1422. doi:10.1136/bjophthalmol-2018-313356.
72. Giorgiutti S, Jacquot R, El Jammal T, et al. Sarcoidosis-related uveitis: a review. *J Clin Med.* 2023;12(9):3194. doi:10.3390/jcm12093194.
73. Cotte P, Pradat P, Kodjikian L, et al. Diagnostic value of lymphopaenia and elevated serum ACE in patients with uveitis. *Br J Ophthalmol.* 2021;105(10):1399–1404. doi:10.1136/bjophthalmol-2020-316563.
74. Groen-Hakan F, Eurelings L, Ten Berge JC, et al. Diagnostic value of serum-soluble interleukin 2 receptor levels vs angiotensin-converting enzyme in patients with sarcoidosis-associated uveitis. *JAMA Ophthalmol.* 2017;135(12):1352. doi:10.1001/jamaophthalmol.2017.4771.
75. Gundlach E, Hoffmann MM, Prasse A, et al. Interleukin-2 receptor and angiotensin-converting enzyme as markers for ocular sarcoidosis. Rosenbaum JT, ed. *PLoS One.* 2016;11(1):e0147258. doi:10.1371/journal.pone.0147258.
76. Chauvelot P, Skanjeti A, Jamilloux Y, et al. 18F-fluorodeoxyglucose positron emission tomography is useful for the diagnosis of intraocular sarcoidosis in patients with a normal CT scan. *Br J Ophthalmol.* 2019;103(11):1650–1655. doi:10.1136/bjophthalmol-2018-313133.
77. Sahin O, Ziaei A, Karaismailoğlu E, et al. The serum angiotensin converting enzyme and lysozyme levels in patients with ocular involvement of autoimmune and infectious diseases. *BMC Ophthalmol.* 2016;16(1):19. doi:10.1186/s12886-016-0194-4.
78. Takahashi T, Azuma A, Abe S, et al. Significance of lymphocytosis in bronchoalveolar lavage in suspected ocular sarcoidosis. *Eur Respir J.* 2001;18(3):515–521. doi:10.1183/09031936.01.99104501.
79. Kefella H, Luther D, Hainline C. Ophthalmic and neuro-ophthalmic manifestations of sarcoidosis. *Curr Opin Ophthalmol.* 2017;28(6):587–594. doi:10.1097/ICU.0000000000000415.
80. Oleñik A, Gonzalo-Suárez B, Revenga M, et al. Use of aqueous humor and flow cytometry in ocular sarcoidosis diagnosis. *Ocul Immunol Inflamm.* 2017;25(4):540–544. doi:10.3109/09273948.2016.1158839.
81. Bui KM, Garcia-Gonzalez JM, Patel SS, et al. Directed conjunctival biopsy and impact of histologic sectioning methodology on the diagnosis of ocular sarcoidosis. *J Ophthalmic Inflamm Infect.* 2014;4(1):8. doi:10.1186/1869-5760-4-8.

82. Blaise P, Fardeau C, Chapelon C, et al. Minor salivary gland biopsy in diagnosing ocular sarcoidosis. *Br J Ophthalmol*. 2011;95(12):1731–1734. doi:10.1136/bjophthalmol-2011-300129.

83. Baughman RP, Teirstein AS, Judson MA, et al. Clinical characteristics of patients in a case control study of sarcoidosis. *Am J Respir Crit Care Med*. 2001;164(10 Pt 1):1885–1889. doi:10.1164/ajrccm.164.10.2104046.

84. Sève P, Pacheco Y, Durupt F, et al. Sarcoidosis: a clinical overview from symptoms to diagnosis. *Cells*. 2021;10(4):766. doi:10.3390/cells10040766.

85. Mihailovic-Vucinic V, Jovanovic D. Pulmonary sarcoidosis. *Clin Chest Med*. 2008;29(3):459–473, viii–ix. doi:10.1016/j.ccm.2008.03.002.

86. Byrne B, Goh A, Izham NF, et al. Systemic evaluation of cutaneous sarcoidosis: 15-year dermatology experience at University Hospital Limerick. *Clin Exp Dermatol*. 2022;47(5):850–857. doi:10.1111/ced.15097.

87. Rao DA, Dellaripa PF. Extrapulmonary manifestations of sarcoidosis. *Rheum Dis Clin North Am*. 2013;39(2):277–297. doi:10.1016/j.rdc.2013.02.007.

88. Caplan A, Rosenbach M, Imadojemu S. Cutaneous sarcoidosis. *Semin Respir Crit Care Med*. 2020;41(5):689–699. doi:10.1055/s-0040-1713130.

89. Wanat KA, Rosenbach M. Cutaneous sarcoidosis. *Clin Chest Med*. 2015;36(4):685–702. doi:10.1016/j.ccm.2015.08.010.

90. Brito-Zerón P, Lower EE, Ramos-Casals M, et al. Hematological involvement in sarcoidosis: from cytopenias to lymphoma. *Expert Rev Clin Immunol*. Published online 2023 Oct. 25:1–12. doi:10.1080/1744666X.2023.2274363.

91. Arish N, Kuint R, Sapir E, et al. Characteristics of sarcoidosis in patients with previous malignancy: causality or coincidence? *Respiration*. 2017;93(4):247–252. doi:10.1159/000455877.

92. Shah HH, Zehra SA, Shahrukh A, et al. Cardiac sarcoidosis: a comprehensive review of risk factors, pathogenesis, diagnosis, clinical manifestations, and treatment strategies. *Front Cardiovasc Med*. 2023;10:1156474. doi:10.3389/fcvm.2023.1156474.

93. Lam CSP, Tolep KA, Metke MP, et al. Coronary sarcoidosis presenting as acute coronary syndrome. *Clin Cardiol*. 2009;32(6):e68–e71. doi:10.1002/clc.20381.

94. Cereceda-Monteoliva N, Rouhani MJ, Maughan EF, et al. Sarcoidosis of the ear, nose and throat: a review of the literature. *Clin Otolaryngol Off J ENT-UK Off J Neth Soc Oto-Rhino-Laryngol Cervico-Facial Surg*. 2021;46(5):935–940. doi:10.1111/coa.13814.

95. Hasbani GE, Uthman I, Jawad AS. Musculoskeletal manifestations of sarcoidosis. *Clin Med Insights Arthritis Musculoskelet Disord*. 2022;15. doi:10.1177/11795441211072475.

96. Krumholz A, Stern BJ. Neurologic manifestations of sarcoidosis. *Handb Clin Neurol*. 2014;119:305–333. doi:10.1016/B978-0-7020-4086-3.00021-7.

97. Ungprasert P, Matteson EL. Neurosarcoidosis. *Rheum Dis Clin N Am*. 2017;43(4):593–606. doi:10.1016/j.rdc.2017.06.008.

98. Freda PU, Silverberg SJ, Post KD, et al. Hypothalamic-pituitary sarcoidosis. *Trends Endocrinol Metab TEM*. 1992;3(9):321–325. doi:10.1016/1043-2760(92)90110-m.

99. Vardhanabhuti V, Venkatanarasimha N, Bhatnagar G, et al. Extra-pulmonary manifestations of sarcoidosis. *Clin Radiol*. 2012;67(3):263–276. doi:10.1016/j.crad.2011.04.018.

100. Farman J, Ramirez G, Rybak B, et al. Gastric sarcoidosis. *Abdom Imaging*. 1997;22(3):248–252. doi:10.1007/s002619900182.

101. Yeboah J, Sharma OP. Co-existence of Crohn's disease, sarcoidosis and malignant lymphomas. *JRSM Short Rep*. 2012;3(2):1–5. doi:10.1258/shorts.2011.011133.

102. Baughman RP, Janovcik J, Ray M, et al. Calcium and vitamin D metabolism in sarcoidosis. *Sarcoidosis Vasc Diffuse Lung Dis Off J WASOG*. 2013;30(2):113–120.

103. Kotwica-Strzałek E, Janicki P, Dociak I, et al. Manifestations of renal involvement in sarcoidosis – case series. *Pol Merkur Lek Organ Pol Tow Lek*. 2022;50(296):124–127.

104. Radosavljević A, Jakšić V, Pezo L, et al. Clinical features of ocular sarcoidosis in patients with biopsy-proven pulmonary sarcoidosis in Serbia. *Ocul Immunol Inflamm*. 2017;25(6):785–789. doi:10.3109/09273948.2016.1167224.

105. Bazewicz M, Heissigerova J, Pavesio C, et al. Ocular sarcoidosis in adults and children: update on clinical manifestation and diagnosis. *J Ophthalmic Inflamm Infect*. 2023;13(1):41. doi:10.1186/s12348-023-00364-z.

106. Rothova A. Ocular involvement in sarcoidosis. *Br J Ophthalmol*. 2000;84(1):110–116. doi:10.1136/bjo.84.1.110.

107. Matsou A, Tsaousis KT. Management of chronic ocular sarcoidosis: challenges and solutions. *Clin Ophthalmol*. 2018;12:519–532. doi:10.2147/OPTH.S128949.

108. Teo HMT, Elner SG, Sassalos TMP, et al. Ciliary body mass as a feature of ocular sarcoidosis. *JAMA Ophthalmol*. 2020;138(3):300. doi:10.1001/jamaophthalmol.2019.5704.

109. De Saint Sauveur G, Gratiot C, Debieb AC, et al. Retinal and pre-retinal nodules: a rare manifestation of probable ocular sarcoidosis. *Am J Ophthalmol Case Rep*. 2022;26:101525. doi:10.1016/j.ajoc.2022.101525.

110. Baş Z, Sajjadi Z, Shields CL. Sarcoid granuloma of the choroid and ciliary body in 50 cases. *Retina*. 2023;43(11):1842–1851. doi:10.1097/IAE.0000000000003925.

111. Agrawal R, Kee AR, Ang L, et al. Tuberculosis or sarcoidosis: opposite ends of the same disease spectrum? *Tuberculosis*. 2016;98:21–26. doi:10.1016/j.tube.2016.01.003.

112. Mahendradas P, Maruyama K, Mizuuchi K, et al. Multimodal imaging in ocular sarcoidosis. *Ocul Immunol Inflamm*. 2020;28(8):1205–1211. doi:10.1080/09273948.2020.1751210.

113. Wolfensberger TJ, Herbort CP. Indocyanine green angiographic features in ocular sarcoidosis. *Ophthalmology*. 1999;106(2):285–289. doi:10.1016/S0161-6420(99)90067-2.

114. Goldberg NR, Jabs DA, Busingye J. Optical coherence tomography imaging of presumed sarcoid retinal and optic nerve nodules. *Ocul Immunol Inflamm*. Published online 2014 Oct. 30:1–4. doi:10.3109/09273948.2014.971972.

115. Mehta H, Sim DA, Keane PA, et al. Structural changes of the choroid in sarcoid- and tuberculosis-related granulomatous uveitis. *Eye*. 2015;29(8):1060–1068. doi:10.1038/eye.2015.65.

116. Takase H, Acharya NR, Babu K, et al. Recommendations for the management of ocular sarcoidosis from the international workshop on ocular sarcoidosis. *Br J Ophthalmol*. 2021;105(11): 1515–1519. doi:10.1136/bjophthalmol-2020-317354.

117. Baughman RP, Lower EE. Treatment of sarcoidosis. *Clin Rev Allergy Immunol*. 2015;49(1):79–92. doi:10.1007/s12016-015-8492-9.

118. Baughman RP, Winget DB, Lower EE. Methotrexate is steroid sparing in acute sarcoidosis: results of a double blind, randomized trial. *Sarcoidosis Vasc Diffuse Lung Dis Off J WASOG*. 2000;17(1):60–66.

119. Lower EE, Baughman RP. Prolonged use of methotrexate for sarcoidosis. *Arch Intern Med*. 1995;155(8):846–851.

120. Vucinic VM. What is the future of methotrexate in sarcoidosis? A study and review. *Curr Opin Pulm Med*. 2002;8(5):470–476. doi:10.1097/00063198-200209000-00022.

121. Hwang DK, Sheu SJ. An update on the diagnosis and management of ocular sarcoidosis. *Curr Opin Ophthalmol*. 2020;31(6):521–531. doi:10.1097/ICU.0000000000000704.

122. Moravan M, Segal BM. Treatment of CNS sarcoidosis with infliximab and mycophenolate mofetil. *Neurology*. 2009;72(4):337–340. doi:10.1212/01.wnl.0000341278.26993.22.

123. Judson MA, Baughman RP, Costabel U, et al. Efficacy of infliximab in extrapulmonary sarcoidosis: results from a randomised trial. *Eur Respir J*. 2008;31(6):1189–1196. doi:10.1183/09031936.00051907.

124. Baughman RP, Drent M, Kavuru M, et al. Infliximab therapy in patients with chronic sarcoidosis and pulmonary involvement. *Am J Respir Crit Care Med*. 2006;174(7):795–802. doi:10.1164/rccm.200603-402OC.

125. Rossman MD, Newman LS, Baughman RP, et al. A double-blinded, randomized, placebo-controlled trial of infliximab in subjects with active pulmonary sarcoidosis. *Sarcoidosis Vasc Diffuse Lung Dis Off J WASOG*. 2006;23(3):201–208.

126. Sweiss NJ, Noth I, Mirsaeidi M, et al. Efficacy results of a 52-week trial of adalimumab in the treatment of refractory sarcoidosis. *Sarcoidosis Vasc Diffuse Lung Dis Off J WASOG*. 2014;31(1):46–54.

127. Jaffe GJ, Dick AD, Brézin AP, et al. Adalimumab in patients with active noninfectious uveitis. *N Engl J Med*. 2016;375(10):932–943. doi:10.1056/NEJMoa1509852.

128. Nguyen QD, Merrill PT, Jaffe GJ, et al. Adalimumab for prevention of uveitic flare in patients with inactive non-infectious uveitis controlled by corticosteroids (VISUAL II): a multicentre, double-masked, randomised, placebo-controlled phase 3 trial. *The Lancet*. 2016;388(10050): 1183–1192. doi:10.1016/S0140-6736(16)31339-3.

129. Kim JS, Knickelbein JE, Nussenblatt RB, et al. Clinical trials in noninfectious uveitis. *Int Ophthalmol Clin*. 2015;55(3):79–110. doi:10.1097/IIO.0000000000000070.

130. Utz JP, Limper AH, Kalra S, et al. Etanercept for the treatment of stage II and III progressive pulmonary sarcoidosis. *Chest*. 2003;124(1):177–185. doi:10.1378/chest.124.1.177.

131. Judson MA, Baughman RP, Costabel U, et al. Safety and efficacy of ustekinumab or golimumab in patients with chronic sarcoidosis. *Eur Respir J*. 2014;44(5):1296–1307. doi:10.1183/09031936.00000914.

132. Sweiss NJ, Lower EE, Mirsaeidi M, et al. Rituximab in the treatment of refractory pulmonary sarcoidosis. *Eur Respir J*. 2014;43(5):1525–1528. doi:10.1183/09031936.00224513.

133. El Jammal T, Jamilloux Y, Gerfaud-Valentin M, et al. Refractory sarcoidosis: a review. *Ther Clin Risk Manag*. 2020;16:323–345. doi:10.2147/TCRM.S192922.

134. Rochepeau C, Jamilloux Y, Kerever S, et al. Long-term visual and systemic prognoses of 83 cases of biopsy-proven sarcoid uveitis. *Br J Ophthalmol*. 2017;101(7):856–861. doi:10.1136/bjophthalmol-2016-309767.

135. Ma SP, Rogers SL, Hall AJ, et al. Sarcoidosis-related uveitis: clinical presentation, disease course, and rates of systemic disease progression after uveitis diagnosis. *Am J Ophthalmol*. 2019;198:30–36. doi:10.1016/j.ajo.2018.09.013.

136. Paovic J, Paovic P, Sredovic V, Jovanovic S. Clinical manifestations, complications and treatment of ocular sarcoidosis: correlation between visual efficiency and macular edema as seen on optical coherence tomography. *Semin Ophthalmol*. Published online 2016 Sept. 14:1–8. doi:10.1080/08820538.2016.1206576.

137. Suzuki K, Ishihara M, Namba K, et al. Clinical features of ocular sarcoidosis: severe, refractory, and prolonged inflammation. *Jpn J Ophthalmol*. 2022;66(5):447–454. doi:10.1007/s10384-022-00927-y.

138. Mañá J, Rubio-Rivas M, Villalba N, et al. Multidisciplinary approach and long-term follow-up in a series of 640 consecutive patients with sarcoidosis: cohort study of a 40-year clinical experience at a tertiary referral center in Barcelona, Spain. *Medicine (Baltimore)*. 2017;96(29):e7595. doi:10.1097/MD.0000000000007595.

139. Judson MA, Baughman RP, Thompson BW, et al. Two year prognosis of sarcoidosis: the ACCESS experience. *Sarcoidosis Vasc Diffuse Lung Dis Off J WASOG*. 2003;20(3):204–211.

140. Neville E, Walker AN, James DG. Prognostic factors predicting the outcome of sarcoidosis: an analysis of 818 patients. *Q J Med*. 1983;52(208):525–533.

141. Nagai S, Handa T, Ito Y, et al. Outcome of sarcoidosis. *Clin Chest Med*. 2008;29(3):565–574. doi:10.1016/j.ccm.2008.03.006.

142. Gottlieb JE, Israel HL, Steiner RM, et al. Outcome in sarcoidosis. *Chest*. 1997;111(3):623–631. doi:10.1378/chest.111.3.623.

143. Baughman RP, Lower EE. Features of sarcoidosis associated with chronic disease. *Sarcoidosis Vasc Diffuse Lung Dis Off J WASOG*. 2015;31(4):275–281.

144. Kirkil G, Lower EE, Baughman RP. Predictors of mortality in pulmonary sarcoidosis. *Chest*. 2018;153(1):105–113. doi:10.1016/j.chest.2017.07.008.

8 Ophthalmologic Disease in Systemic Lupus Erythematosus and Antiphospholipid Syndrome

Shivani Garg, Julia A. Pulliam, Rajiv Gupta, and Lynn M. Hassman

8.1 BACKGROUND ON SYSTEMIC LUPUS ERYTHEMATOSUS (SLE OR LUPUS)

Systemic lupus erythematosus (SLE or lupus) is a life-threatening autoimmune disease that can have deleterious effects on many systems and organs of the body, including the eyes.[1–3] SLE is a chronic autoimmune disease and often presents with a relapsing clinical course.[1, 4, 5] SLE, or lupus, was first described in 1833 with the key manifestation of erythematous rashes, and the first biopsy of skin lesions to understand the underlying pathology was performed in 1872.[6] In 1929, the first description of ocular complications of SLE was noted.[7–9] In 1933, Semon and Wolff described the histopathological features of choroiditis and subretinal fluid associated with SLE.[9] It is estimated that as many as one-third of SLE patients experience ophthalmic symptoms ranging from relatively mild to severe and vision-threatening.[7, 8, 10, 11] Ocular involvement often parallels systemic disease activity and is occasionally the first recognized manifestation of lupus.[7, 8, 10, 11]

8.2 EPIDEMIOLOGY

The prevalence of SLE in the population is 20 to 150 per 100,000.[2–5, 12] SLE prevalence differs between age, gender, geographic, and racial distributions.[3, 4, 13–16] The female-to-male ratio is close to 9:1, and the estimated prevalence is 1/1,000 among women of reproductive age.[3, 4, 13–16] Moreover, lupus is more common in Black, Hispanic, Asian, Native American, and Alaskan Native women than White women.[17] Lupus prevalence ranges from 40 to 400 per 100,000 in people of Black racial group, with the highest in women of Black race.[13, 17, 18] Ocular disease affects one-third of patients with SLE. No specific data on difference in ocular manifestations by race, geographic, or gender distributions have been reported thus far.

8.3 ETIOLOGY AND TRIGGERS

Lupus is a multifactorial disease with unknown etiology. Genetic, immunologic, social, and environmental factors play a role. Familial rates and high concordance in identical twins suggest a genetic contribution, although there is no obvious pattern of inheritance.[19] Women are 9 to 10 times more at risk of developing lupus, and the risk of lupus is 14 times higher in men with Klinefelter syndrome (a.k.a. 47, XXY). This suggests an association with genes on the X chromosome, although over 90 genetic loci including on autosomes have been associated with lupus, most affecting the immune system. Additionally, estrogens increase the production of B cell activation factor and modulate other proinflammatory cells in SLE. While a causal association between oral contraceptives and lupus flares has not been established, hormonal oral contraceptives are often avoided in severe lupus.[20] Environmental triggers of lupus include medications, ultraviolet rays and sun exposure, smoking, and viral infections.[21, 22] Drug-induced lupus, most commonly due to procainamide, hydralazine, and quinidine, usually presents with skin and joint disease and rarely with renal and CNS manifestations.[23]

8.4 PATHOGENESIS

In SLE, there is dysregulation of the immune system at multiple levels. Loss of immunologic self-tolerance occurs after cell damage caused by infectious and environmental triggers exposes self-antigens, activating T and B cells. T cells activate autoreactive B cells that lead to autoantibody production, which is a hallmark of SLE. These autoantibodies are pathogenic and cause organ damage through immune-complex deposition, complement activation, and altered cell function leading to apoptosis. Activated B cells can also serve as antigen-presenting cells to activate T cells, creating a loop that propagates inflammation. These important steps, along with the production of cytokines such as tumor necrosis factor (TNF)-α, interferon (INF)-γ, interleukin (IL)-10, and B-lymphocyte stimulator, lead to the mass production of autoantibodies that deposit in tissues as immune complexes and activate complement. This process results in more cell death, triggering chronic and relapsing inflammation in SLE.

8.5 OCULAR DISEASE PRESENTATION

Ocular manifestations affect 33% to 50% of patients with SLE.[7, 8, 10, 11] These can vary, ranging from mild ocular surface irritation in keratoconjunctivitis sicca to vision-threatening retinal vasculopathy.[24] Several ocular manifestations like dry eye, retinopathy, and choroidopathy have been linked with specific systemic manifestations like lupus nephritis or CNS disease. Furthermore, the presence

DOI: 10.1201/9781003453710-8

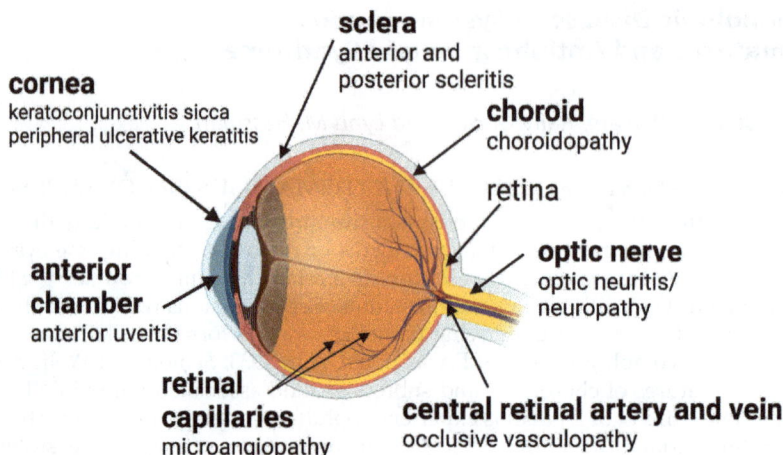

Figure 8.1   Major vision-threatening ophthalmic manifestations of SLE.

Table 8.1 Common Ocular Manifestations in SLE

Ocular Structure	Ocular Manifestations in SLE	Prevalence in SLE
Orbit	■ Myositis	■ Rare
	■ Panniculitis	■ Rare
	■ Other/Nonspecific orbital inflammation	■ Rare
Eyelids	■ Discoid rash	■ Uncommon: 6% of all discoid lupus cases
	■ Blepharitis	■ Common
Anterior Segment	■ Keratoconjunctivitis sicca	■ Common: 25–30%
	■ Peripheral ulcerative keratitis	■ Rare
	■ Chemosis	■ Rare, possibly more common in nephrotic syndrome
	■ Cicatrizing conjunctivitis	■ Rare
	■ Episcleritis	■ Somewhat common
	■ Anterior scleritis	■ Uncommon, 0–2%
	■ Anterior uveitis	■ Uncommon, 0–2.9%
Posterior Segment	■ Retinal microangiopathy	■ Common up to 30%
	■ Occlusive retinal vasculopathy	■ Rare, associated with APS
	■ Choroidopathy	■ Severe cases are rare
	■ Posterior scleritis	■ Uncommon
Central Nervous System	■ Optic neuritis/Neuropathy	■ 0–2.3%
	■ Other cranial Neuropathy	■ 7–12.7%

of ocular manifestations is often correlated with the severity of SLE in other organs. Table 8.1 lists common and uncommon ocular manifestations of SLE.[7, 8, 10, 11, 24, 25] Figure 8.1 is a diagram of the anatomic location of each ocular manifestation.

8.6 GENERAL TREATMENT PARADIGMS

Since the ocular complications of SLE are generally associated with active systemic disease, control of the systemic disease often leads to the resolution of ocular manifestations. According to the 2023 European Union League Against Rheumatism (EULAR) SLE Treatment Guidelines,[26] general management of SLE should include hydroxychloroquine. Even if ocular manifestation is the first presentation of SLE, hydroxychloroquine should be started in all patients, as it reduces the risk of organ damage by 73% and reduces risk of flares by 46%.[27–32] Moreover, the use of hydroxychloroquine increases survival in patients with SLE by eightfold.[33]

Hydroxychloroquine can damage the central retina, and its use carries a risk for permanent vision loss, particularly when used at high doses or in patients with renal compromise, as well as in the setting of pre-existing retinal pathology or with concomitant use of tamoxifen. High-definition imaging of the retina using optical coherence tomography (OCT) is sensitive to detect subtle retinal damage; however, this damage is irreversible. A baseline exam and OCT should be performed before starting hydroxychloroquine to evaluate for pre-existing pathology. Additionally, annual screening for toxicity should be performed after 5 years of therapy. When dosed at less than 5 mg/kg/day actual body weight, the risk for retinal toxicity is less than 2% for up to 10 years.[34, 35] However, recent studies have shown that doses below 5 mg/kg/day could increase risk of SLE flares by 2× to 6×.[31, 32] Therefore, the decision to continue or stop therapy should involve a detailed discussion of the low risks and the lifesaving benefits between the patient, rheumatologist, and ophthalmologist.[36] Additionally, a consideration to monitor hydroxychloroquine blood levels to guide a safe and effective dose could be considered during routine lupus visits.[26, 30, 37, 38]

Other medications may be recommended based on the severity and risk for vision loss, such as severe ocular manifestations, such as lupus retinopathy. Addition of steroid-sparing agents should involve a discussion between the ophthalmologist and rheumatologist. Commonly prescribed therapies include cyclophosphamide, mycophenolate, belimumab, anifrolumab, rituximab, and plasmapheresis. Table 8.2 highlights vision-threatening ocular manifestations, complications, and the recommended treatment paradigms.

Table 8.2 Vision-Threatening Ocular Manifestations in SLE and Common Treatments

Ocular Manifestation	Presentations & Complications	Recommended Treatment
Keratoconjunctivitis sicca (KCS)	*Presentation*: When severe, causes pain and significant blurring, redness *Complications*: Corneal and conjunctival scaring resulting in loss of vision	Aggressive lubrication, topical steroids, and possibly topical cyclosporine, contact lenses, amniotic membrane implants. May be a role for other topical anti-inflammatory therapy or autologous serum tears.
Cicatrizing conjunctivitis	*Presentation*: Pain, redness, blurring *Complications*: Conjunctival scaring resulting in inability to close the eyelids	Local and systemic corticosteroids, treatment of discoid lupus. Steroid-sparing immunosuppression such as mycophenolate, rituximab, cyclophosphamide.
Peripheral ulcerative keratitis (PUK)	*Presentation*: Pain, blurring, tearing, redness of eye, foreign body sensation, corneal thinning often associated with adjacent scleritis *Complication*: Corneal perforation	*Treatment*: High-dose prednisone (1 mg/kg/day) and immunosuppressive medications such as methotrexate, cyclophosphamide, rituximab. Surgical intervention may be needed to preserve the integrity of the globe.
Anterior scleritis	*Presentation*: Severe boring pain that wakes the patient up, red or violaceous discoloration of the eye, excessive tearing *Complications*: Severe scleral thinning and globe rupture	*Treatment*: High-dose prednisone (1 mg/kg/day) followed by slow taper over 4–6 months. Steroid-sparing immunosuppression such as mycophenolate, rituximab, cyclophosphamide. Surgical intervention may be needed to preserve the integrity of the globe.
Posterior scleritis	*Presentation*: Pain, vision loss is more significant, discoloration of the anterior sclera may be absent *Complications*: Retinal detachment, retinal atrophy, optic nerve atrophy	*Treatment*: High-dose prednisone (1 mg/kg/day) followed by slow taper over 4–6 months. Steroid-sparing immunosuppression such as mycophenolate, rituximab, cyclophosphamide. Surgical intervention may be needed to resolve chronic retinal detachment.

Table 8.2 (*Continued*) Vision-Threatening Ocular Manifestations in SLE and Common Treatments

Ocular Manifestation	Presentations & Complications	Recommended Treatment
Occlusive retinal vasculopathy, vasculitis	*Presentation*: Monocular or binocular partial or complete vision loss *Complications*: Retinal infarcts or ischemia, retinal neovascularization, retinal detachment	*Treatment*: Immediate therapy is recommended to prevent permanent vision loss. *Treatment*: High-dose prednisone (1 mg/kg/day) followed by slow taper over 4–6 months. A higher dose of steroids (up to 2 mg/kg/day) or methylprednisolone could be considered. Steroid-sparing immunosuppression such as mycophenolate, rituximab, cyclophosphamide. In the setting of antiphospholipid antibody syndrome, anti-platelet (aspirin) and/or anticoagulation (warfarin) is recommended along with blood pressure control. Intravitreal injections, retinal laser photocoagulation, or surgical intervention may be required to treat or prevent complications of retinal neovascularization.
Choroidopathy	*Presentation*: Loss of vision *Complications*: Retinal atrophy and permanent blind spots	*Treatment*: Trial of corticosteroids, control of blood pressure and lupus-specific steroid-sparing immune suppression.
Optic neuritis/Neuropathy	*Presentation*: Loss of vision and/or color vision, afferent pupillary defect, visual field defects, pain signifies optic neuritis *Complications*: Optic nerve atrophy	*Treatment*: Immediate treatment of optic neuritis with intravenous methylprednisolone (1 g/day for 3 days) followed by high doses of prednisone (1 mg/kg/day) are recommended. Immunosuppressive therapy (cyclophosphamide) could be considered in refractory cases.

8.7 DISEASES OF THE ANTERIOR SEGMENT

SLE-associated inflammatory diseases affecting the external surface of the eye include relatively common keratoconjunctivitis sicca and episcleritis, as well as less common scleritis and severe cicatrizing conjunctivitis. Anterior uveitis, which refers to inflammation located primarily in the anterior compartment of the immune-privileged intraocular space, can also occur in SLE. Each of these conditions can range from mild ocular surface irritation to vision-threatening disease.

8.8 KERATOCONJUNCTIVITIS SICCA

Keratoconjunctivitis sicca (KCS) refers to desiccation-related damage to the cornea and conjunctiva, and the term was initially applied to cases of primary or secondary Sjögren's syndrome. The term KCS is often applied in the absence of a concrete diagnosis of Sjögren's, both because many ophthalmologists do not test for Sjögren's and because the disease can occur in the absence of serologic evidence of Sjögren's. The pathophysiology involves lymphocytic infiltration of the exocrine glands leading to lacrimal gland scarring.[7, 8]

8.8.1 Prevalence

Keratoconjunctivitis sicca is the most common ocular manifestation of SLE, presenting in approximately 25% to 35% of the patients,[39, 40] while secondary Sjögren's, or polyautoimmunity in Sjögren's, is recognized in only 14% of patients with SLE.[7, 8] Dry eye disease is very common in the general population, and the prevalence of Sjögren's disease amongst patients presenting with dry eye disease is at least 10%.[41]

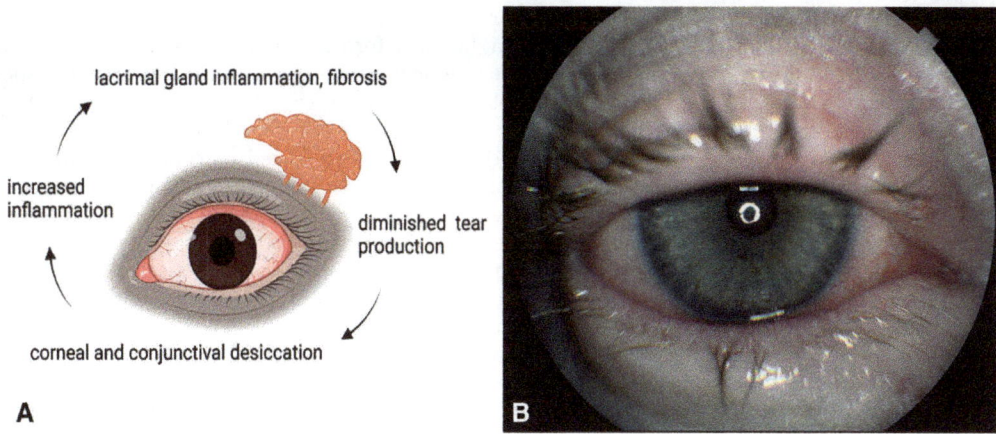

Figure 8.2 Keratoconjunctivitis sicca. (A) Lymphocytic infiltration of the lacrimal gland leads to scarring and atrophy, which reduces tear production. Desiccation of the ocular surface causes loss of mucosal barrier integrity and stimulates inflammation. Soluble inflammatory mediators potentiates lacrimal gland inflammation and atrophy. (B) Eyelid edema, conjunctival hyperemia, and corneal epithelial disruption in a patient with keratoconjunctivitis sicca.

8.8.2 Presentation

Glandular inflammation leads to lacrimal gland scarring and atrophy that results in diminished aqueous tear production. Ocular surface dryness causes irritation, conjunctival redness, and a burning sensation. Ocular surface desiccation also leads to inflammation of the cornea and conjunctiva and results in disruption of the normal epithelial barriers (Figure 8.2). Clinically, punctate epithelial erosions are visible on the cornea and can be accompanied by filaments composed of epithelium, mucus, and cellular debris. Uncontrolled inflammation of the cornea can lead to scarring that impairs vision, while scarring of the conjunctiva, termed cicatrization, can result in foreshortening of the conjunctival lining of the eyelid and inability to close the eyelid, or lagophthalmos, which leads to further desiccation.

8.8.3 Diagnosis

The Schirmer's test, in which tear production is measured as the amount of fluid that wicks along a strip of filter paper applied to the patient's eyelid, is specific for KCS associated with Sjögren's syndrome when less than 5 mm of filter paper is wetted over 5 minutes.[42] This test is not as sensitive as visual assessment of the epithelial damage using either fluorescein staining of the cornea or lissamine green staining of the conjunctiva. Additionally, the corneal fluorescein staining method can be used to confirm reduced tear production.[24] Importantly, serologic testing for anti-SSA/Ro and/or anti-SSB/La antibodies should be performed in patients with suspicion of keratoconjunctivitis sicca, even though Sjögren's syndrome can occur in the absence of these antibodies. Given the potential for systemic morbidity-associated Sjögren's syndrome, ophthalmologists should have a low threshold for referring patients with KCS to a rheumatologist for formal evaluation of Sjögren's disease and lupus.

8.8.4 Management

Treatment for keratoconjunctivitis sicca is aimed at minimizing desiccation, reducing inflammation, and supporting corneal healing. Aqueous tear production can be replaced, ideally with preservative-free artificial tears, and tear loss can be reduced by occlusion of the lacrimal ducts with punctal plugs. Pilocarpine is a cholinergic parasympathetic agonist used to stimulate exocrine secretion. While pilocarpine has some demonstrated efficacy in relieving oral symptoms of Sjögren's, its objective benefits to ocular surface disease are minimal. Significant side effects, particularly sweating and nausea, can limit the use of this drug.

Short courses of low-dose topical steroids can be used to reduce inflammation. While 0.05% cyclosporine has been extensively marketed for dry eye disease, the literature is fraught with poorly designed and reported studies, and a major Cochrane review did not find evidence for its efficacy among 30 randomized controlled trials.[43] Newer higher dose formulations of up to 2% cyclosporine are less studied, but preliminary analysis suggests they may prove more effective at reducing subjective discomfort as well as desiccation-related ocular surface damage. Newer anti-inflammatory therapies include tacrolimus as well as lifitegrast, an inhibitor of lymphocyte function–associated antigen intracellular adhesion molecule 1 (LFA-1), which hinders T cell recruitment. Lifitegrast may provide a modest improvement in desiccation-related corneal damage in post-hoc analysis.[44] Importantly, these topical therapies often take many weeks to provide any benefit and can cause ocular discomfort. While oral hydroxychloroquine is an effective anti-inflammatory therapy in systemic SLE, data on the benefit of hydroxychloroquine specifically for dry eye disease are mixed, although several prospective trials have revealed modest objective improvements in desiccation-related damage.[41, 45] The benefits of hydroxychloroquine to KCS may be secondary to control of underlying SLE.

Autologous serum tears prepared by specialty laboratories from patients' own serum contain poorly defined growth factors and anti-inflammatory mediators that are believed to reduce inflammation and promote corneal healing and have been used with mixed benefit in severe dry eye disease. In cases of severe corneal disease, bandage contact or scleral lenses or amniotic membranes can be placed on the ocular surface to reduce pain and promote corneal healing. Additional discussion of the ocular manifestations of Sjögren's disease is available in Chapter 10.

8.8.5 Prognosis

With adequate ophthalmic intervention, often by a dry eye disease specialist, SLE-related KCS can be managed. However, severe disease may lead to corneal and conjunctival scarring and/or thinning. In extreme cases, the compromised epithelial barrier increases the risk of fungal and bacterial infections that can progress to corneal ulceration and perforation.

8.9 PERIPHERAL ULCERATIVE KERATITIS (PUK)

PUK is a crescentic peripheral corneal lesion in which inflammation drives tissue destruction and thinning of the tissue. The pathophysiology is not fully understood. Collagenases produced by neutrophils likely play a key role in the rapid destruction of corneal tissue. Biopsy of adjacent scleral tissue shows vascular inflammation, suggesting that the pathophysiology may be related to vasculitis. Based on the strong association with systemic autoimmune disease activity, the mechanisms are thought to be related to both immune complexes and T cells.[46, 47]

8.9.1 Disease Presentation

PUK occurs in the peripheral cornea within 2 mm from the limbus and can be accompanied by adjacent necrotizing scleritis. Severe disease progresses to corneal melt, in which the tissue thins to the point of perforation.

8.9.2 Prevalence

PUK is quite rare, but when present, it is commonly associated with systemic autoimmunity and usually reflects the presence of severe systemic vasculitis.[46, 47] Other vasculitis and connective tissue diseases commonly associated with PUK, including rheumatoid arthritis and antineutrophil cytoplasmic antibodies–associated vasculitis, may be more common causes of PUK and should be ruled out.[46–48] Finally, infectious agents such as varicella zoster can cause PUK-like corneal thinning associated with scleritis and should be considered, especially in immune-compromised patients.

8.9.3 Treatment

Given the high risk for visual disability, high-dose corticosteroids are the cornerstone of therapy, and often, steroid-sparing immune suppression is required to wean corticosteroids to an acceptable dose. Systemic immunosuppressive therapy such as methotrexate, mycophenolate, or cyclophosphamide could be used as a steroid-sparing agent.[46, 47] Other systemic biologic therapy approved for SLE such as rituximab or belimumab could be considered.[26, 46, 47] Surgical repair or prevention of corneal perforation is required in some cases and includes tissue adhesives, as well as penetrating keratoplasty, lamellar grafts, and amniotic membrane transplantation.[7, 8, 49] Despite improvement in graft survival with cytotoxic therapy, the outcomes of penetrating keratoplasty for PUK are disappointing.

Of note, active SLE should be considered a contraindication for the refractive surgeries that ablate corneal layers, including photorefractive keratectomy (PRK) and laser-assisted in situ keratomileusis

(LASIK) due to the unpredictable reaction of corneal tissue to the laser ablation and poor epithelial healing.[50, 51]

8.10 INTERSTITIAL KERATITIS

Interstitial keratitis (IK) is non-ulcerative inflammation and vascularization of the corneal stroma. It presents with light sensitivity and pain. IK is a rare manifestation of SLE and is more commonly caused by infections including herpesviruses and syphilis. Treatment in SLE requires control of underlying disease as well as topical corticosteroids.

8.11 CICATRIZING CONJUNCTIVITIS

8.11.1 Prevalence

Cicatrizing conjunctivitis is a rare manifestation of SLE, most often associated with discoid lupus. The pathophysiology involves linear deposition of immune complexes at the basement membrane,[52] which have also been seen in patients without clinical disease.[53, 54]

8.11.2 Disease Presentation

Symptoms of cicatrizing conjunctivitis can be mild, including irritation, tearing, and redness of the eye and eyelid. Progressive disease can cause scarring and adhesions between the palpebral and bulbar conjunctival (symblepharon), leading to contraction of the eyelids. Multiple case reports of severe cicatrizing conjunctivitis, similar in appearance to ocular mucous membrane pemphigoid (MMP) disease, have been associated with discoid lupus.[55] This disease can occur in the absence of discoid rash on the eyelids (Figure 8.3), and thus, clinicians should ask about rashes on sun-exposed skin in patients presenting with cicatrizing conjunctivitis.

8.11.3 Treatment

In milder cases, topical or intralesional steroids are warranted, along with systemic steroids and hydroxychloroquine to treat the underlying discoid lupus. In severe or recalcitrant cases, immunosuppressive agents such as methotrexate, mycophenolate, or azathioprine could be considered, along with biologics with good response in discoid lupus, such as belimumab or anifrolumab.[26, 56, 57] If a symblepharon is present, surgical intervention might be required.

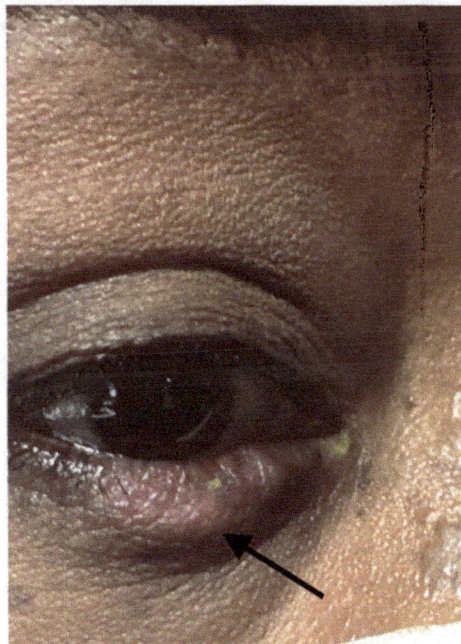

Figure 8.3 Discoid rash of the lower eyelid.

8.11.4 Prognosis

Chronic scarring and hazy vision due to scarring is possible. Aggressive treatment of cutaneous lesions is recommended.

8.12 EPISCLERITIS

Episcleritis is inflammation of the superficial conjunctival vessels. It is relatively common in the general population and affects up to 28% of patients with lupus.[54] Episcleritis generally causes mild to moderate ocular discomfort, redness, and tearing and responds to low-dose topical steroids or non-steroidal anti-inflammatory therapy. It is not associated with a risk for scleral perforation.

8.13 ANTERIOR SCLERITIS

Scleritis refers to inflammation in the sclera, the tough white outer wall of the eye that lies just beneath the conjunctiva. Anterior scleritis is visible as violaceous erythema upon inspection with eyelids raised.

8.13.1 Prevalence

The prevalence of scleritis in SLE is between 1.7%[58] and 3% of patients.[59] While 50% of patients presenting with scleritis have an underlying systemic autoimmune disease, SLE is a less common cause compared to RA and ANCA-associated vasculitis.

8.13.2 Presentation

It is critical to differentiate episcleritis from scleritis. Patients with scleritis typically present with severe, boring eye pain, which wakes them up at night, along with significant redness and often photophobia.

Anterior scleritis can be either diffuse or nodular and may present with PUK. Either can progress if untreated to a necrotizing form with a high risk for perforation.

Scleritis can be the presenting manifestation of SLE and is often correlated with systemic activity of SLE. Like PUK, anterior scleritis can be a manifestation of infections such as varicella zoster, particularly in elderly or immune-compromised patients (Figure 8.4).

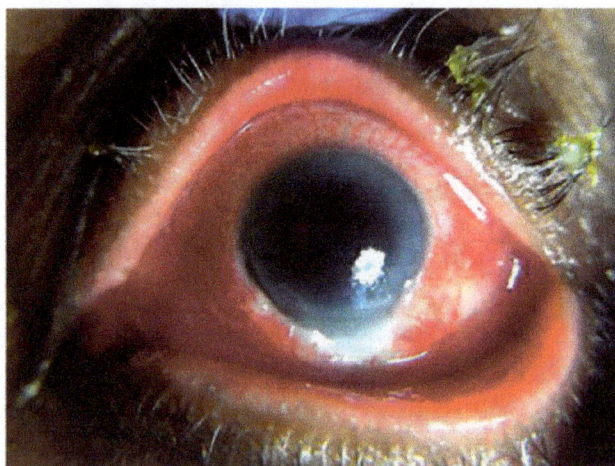

Figure 8.4 Scleritis and peripheral ulcerative keratitis. Diffuse deep erythema of the sclera caused areas of white ischemia near the corneal limbus; peripheral corneal ulceration and thinning from 4:30–9:00, adjacent to an area of scleral ulceration; and thinning inferiorly. This patient had hydralazine-induced lupus, which was being successfully treated with high-dose prednisone, mycophenolate, and rituximab when this unilateral scleritis presented. Because the underlying disease was inactive and she was significantly immune compromised, infectious etiology was suspected. Varicella zoster was identified as the causative agent by polymerase chain reaction from a conjunctival swab.

8.13.3 Diagnosis

Topical application of 10% phenylephrine temporarily blanches the episcleral vessels and can be used to differentiate scleritis from episcleritis (see Chapter 3, Figure 3.1).

8.13.4 Management

Because scleral disease suggests that SLE is active, treatment requires the same systemic approach (including high doses of steroids and immunosuppressive drugs) that is employed in all situations of active SLE. Scleritis should be considered an organ-threatening manifestation of SLE. It is also relatively recalcitrant to therapy, possibly due to the poor vascular supply, and carries a high risk for visual morbidity with disease recurrence. Thus, scleritis should be treated with high-dose corticosteroids, which must be tapered slowly over 3 to 4 months, as well as steroid-sparing immunosuppressive therapies, such as azathioprine, methotrexate, mycophenolate mofetil, tacrolimus, cyclophosphamide, or rituximab.[26, 56]

8.13.5 Prognosis

Immediate diagnosis and treatment are necessary to prevent vision loss and globe rupture.

8.14 UVEITIS

Uveitis is inflammation that occurs within the immune-privileged intraocular space. While the uvea refers specifically to the iris, ciliary body, and choroid, use of the term "uveitis" has broadened to include inflammation of the intraocular space. While the uveal tissues are affected by most forms of intraocular inflammation, they may not be the primary tissue involved in specific forms of uveitis.

8.14.1 Prevalence

Anterior segment uveitis is the most common form of noninfectious intraocular inflammation, with a US prevalence of 100/100,000 patients. Of these cases, only 11% are associated with any systemic autoimmune disease, and the prevalence of SLE as a cause of uveitis is estimated to be as low as 0.47% (95% CI 0.41–0.53%).[60]

The incidence of uveitis among patients with SLE may be declining over time, possibly the result of improved therapy. While a tertiary care center–based study from the 1990s noted the prevalence of uveitis at 4.8%,[61] a more recent systematic review estimated its prevalence at 0% to 2.9%.[62]

8.14.2 Presentation

Anterior uveitis associated with SLE is typically a bilateral, anterior, non-granulomatous uveitis, which may present with progressive vison loss and floaters, or with significant light sensitivity and eye redness. Posterior segment involvement with granulomatous inflammation has also been reported in SLE. Tubulointerstitial nephritis and uveitis (TINU) syndrome is a rare immune-mediated disorder involving both the kidney and the eye and sometimes is associated with immune-related diseases, such as SLE.[7, 8]

8.14.3 Diagnosis

SLE should be considered a rare cause of uveitis, and other causes, particularly syphilis, should be ruled out before uveitis is considered to be a manifestation of SLE. Furthermore, routine ANA, given its low positive predictive value for SLE, should not be ordered in all patients with uveitis. ANA test alone has a low positive predictive value for SLE; therefore, if clinical suspicion for SLE is high, specific serologies, including extranuclear antibody panel, complement activity, and double-stranded DNA antibody, are recommended.

8.15 DISEASES OF THE POSTERIOR SEGMENT

Inflammation of the posterior segment, comprised of the vitreous, retina, retinal vasculature, and choroid, is referred to as noninfectious intermediate, posterior, and panuveitis (NIPPU) and collectively account for 20% of all noninfectious uveitis. Most cases of posterior uveitis have a robust cellular infiltrate that is visible upon examination. This type of presentation is rare in SLE; rather, posterior segment disease more commonly involves inflammatory or occlusive disease of the blood vessels supplying the retina, choroid, and optic nerve. Posterior segment involvement has a high potential for permanent devastating impact on visual prognosis and is also associated with poor systemic disease control.

8.16 LUPUS RETINOPATHY

Because an overt inflammatory cell infiltrate is rarely seen on ophthalmic examination or histologically, the terms "retinal vasculopathy" and "retinopathy" are applied to encompass both direct inflammation of the retinal vessels and the effects of systemic inflammation on the retinal vessels.

8.16.1 Prevalence

The prevalence of lupus retinopathy ranges from 3% to 29%, depending on the population studied and the activity of the disease. Lupus retinopathy is more common in patients with chronically active systemic lupus, with estimates as high as 50% before the advent of corticosteroid therapy.[7, 8, 24, 59]

8.16.2 Pathophysiology

Immune complex deposition in retinal vessels leads to complement activation and subsequent release of inflammatory mediators. The resulting endothelial cell necrosis, as well as aggregation of complement, platelets, and inflammatory cells, leads to nonperfusion and retinal ischemia. This process most commonly occurs in small retinal capillaries, causing microangiopathy. Antiphospholipid antibodies are present in 40% to 80% of patients with SLE and as high as 86% in patients with retinopathy.[63] These antiphospholipid antibodies attach to endothelium of retinal vessels, augment the cascade of immune complex deposition and complement activation, and trigger further thrombosis and occlusive vasculopathy, leading to catastrophic occlusion of larger retinal arteries and veins.[64–66]

While ocular tissue biopsies are not practical, post-mortem histopathological findings include perivascular lymphocytic infiltrates, endothelial swelling, and thrombus formation, causing occlusion of retinal and choroidal vessels, as well as immune complex deposits on the vessels and rare fibrinoid degeneration with necrosis.[67]

8.16.3 Presentation

Microangiopathy occurs in >90% of lupus retinopathy cases and is evidenced by soft exudates, microaneurysms, and small infarcts in the retinal nerve fiber layer (cotton-wool spots) in the absence of major vascular occlusions.[64, 65] These cases are generally asymptomatic, and the findings may be transient. Retinal artery or vein occlusions are less common but cause new-onset loss of vision, either centrally or peripherally. While these occlusions can occasionally be occult with only transient obscurations, any vision loss in a patient with SLE warrants immediate ophthalmic examination. Frank retinal vasculitis with perivascular exudation is rare in SLE. Widespread occlusive vasculopathy is also quite rare and should prompt evaluation for associated APS.

8.16.4 Diagnosis

On fundus examination, the classic finding in SLE retinopathy is the cotton-wool spot, an ischemic infarct in the retinal nerve fiber layer, which may be isolated or may be seen in association with areas of retinal edema, ischemia, hard exudates, and hemorrhages.[67] Various abnormalities of the retinal vasculature, such as vascular sheathing, arterial narrowing, capillary and venous dilatation, tortuosity, microaneurysms, and venous engorgement, have been described. Rarely, frank vasculitis can be seen in SLE as dense perivascular infiltrates.

Fluorescein angiography is a minimally invasive test performed in clinic that can demonstrate retinal capillary dilatation and microaneurysms in asymptomatic patients with mild to moderate disease activity as well as areas of large-vessel thrombosis and non-perfusion or focal vascular leakage in severe occlusive retinopathy or vasculitis (Figure 8.5). Ocular coherence tomography (OCT) is used to monitor the structural changes in the central retina or macula.

Systemic tests including ANA test, extranuclear antibody panel, complement activity testing, and double-stranded DNA antibody is recommended. Inflammatory markers such as sedimentation rate and C-reactive protein should be done. Additionally, antiphospholipid antibody panel including anticardiolipin antibodies (IgG, IgM, IgA), beta-2 glycoprotein antibodies (IgG, IgM, IgA), and lupus anticoagulant testing should be performed at baseline and then repeated after 12 weeks to confirm true positivity. Other systemic diseases, such as Behçet disease, sarcoidosis, Lyme disease, diabetes, hypertensive retinopathy, and syphilis, that can mimic retinopathy should be ruled out.

8.16.5 Management

Retinal vascular disease in SLE parallels systemic disease activity, and thus effective treatment of the systemic disease, along with simultaneous control of any associated systemic hypertension, can ameliorate microangiopathy and may reduce the risk for catastrophic occlusive disease.

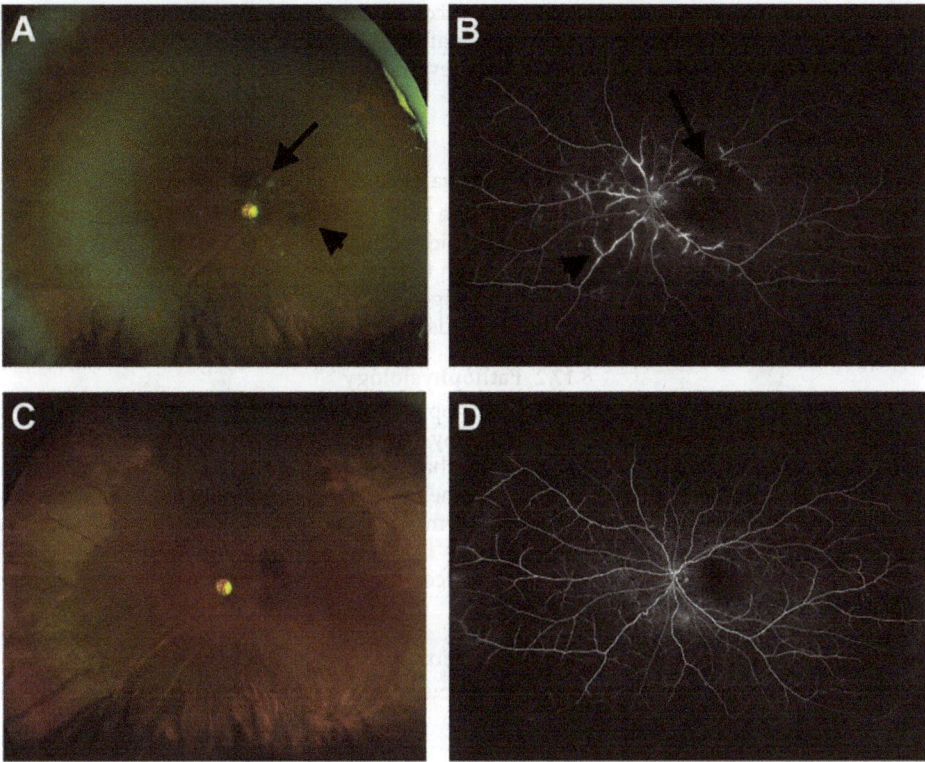

Figure 8.5 Lupus retinal vasculopathy. A 23-year-old female with a 10-year history of SLE with nephritis, cutaneous lesions, and renal vein thrombosis who was treated with prednisone and mycophenolate but had self-discontinued her anticoagulation one year prior presented with progressive decrease in central vision bilaterally. (A) Fundus examination showed macular edema (arrowhead), retinal infarcts (cotton-wool spots, arrow), and hard exudates. (B) Fluorescein angiography revealed focal leakage (arrowhead) and occlusion (arrow) of the arterioles and venules indicating occlusive vasculitis. She was treated with high-dose corticosteroids, cyclophosphamide, and rituximab which resulted in resolution of the retinal edema and infarcts (C) and retinal vasculitis with reperfusion of the occluded segments (D).

For severe occlusive retinal vasculopathy, initial empiric treatment with high-dose oral corticosteroids, with or without initial pulse with intravenous corticosteroids, is standard therapy. Patients may not exhibit clinical improvement until 3 to 4 weeks following initiation of therapy, and vascular occlusions often do not re-perfuse. The goal of therapy in these cases should be to prevent further occlusive disease. Given the sparsity of cases of severe occlusive disease, there is not a validated regimen. However, both cyclophosphamide and rituximab have found success in cases of severe retinal vasculitis,[68, 69] while methotrexate, mycophenolate, azathioprine and cyclosporine can be effective in less severe cases.[7, 8, 69] Plasma exchange could be considered as well.[70] Antiplatelet treatment (aspirin) and anticoagulation (warfarin), in combination with immunosuppression, may have a role in limiting the progression of the vaso-occlusive retinopathy, especially in the presence of antiphospholipid antibodies.[64]

Retinal ischemia can result in retinal neovascularization and associated bleeding, fibrosis, and retinal detachment. Injectable therapies targeting vascular endothelial growth factor as well as retinal photocoagulation may be used to prevent such complications, while surgical interventions may be required to treat them.

8.16.6 Prognosis

Most cases of SLE-associated retinopathy involve only microangiography, which responds well to systemic therapy and generally portends a good visual prognosis. However, retinopathy is a marker of decreased survival and worse SLE systemic outcomes compared to patients with SLE without retinopathy.[71] While rare, severe occlusive retinopathy has a poor prognosis, with most patients suffering permanent vision loss and some cases developing ischemic complications that result in further vision loss.

8.17 LUPUS CHOROIDOPATHY

8.17.1 Prevalence

The choroid is a highly vascular layer between the sclera and the retina that provides perfusion and thermoregulation to the outer retina. SLE choroidopathy is characterized by a microangiopathy leading to capillary vaso-occlusions and is common in patients with lupus nephritis, thus suggesting a relationship between LN and choroidal changes.[72, 73] Choroidopathy is also associated with systemic disease activity, particularly lupus nephritis.

8.17.2 Pathophysiology

Due to a paucity of histologic specimens, the pathophysiology of SLE choroidopathy is unknown, but mechanisms similar to those driving retinopathy are hypothesized, with immune complex and thrombus deposition leading to microangiopathy that may progress to larger occlusions. In addition, uncontrolled hypertension is thought to further constrict choroidal blood flow and increase the ischemia. The retinal pigment epithelial cells form one aspect of the blood–retinal barrier. When the choroidal circulation is disrupted significantly in SLE choroidopathy, the RPE are unable to sufficiently maintain this barrier, and serous fluid accumulates in the subretinal space, resulting in retinal detachment and loss of vision.

8.17.3 Presentation

While many patients experience loss of vision, some may present with surprisingly good visual acuity despite choroidal ischemia.

8.17.4 Diagnosis

Fundoscopic manifestations are generally observed as single or multiple areas of serous elevation of the RPE and sensory retina associated with RPE mottling. Fluorescein angiography can reveal delayed choroidal filling as well as focal areas of leakage through the RPE. Indocyanine green angiography is more sensitive for assessing the choroidal circulation and can highlight areas of either choroidal infarction (hypofluorescence, Figure 8.6) or immune cell aggregation (hyperfluorescence).[74] Optical coherence tomography is the most sensitive way to assess the extent of subretinal fluid accumulations and their response to treatment. Extended-depth optical coherence tomography

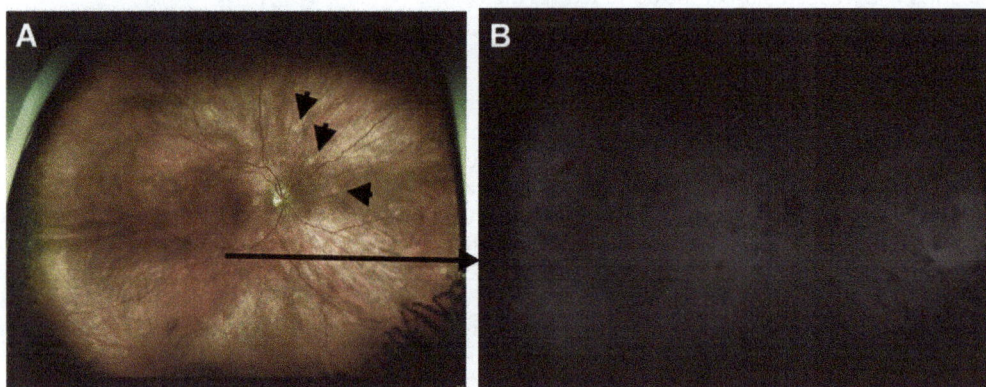

Figure 8.6 Lupus choroidopathy. A 39-year-old female with a history of autoimmune hepatitis, eclampsia, difficult-to-control hypertension, oral ulcers, joint pain, and folliculitis presented with mild blurring. In addition to mild anterior uveitis, examination showed scattered faint hypopigmented lesions (A: examples arrowheads) that were hypofluorescent on indocyanine green angiography (B: example arrow), indicating focal choroidal infarcts/lesions. Serology was positive for ANA, speckled pattern, and dsDNA, and she was ultimately diagnosed with SLE.

allows sensitive measurement of choroidal thickness, which may allow a non-invasive assessment of choroidal involvement. The qualitative and quantitative evaluations of OCT are also beneficial in the diagnosis and monitoring of lupus choroidopathy.

8.17.5 Treatment

Large serous accumulations of subretinal fluid can be managed initially with local or systemic corticosteroids. Control of SLE, nephritis, and associated hypertension is important in the long-term management of SLE choroidopathy. The optimal immunosuppressive therapy for SLE choroidopathy is not clear. Anecdotal evidence supports the use of immunosuppressors including azathioprine, cyclosporine, and cyclophosphamide. Local therapies including focal laser and photodynamic therapy and surgery can be used to resolve persistent subretinal fluid accumulation.

8.17.6 Prognosis

Lupus choroidopathy usually has a relatively good ocular prognosis when systemic immunosuppressive treatment is used to control underlying SLE. The main complications of lupus choroidopathy are choroidal ischemia causing adjacent retinal atrophy as well as rare cases of secondary angle closure glaucoma due to choroidal effusion.

8.18 POSTERIOR SCLERITIS

8.18.1 Prevalence

The prevalence of scleritis in SLE is between 1.7%[58] and 3% of patients.[59]

8.18.2 Presentation

Posterior scleritis causes blurred vision and may also cause eyelid swelling, pain, diplopia, restricted eye movements, and proptosis.[10] It may present concomitantly with anterior scleritis.

8.18.3 Diagnosis

Fluorescein angiography shows optic nerve hyperfluorescence and early scattered pinpoint leakage and may show late pooling of the dye into focal serous retinal detachments. Focal posterior nodules can be seen in some cases. Ophthalmic ultrasound and optical coherence tomography can also be used to image the serous fluid accumulations in posterior scleritis. Computed tomography (CT) and magnetic resonance (MR) imaging will show focal enhancement of the sclera.[75]

8.18.4 Treatment

Like anterior scleritis, posterior scleritis should be treated with high-dose corticosteroids, which must be tapered slowly over 3 to 4 months, as well as steroid-sparing immunosuppressive therapies, such as azathioprine, methotrexate, mycophenolate mofetil, tacrolimus, cyclophosphamide, or rituximab.[26, 56] Local steroid injections can also be used to reduce system corticosteroid burden.

8.18.5 Prognosis

Posterior scleritis is responsive to corticosteroids, and reasonable recovery of vision occurs in most cases.

8.19 OPTIC NEUROPATHY AND OPTIC NEURITIS

Optic neuritis refers to localized inflammation of the optic nerve, which can be seen in either the intraocular or retrobulbar portions of the nerve. Optic neuropathy refers to damage to the nerve that can result from multiple pathologic processes, including primary optic neuritis and ischemic injury resulting from occlusion of the nerve's vascular supply.

8.19.1 Prevalence

SLE is a rare cause of optic neuritis or optic neuropathy. Similarly, optic nerve disease is a rare manifestation of SLE, occurring in around 1% of SLE patients.[11, 71]

8.19.2 Pathophysiology

Optic nerve involvement in patients with SLE includes both optic neuritis and ischemic optic neuropathy.[76] Optic neuropathy in SLE may result from vaso-occlusive disease caused by antiphospholipid antibody antibodies. In other cases, SLE-associated optic neuritis overlaps with neuromyelitis optica spectrum disorders (NMOSDs).[77, 78] NMOSDs are characterized by a combination of optic neuritis and transverse myelitis. Associated anti-aquaporin-4 antibodies cause tissue destruction by inducing complement activation and are associated with a relapsing course of myelitis and optic neuritis, with a high incidence of blindness and paresis.[77, 78]

8.19.3 Presentation

Optic neuropathy or neuritis usually presents as an acute visual loss, which can be followed by progressive visual deterioration. Vision loss is often acutely more severe in optic neuritis. Optic neuritis presents with pain and impairment of color vision (dyschromatopsia), whereas these are less common features in ischemic optic neuropathy. Ischemic optic neuropathy often presents with permanent altitudinal visual field defects. However, complete visual loss may also occur.[79] On the other hand, in optic neuritis, visual field defects are often central or paracentral scotomas, and visual recovery is more likely.

8.19.4 Diagnosis

Clinical signs include an afferent pupillary defect when the disease is unilateral as well as optic disc swelling or pallor. Disc edema or pallor may not be seen on exam when only the retrobulbar optic nerve is involved.

In optic neuritis, fluorescein angiography demonstrates vasodilation of the peripapillary capillaries and hyperfluorescent dye leakage during the late phases of the exam. In some cases of ischemic optic neuropathy, an incomplete capillary and choroidal filling may indicate impaired perfusion of the shared vascular supply to the optic nerve and choroid.[11, 71, 77–79] If retrobulbar lesions are present, fundoscopic examination and fluorescein angiography may be normal. MRI with gadolinium shows enlargement and enhancement of the optic nerve in cases of optic neuritis.[11, 71]

8.19.5 Treatment

Optic neuritis typically responds dramatically to corticosteroid treatment. Early diagnosis and prompt treatment with high-dose corticosteroids are associated with better visual outcomes. Usually, a pulse steroid therapy (up to 1 g per day for 3 days), followed by high doses of steroids (up to 1 mg/kg/day) tapered over time, results in at least partial visual recovery.[7, 8, 71, 80, 81] Some cases require steroid-sparing immunosuppressive agents such as cyclophosphamide, cyclosporine, methotrexate, and azathioprine.[82, 83] Ischemic optic neuropathy is usually observed. However, due to the likely role of systemic vasculopathy and/or antiphospholipid antibodies in SLE-associated optic neuropathy, trial of corticosteroids is warranted and may result in visual improvement.[79]

8.19.6 Prognosis

Visual recovery is variable in most patients and can range anywhere from full recovery to count-fingers vision, likely reflecting the heterogeneous pathophysiology underlying SLE-associated optic nerve disease. Idiopathic optic neuritis generally has a good prognosis with appropriate treatment, and 87% of patients recovered to better than 20/25 at 5 years of follow-up.[84] In SLE-associated optic neuritis, the prognosis may be worse, with only 50% of patients experiencing recovery to 20/25 or better and 37.5% left legally blind with a visual acuity worse than 20/200.[85] Other optic neuropathy in SLE has a variable response to treatment, and visual field defects may persist.

8.20 ORBITAL DISEASE

Orbital involvement in SLE is uncommon and includes inflammation of extraocular muscles (inflammatory myositis), subcutaneous fat (panniculitis), or an infiltrating inflammatory mass.[86, 87] Presenting symptoms include pain, proptosis, diplopia, and restricted eye movement. One case report described Brown syndrome and development of vertical diplopia due to a transient tenosynovitis affecting the superior oblique tendon.[88] Systemic corticosteroids, as well as treatment of underlying SLE with hydroxychloroquine, and steroid-sparing agents are recommended.

8.21 SUMMARY

Up to 30% of patients with SLE present with ocular manifestations, and these may represent the earliest recognized disease manifestation in SLE. Keratoconjunctivitis sicca is the most common ocular manifestation and varies from mild to vision threatening. Other vision-threatening ocular manifestations include lupus retinopathy as well as rarer optic neuropathy, peripheral ulcerative keratitis, and scleritis. Ophthalmic manifestations of SLE require urgent ophthalmic evaluation, timely diagnosis with specific testing, and immediate systemic immunosuppressive treatment for vision-threatening disease.

REFERENCES

1. Preble JM, Silpa-Archa S, Foster CS. Ocular involvement in systemic lupus erythematosus. *Curr Opin Ophthalmol.* 2015;26(6).
2. Mills JA. Systemic lupus erythematosus. *N Engl J Med.* 1994;330(26):1871–1879.
3. Pons-Estel GJ, Alarcón GS, Scofield L, et al. Understanding the epidemiology and progression of systemic lupus erythematosus. *Semin Arthritis Rheum.* 2010;39(4):257–268.
4. Chakravarty EF, Bush TM, Manzi S, et al. Prevalence of adult systemic lupus erythematosus in California and Pennsylvania in 2000: estimates obtained using hospitalization data. *Arthritis Rheum.* 2007;56(6):2092–2094.
5. Lawrence RC, Helmick CG, Arnett FC, et al. Estimates of the prevalence of arthritis and selected musculoskeletal disorders in the United States. *Arthritis Rheum.* 1998;41(5):778–799.
6. Hebra F, Kaposi M. *On diseases of the skin, including the exanthemata.* London: The New Sydenham Society, 1875.
7. Peponis V, Kyttaris VC, Chalkiadakis SE, et al. Review: ocular side effects of anti-rheumatic medications: what a rheumatologist should know. *Lupus.* 2010;19(6):675–682.
8. Peponis V, Kyttaris VC, Tyradellis C, et al. Ocular manifestations of systemic lupus erythematosus: a clinical review. *Lupus.* 2006;15(1):3–12.
9. Semon HC, Wolff E. Acute lupus erythematosus, with fundus lesions. *Proc R Soc Med.* 1933;27(2):153–157.
10. Palejwala NV, Walia HS, Yeh S. Ocular manifestations of systemic lupus erythematosus: a review of the literature. *Autoimmune Dis.* 2012;2012:290898.
11. Sivaraj RR, Durrani OM, Denniston AK, et al. Ocular manifestations of systemic lupus erythematosus. *Rheumatology.* 2007;46(12):1757–1762.
12. Ward MM. Prevalence of physician-diagnosed systemic lupus erythematosus in the United States: results from the third national health and nutrition examination survey. *J Womens Health (Larchmt).* 2004;13(6):713–718.
13. Lim SS, Bayakly AR, Helmick CG, et al. The incidence and prevalence of systemic lupus erythematosus, 2002–2004: the Georgia Lupus registry. *Arthritis Rheumatol.* 2014;66(2):357–368.
14. Feldman CH, Hiraki LT, Liu J, et al. Epidemiology and sociodemographics of systemic lupus erythematosus and lupus nephritis among US adults with Medicaid coverage, 2000–2004. *Arthritis Rheum.* 2013;65(3):753–763.
15. Mok CC. Epidemiology and survival of systemic lupus erythematosus in Hong Kong Chinese. *Lupus.* 2011;20(7):767–771.
16. Helmick CG, Felson DT, Lawrence RC, et al. Estimates of the prevalence of arthritis and other rheumatic conditions in the United States: part I. *Arthritis Rheum.* 2008;58(1):15–25.
17. Izmirly PM, Parton H, Wang L, et al. Prevalence of systemic lupus erythematosus in the United States: estimates from a meta-analysis of the Centers for Disease Control and Prevention national lupus registries. *Arthritis Rheum.* 2021;73(6):991–996.
18. CfDCa Prevention. *Systemic lupus erythematosus (SLE).* Updated 2022 Jul. 5. https://www.cdc.gov/lupus/facts/detailed.html. Accessed 30 Nov. 2023.
19. Block SR, Winfield JB, Lockshin MD, et al. Studies of twins with systemic lupus erythematosus. A review of the literature and presentation of 12 additional sets. *Am J Med.* 1975;59(4):533–552.
20. Petri M, Kim MY, Kalunian KC, et al. Combined oral contraceptives in women with systemic lupus erythematosus. *N Engl J Med.* 2005;353(24):2550–2558.
21. Esen BA, Yılmaz G, Uzun S, et al. Serologic response to Epstein-Barr virus antigens in patients with systemic lupus erythematosus: a controlled study. *Rheumatol Int.* 2012;32(1):79–83.
22. Costenbader KH, Karlson EW. Cigarette smoking and systemic lupus erythematosus: a smoking gun? *Autoimmunity.* 2005;38(7):541–547.
23. Rubin R. *Drug induced lupus.* Philadelphia, PA: Lippincott Williams & Wilkins, 2002.
24. Dammacco R. Systemic lupus erythematosus and ocular involvement: an overview. *Clin Exp Med.* 2018;18(2):135–149.
25. Silpa-Archa S, Lee JJ, Foster CS. Ocular manifestations in systemic lupus erythematosus. *Br J Ophthalmol.* 2015;100.
26. Antonis F, Myrto K, Jeanette A, et al. EULAR recommendations for the management of systemic lupus erythematosus: 2023 update. *Ann Rheum Dis.* 2023:ard-2023-224762.
27. Petri M, Purvey S, Fang H, et al. Predictors of organ damage in systemic lupus erythematosus: the Hopkins Lupus cohort. *Arthritis Rheum.* 2012;64(12):4021–4028.

28. Ruiz-Irastorza G, Ramos-Casals M, Brito-Zeron P, et al. Clinical efficacy and side effects of antimalarials in systemic lupus erythematosus: a systematic review. *Ann Rheum Dis.* 2010;69(1):20–28.

29. Fasano S, Messiniti V, Iudici M, et al. Hydroxychloroquine daily dose, hydroxychloroquine blood levels and the risk of flares in patients with systemic lupus erythematosus. *Lupus Sci Med.* 2023;10(1):e000841.

30. Garg S, Chewning B, Hutson P, et al. A reference range of hydroxychloroquine blood levels that can reduce odds of active lupus and prevent flares. *Arthritis Care Res (Hoboken).* 2023;76(2):241–250. doi:10.1002/acr.25228. Epub 2023 Nov 28. PMID: 37667434 PMCID: PMC11078155.

31. Almeida-Brasil CC, Hanly JG, Urowitz M, et al. Flares after hydroxychloroquine reduction or discontinuation: results from the Systemic Lupus International Collaborating Clinics (SLICC) inception cohort. *Ann Rheum Dis.* 2022;81(3):370.

32. Jorge AM, Mancini C, Zhou B, et al. Hydroxychloroquine dose per ophthalmology guidelines and the risk of systemic lupus erythematosus flares. *JAMA.* 2022.;328(14):1458–1460. doi:10.1001/jama.2022.13591. PMID: 36112387, PMCID: PMC9554698.

33. Alarcon GS, McGwin G, Bertoli AM, et al. Effect of hydroxychloroquine on the survival of patients with systemic lupus erythematosus: data from LUMINA, a multiethnic US cohort (LUMINA L). *Ann Rheum Dis.* 2007;66(9):1168–1172.

34. Melles RB, Marmor MF. The risk of toxic retinopathy in patients on long-term hydroxychloroquine therapy. *JAMA Ophthalmol.* 2014;132(12):1453–1460.

35. Marmor MF. Comparison of screening procedures in hydroxychloroquine toxicity. *Arch Ophthalmol.* 2012;130(4):461–469.

36. Garg S, Ferguson S, Chewning B, et al. Clarifying misbeliefs about hydroxychloroquine (HCQ): developing the HCQ benefits versus harm decision aid (HCQ-SAFE) per low health literacy standards. *Lupus Sci Med.* 2023;10(2).

37. Garg S, Unnithan R, Hansen KE, et al. The clinical significance of monitoring hydroxychloroquine levels in patients with systemic lupus erythematosus: a systematic review and meta-analysis. *Arthritis Care Res (Hoboken).* 2020;73(5):707–716. doi:10.1002/acr.24155. Epub 2021 Mar 30. PMID: 32004406.

38. Petri M, Elkhalifa M, Li J, et al. Hydroxychloroquine blood levels predict hydroxychloroquine retinopathy. *Arthritis Rheumatol.* 2020;72(3):448–453.

39. Wang L, Xie Y, Deng Y. Prevalence of dry eye in patients with systemic lupus erythematosus: a meta-analysis. *BMJ Open.* 2021;11(9):e047081.

40. Luboń W, Luboń M, Kotyla P, et al. Understanding ocular findings and manifestations of systemic lupus erythematosus: update review of the literature. *Int J Mol Sci.* 2022;23(20).

41. Akpek EK, Lindsley KB, Adyanthaya RS, et al. Treatment of Sjögren's syndrome-associated dry eye an evidence-based review. *Ophthalmology.* 2011;118(7):1242–1252.

42. Brott NR, Ronquillo Y. Schirmer test. In: *StatPearls.* Treasure Island, FL: StatPearls Publishing LLC, 2023. Copyright © 2023.

43. de Paiva CS, Pflugfelder SC, Ng SM, et al. Topical cyclosporine A therapy for dry eye syndrome. *Cochrane Database Syst Rev.* 2019;9.

44. Holland EJ, Jackson MA, Donnenfeld E, et al. Efficacy of lifitegrast ophthalmic solution, 5.0%, in patients with moderate to severe dry eye disease: a post hoc analysis of 2 randomized clinical trials. *JAMA Ophthalmol.* 2021;139(11):1200–1208.

45. Brito-Zerón P, Retamozo S, Kostov B, et al. Efficacy and safety of topical and systemic medications: a systematic literature review informing the EULAR recommendations for the management of Sjögren's syndrome. *RMD Open.* 2019;5(2):e001064.

46. Messmer EM, Foster CS. Vasculitic peripheral ulcerative keratitis. *Surv Ophthalmol.* 1999;43(5):379–396.

47. Cao Y, Zhang W, Wu J, et al. Peripheral ulcerative keratitis associated with autoimmune disease: pathogenesis and treatment. *J Ophthalmol.* 2017;2017:7298026.

48. Galor A, Thorne JE. Scleritis and peripheral ulcerative keratitis. *Vasculitis.* 2007;33(4):835–854.

49. Lu CW, Zhou DD, Wang J, et al. Surgical treatment of peripheral ulcerative keratitis and necrotizing scleritis in granulomatosis with polyangiitis. *Saudi Med J.* 2016;37(2):205–207.

50. Stein R. Photorefractive keratectomy. *Int Ophthalmol Clin.* 2000;40(3):35–56.

51. Cua IY, Pepose JS. Late corneal scarring after photorefractive keratectomy concurrent with development of systemic lupus erythematosus. *J Refract Surg.* 2002;18(6):750–752.

52. Firth AY. Pupillary responses in amblyopia. *Br J Ophthalmol.* 1990;74(11):676–680.

53. Burge SM, Frith PA, Millard PR, et al. The lupus band test in oral mucosa, conjunctiva and skin. *Br J Dermatol.* 1989;121(6):743–752.
54. Frith P, Burge SM, Millard PR, et al. External ocular findings in lupus erythematosus: a clinical and immunopathological study. *Br J Ophthalmol.* 1990;74(3):163–167.
55. Thorne JE, Anhalt GJ, Jabs DA. Ocular mucous membrane pemphigoid. *Dermatol Ther.* 2002;15(4):389–396.
56. Fanouriakis A, Kostopoulou M, Cheema K, et al. 2019 Update of the Joint European League Against Rheumatism and European Renal Association – European Dialysis and Transplant Association (EULAR/ERA-EDTA) recommendations for the management of lupus nephritis. *Ann Rheum Dis.* 2020;79(6):713–723.
57. Fanouriakis A, Kostopoulou M, Alunno A, et al. 2019 update of the EULAR recommendations for the management of systemic lupus erythematosus. *Ann Rheum Dis.* 2019;78(6):736.
58. Hsu CS, Hsu CW, Lu MC, et al. Risks of ophthalmic disorders in patients with systemic lupus erythematosus – a secondary cohort analysis of population-based claims data. *BMC Ophthalmol.* 2020;20(1):96.
59. Dammacco R, Procaccio P, Racanelli V, et al. Ocular involvement in systemic lupus erythematosus: the experience of two tertiary referral centers. *Ocul Immunol Inflamm.* 2018;26(8):1154–1165.
60. Gallagher K, Viswanathan A, Okhravi N. Association of systemic lupus erythematosus with uveitis. *JAMA Ophthalmol.* 2015;133(10):1190–1193.
61. Rodriguez A, Calonge M, Pedroza-Seres M, et al. Referral patterns of uveitis in a tertiary eye care center. *Arch Ophthalmol.* 1996;114(5):593–599.
62. Jawahar N, Walker JK, Murray PI, et al. Epidemiology of disease-activity related ophthalmological manifestations in systemic lupus erythematosus: a systematic review. *Lupus.* 2021;30(14):2191–2203.
63. Montehermoso A, Cervera R, Font J, et al. Association of antiphospholipid antibodies with retinal vascular disease in systemic lupus erythematosus. *Semin Arthritis Rheum.* 1999;28(5):326–332.
64. Seth G, Chengappa KG, Misra DP, et al. Lupus retinopathy: a marker of active systemic lupus erythematosus. *Rheumatol Int.* 2018;38(8):1495–1501.
65. Stafford-Brady FJ, Urowitz MB, Gladman DD, et al. Lupus retinopathy: patterns, associations, and prognosis. *Arthritis Rheum.* 1988;31(9):1105–1110.
66. Ushiyama O, Ushiyama K, Koarada S, et al. Retinal disease in patients with systemic lupus erythematosus. *Ann Rheum Dis.* 2000;59(9):705–708.
67. Au A, O'Day J. Review of severe vaso-occlusive retinopathy in systemic lupus erythematosus and the antiphospholipid syndrome: associations, visual outcomes, complications and treatment. *Clin Exp Ophthalmol.* 2004;32(1):87–100.
68. Hickman RA, Denniston AK, Yee CS, et al. Bilateral retinal vasculitis in a patient with systemic lupus erythematosus and its remission with rituximab therapy. *Lupus.* 2010;19(3):327–329.
69. Neumann R, Foster CS. Corticosteroid-sparing strategies in the treatment of retinal vasculitis in systemic lupus erythematosus. *Retina.* 1995;15(3):201–212.
70. Papadaki TG, Zacharopoulos IP, Papaliodis G, et al. Plasmapheresis for lupus retinal vasculitis. *Arch Ophthalmol.* 2006;124(11):1654–1656.
71. de Andrade FA, Guimarães Moreira Balbi G, Bortoloti de Azevedo LG, et al. Neuro-ophthalmologic manifestations in systemic lupus erythematosus. *Lupus.* 2017;26(5):522–528.
72. Baglio V, Gharbiya M, Balacco-Gabrieli C, et al. Choroidopathy in patients with systemic lupus erythematosus with or without nephropathy. *J Nephrol.* 2011;24(4):522–529.
73. Schwartz MM, Roberts JL. Membranous and vascular choroidopathy: two patterns of immune deposits in systemic lupus erythematosus. *Clin Immunol Immunopathol.* 1983;29(3):369–380.
74. Gharbiya M, Bozzoni-Pantaleoni F, Augello F, et al. Indocyanine green angiographic findings in systemic lupus erythematosus choroidopathy. *Am J Ophthalmol.* 2002;134(2):286–290.
75. Diogo MC, Jager MJ, Ferreira TA. CT and MR imaging in the diagnosis of scleritis. *AJNR Am J Neuroradiol.* 2016;37(12):2334–2339.
76. Feinglass EJ, Arnett FC, Dorsch CA, et al. Neuropsychiatric manifestations of systemic lupus erythematosus: diagnosis, clinical spectrum, and relationship to other features of the disease. *Medicine (Baltimore).* 1976;55(4):323–339.
77. Sergio P, Mariana B, Alberto O, et al. Association of neuromyelitis optic (NMO) with autoimmune disorders: report of two cases and review of the literature. *Clin Rheumatol.* 2010;29(11):1335–1338.

78. Birnbaum J, Kerr D. Optic neuritis and recurrent myelitis in a woman with systemic lupus erythematosus. *Nat Clin Pract Rheumatol.* 2008;4(7):381–386.

79. Jabs DA, Miller NR, Newman SA, et al. Optic neuropathy in systemic lupus erythematosus. *Arch Ophthalmol.* 1986;104(4):564–568.

80. Smith SM, Westermeyer HD, Mariani CL, et al. *Optic neuritis*, volume 1, 6th edn. Philadelphia, PA: Lippincott Williams & Wilkins, 2005.

81. Borruat FX, Prado T, Strominger M, et al. Neuro-ophthalmologic complications of disseminated lupus erythematosus. *Klin Monbl Augenheilkd.* 1994;204(5):403–406.

82. Rosenbaum JT, Simpson J, Neuwelt CM. Successful treatment of optic neuropathy in association with systemic lupus erythematosus using intravenous cyclophosphamide. *Br J Ophthalmol.* 1997;81(2):130–132.

83. Myers TD, Smith JR, Wertheim MS, et al. Use of corticosteroid sparing systemic immunosuppression for treatment of corticosteroid dependent optic neuritis not associated with demyelinating disease. *Br J Ophthalmol.* 2004;88(5):673–680.

84. The Clinical Profile of Optic Neuritis. Experience of the optic neuritis treatment trial: optic neuritis study group. *Arch Ophthalmol.* 1991;109(12):1673–1678.

85. Lin YC, Wang AG, Yen MY. Systemic lupus erythematosus-associated optic neuritis: clinical experience and literature review. *Acta Ophthalmol.* 2009;87(2):204–210.

86. Serop S, Vianna RN, Claeys M, et al. Orbital myositis secondary to systemic lupus erythematosus. *Acta Ophthalmol (Copenh).* 1994;72(4):520–523.

87. Stavrou P, Murray PI, Batta K, et al. Acute ocular ischaemia and orbital inflammation associated with systemic lupus erythematosus. *Br J Ophthalmol.* 2002;86:474–475, England.

88. Whitefield L, Isenberg DA, Brazier DJ, et al. Acquired Brown's syndrome in systemic lupus erythematosus. *Br J Rheumatol.* 1995;34(11):1092–1094.

9 Ophthalmologic Disease in Behçet's Syndrome

Ilknur Tugal-Tutkun and Yusuf Yazici

9.1 INTRODUCTION

Behçet syndrome (BS) is a recurrent inflammatory multiorgan illness, a systemic vasculopathy that predominantly affects veins over arteries, leading to manifestations in the skin, mucosa, eyes, joints, lungs, and the gastrointestinal and central nervous systems.[1] The prevalence of BS has a unique geographic distribution, and it is more prevalent around the Mediterranean and Far East than the rest of the world. In general, men have a more severe disease course than women, and the disease severity commonly declines over time.

There is evidence to suggest that different organ manifestations occur together in clinical phenotypes such as arthritis/acne/enthesitis or vascular clusters.[2, 3] Currently, there is not sufficient information as to whether these different clusters represent different disease mechanisms.

BS tends to have waning disease activity over time, which greatly impacts how we approach treatment. Most patients tend to do well with treatment and time and early, aggressive treatment that matches the systemic involvement is the current norm. There is an opportunity to decrease or stop some of the medications used to treat BS over time, allowing patients to achieve remission and stay in remission with no or minimal drug use. However, as a sizeable portion of patients can have serious morbidity, especially with eye and CNS involvement, treatment needs to be individualized and disease activity monitored closely.

9.2 EPIDEMIOLOGY

BS was first described by Hulusi Behçet, a Turkish dermatologist. Patients are most commonly from the Middle East, the Mediterranean region, and the Far East, with Japan and South Korea leading the list. It is most prevalent in Turkey, with a prevalence of 1 in 250 adults;[4] it is rare in northern Europe and Africa. It is relatively rare before the late teens and after age 50 and is most commonly seen in patients in their second and third decades.

Males and females are equally affected, but males frequently have more severe disease and poorer outcomes.[5] Some manifestations may show regional differences; for example, gastrointestinal involvement, rare in Turkey, is more common in Japan and is seen in about 30% of patients in the United States.[6]

Pathergy (subcutaneous skin hyperactivity to needle prick) is more common in the Middle East than in the United States and northern Europe.

9.3 DIAGNOSIS

The diagnosis of BS is based on a compilation of clinical signs and symptoms; there are no specific laboratory, imaging, or biopsy findings to definitively establish the diagnosis of BS. Findings from these tests are utilized in ruling out other conditions that may mimic BS. Several classification or diagnostic criteria have been developed to help clinicians in everyday patient care and in conducting studies to better understand this complex condition.

The International Study Group (ISG) Criteria[7] is the most widely used criteria for both clinical care and research studies. A newer set of criteria called the International Criteria for Behçet's Disease (ICBD) for classification and/or diagnosis of BS has been developed.[8] However, the new ICBD criteria have worse specificity than the ISG criteria, a major issue, as this leads to more people being given a diagnosis when they do not have the disease, a problem especially when the pretest probability is low, which is the case in most parts of the world for BS.[9] One useful set of criteria, especially in areas where gastrointestinal (GI) involvement is more common, is the Japanese criteria,[10] which takes into account GI involvement in addition to other manifestations, such as epididymitis and arthritis, to be included in the diagnosis. Also, the Japanese criteria divides the diagnosis into 'complete' and 'incomplete' groups, which can also be helpful in parts of the world where the prevalence is low or in the case of early phases of the disease when all the symptoms have not yet manifested. Table 9.1 provides a summary overview of these more commonly used criteria.

Imaging may help in identifying the extent of organ involvement in BS. Doppler ultrasonography is helpful in diagnosing venous thrombosis and arterial aneurysms in the extremities and in determining whether the thrombosis is acute, subacute, or chronic. Computerized tomography (CT) and CT-angiograms of the chest and abdomen are usually needed to diagnose larger, proximal vessel involvement. Cranial MRI and MR angiography are useful for diagnosing nervous system

DOI: 10.1201/9781003453710-9

Table 9.1 Comparison of Commonly Used Classification/Diagnostic Criteria for BS

ISG	ICBD: Scoring 4 or More Points	Japanese: Complete or Incomplete Type	
Oral ulcers	■ Ocular lesions: 2 points	Major symptoms	■ Oral ulcer
Plus 2 out of 4 from below:	■ Genital aphthosis: 2 points		■ Genital ulcer
■ Recurrent genital ulcers	■ Oral aphthosis: 2 points		■ Skin lesion
■ Skin lesions	■ Skin lesions: 1 point		■ Ocular lesion
■ Eye lesions	■ Neurological manifestations: 1 point	Minor symptoms	■ Arthritis
■ Pathergy	■ Vascular manifestations: 1 point		■ Epididymitis
	■ Pathergy: 1 point (optional)		■ GI lesion
			■ Vascular lesion
			■ CNS lesion
			■ Arthritis
		Complete type	4 major symptoms
		Incomplete type	3 major or 2 major + 2 minor or Ocular + 1 major or Ocular + 2 minor

involvement. As for laboratory testing, although several biomarkers have been studied, the only ones that may be useful are acute phase reactants, which can be elevated during active vascular and gastrointestinal involvement as well as amyloidosis.

9.4 PATHOGENESIS

Pathogenetic mechanisms underlying BS are not known. However, current knowledge suggests the role of environmental factors including infections that activate the adaptive immune system in the presence of an active innate immune system, driven by a complex genetic background. The strongest genetic association is with HLA B*51, and carrying HLA-B5/B*51 alleles increases the risk of developing BS more than 5 times.[11] Approximately 50% of the patients carry the allele HLA-B*51, although its importance in disease causality seems to be overrated. Much emphasis has been made on altered antigen presentation by HLA–B*51 to the immunoinflammatory cascade in epistasis with mutations in endoplasmic reticulum amino peptidase 1 (ERAP1).[12] The epistasis with ERAP1, which trims peptides that can be loaded onto MHC-1 and the increased risk for developing BS in individuals carrying the ERAP1-Hap10 variant, have been noted. However, considering the proportion of patients who express HLA–B*51, this important observation would explain the disease mechanism in only a portion of the patients. Many patients with severe BS, especially in Europe and the United States, do not carry HLA–B*51. Microorganisms including streptococci and herpes simplex virus were also thought to play a role as environmental triggers through molecular mimicry.[13] Studies on the saliva and the gut microbiome of active BS patients have shown differences from inactive BS patients and healthy and diseased controls, suggesting a potential role of the microbiome in the pathogenesis of BS.[14]

9.5 CLINICAL MANIFESTATIONS

9.5.1 Mucocutaneous Involvement

Various mucocutaneous manifestations, such as oral and genital ulcers and skin lesions, are the most common clinical presentation of BS. These lesions are not highly specific for BS by themselves, but the recurrent nature, occurrence of different types of lesions in the same patient, and the presence of organ involvement may help with the diagnosis. Oral ulcers are seen in virtually all patients and are commonly the first manifestation. They can be present years before other findings of BS develop. They are usually multiple. Unlike herpes ulcers, these lesions are virtually always in the moist mucosal surfaces inside the mouth and do not occur on the outer surfaces of the lips. They are not distinguishable from ordinary oral ulcers. They tend to last around 1 to 2 weeks and recur unless treated. Only major ulcers, which are rare, scar.[15]

Genital ulcers are the most specific lesions, most commonly occurring on the scrotum or labia; the shaft and the glans penis are usually spared. They are usually larger and deeper and take longer to heal than oral ulcers. These lesions tend to get infected, which potentially interferes with the healing process and leads to scarring. About 80% of BS patients have genital ulcers. Genital ulcers tend to lead to scarring in about two-thirds of patients; scrotal scarring in males is very specific for BS.[16]

The majority of BS patients also have acne-like or papulopustular lesions that are indistinguishable from acne vulgaris. They are seen at the usual acne sites as well as at uncommon sites such as lower extremities. Other skin findings are nodular lesions, which are of two types: erythema nodosum lesions due to panniculitis and superficial vein thromboses. Superficial thrombophlebitis often occurs in men and is associated with deep vein thrombosis, which should trigger workup for other vascular involvement, including pulmonary artery aneurysms.[17]

9.5.2 Vascular Involvement

Some form of vascular involvement is reported in 15% to 30% of the patients and is more frequent among men.[18] Venous thrombosis is more common and tends to occur earlier than arterial involvement. Superficial thrombophlebitis usually presents as recurrent nodular lesions on the lower and, less commonly, upper extremities. Inferior vena cava thrombosis with or without hepatic vein involvement may cause Budd–Chiari syndrome that has a poor prognosis in around half of the patients. Pulmonary artery aneurysms (PAA) occur in up to 3% of patients, and despite this low frequency, they are an important cause of mortality due to massive hemoptysis. It is important to differentiate PAA from pulmonary embolism (PE), as PE may present with hemoptysis too. It would be critical to rule out PE because anticoagulation is the treatment choice in PE, whereas it would be contraindicated in PAA.

9.5.3 Nervous System Involvement

Neurological involvement of BS can be classified into parenchymal and cerebral venous sinus thrombosis.[19] The two rarely occur together. Eighty percent of patients with central nervous system involvement have parenchymal involvement, which is harder to treat and usually has a poor prognosis. It usually presents with cranial nerve findings, dysarthria, unilateral or bilateral corticospinal tract signs with or without weakness, ataxia, and mild confusion. Cerebral venous sinus thrombosis (CVST) occurs in up to 20% of BS patients with neurological involvement. Clinical features of CVST include severe headache, papilledema, and sixth-nerve palsy on neurological examination.

9.5.4 Ocular Involvement

The most common form of ocular involvement in BS is recurrent, bilateral nongranulomatous panuveitis with retinal vasculitis.[20, 21] Although there may be unilateral involvement initially, the other eye is rapidly involved in the majority. In a series of patients with BS uveitis, the disease remained unilateral for more than 5 years in 7%.[20] Isolated anterior uveitis is seen in around 10%,[20, 22, 23] mostly in women,[20, 22] and posterior uveitis in around 30%.[20] Ostrovsky et al. reported that isolated anterior uveitis was seen in 13.5% of eyes at initial presentation, and it was more common (30.6%) in patients with late onset of the disease (>40 years of age) than in juvenile (13.6%) or adult-onset disease (9.5%).[24] On the other hand, in an Egyptian cohort, anterior uveitis was more common in juvenile BS patients (19.2%) than in the older patients (9.3%).[25] Although isolated vitritis has been defined as intermediate uveitis in some reports[24, 26–29] and intermediate uveitis has been included in the classification criteria for BS uveitis,[30] it may be a misnomer, because retinal lesions are transient and may be missed at the time of ocular examinations in early disease. In fact, eyes with diffuse vitritis were classified as posterior uveitis in earlier reports.[20, 23, 31, 32]

Patients may present with symptoms of red eye, ocular pain, and photophobia associated with anterior uveitis. Floaters, visual blurring, or a sudden visual loss are the main symptoms due to inflammation in the posterior segment of the eye.[22] As the clinical course is marked by acute-onset inflammatory episodes and relatively quiescent periods between these 'uveitis attacks,' ocular symptoms will vary with the course and severity of intraocular inflammation.

While the typical onset of disease is with an acute symptomatic uveitis attack of variable severity, patients may also present later in the disease course after several episodes of transient visual blurring or waxing and waning floaters in one or both eyes. Spontaneous resolution of inflammatory episodes is a characteristic feature and a cause of late presentation of patients with mild uveitis attacks in early stages of the disease. A history of recurrent visual blurring that improves spontaneously within a few days to weeks is suggestive of BS uveitis, as such a history would be very atypical of other uveitic entities. With the onset of a severe uveitis attack that may cause a sudden drop in visual acuity even to a light perception level, the patients will immediately seek medical attention.

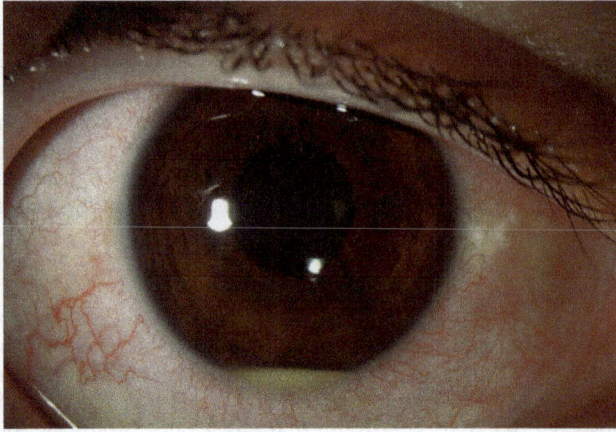

Figure 9.1 Slit lamp photograph of the right eye of a patient with BS uveitis shows mild conjunctival hyperemia and a smooth-layered hypopyon.

9.6 OCULAR FINDINGS

Recurrent acute anterior segment inflammation is characterized by nongranulomatous features, including corneal endothelial dusting, freely circulating anterior chamber cells, and absence of iris nodules.[20, 22, 33] A disproportionately mild conjunctival hyperemia is a common finding even in eyes with a hypopyon, which has been reported in 12% to 34% of eyes in large cohorts.[20, 22, 33] The presence of a hypopyon is usually an indicator of severe panuveitis; i.e., severe posterior segment inflammation as well. A smooth-layered shifting hypopyon is typically seen due to the absence of a fibrinous reaction, and the hypopyon forms and dissolves rapidly (Figure 9.1). Such characteristics of BS hypopyon help to differentiate it from the sticky hypopyon with fibrinous reaction typically seen in HLA-B27-associated acute anterior uveitis.[21] Although anterior segment inflammation is rapidly controlled by topical corticosteroids and the anterior segment is not chronically inflamed in BS uveitis, severe attacks that are not timely treated may cause formation of posterior synechiae, adhesions of the pupil to the anterior lens surface. The intraocular pressure may be normal or slightly decreased during attacks. A hypertensive anterior uveitis is never seen in BS, which is an important differentiating feature from viral anterior uveitis.[21]

Posterior segment inflammation is characterized by diffuse vitritis, optic disc inflammation, retinal infiltrates, diffuse sheathing of especially retinal veins, and occlusive retinal periphlebitis.[20, 21, 22, 33] A dense vitreous haze may obscure fundus details at the onset of severe attacks. With gradual resolution of diffuse vitritis, a number of small white precipitates may appear inferiorly, usually in a linear pattern, on the surface of the retina and disappear within a few weeks without any sequelae.[21] Such inferior precipitates have been described in infectious uveitis[34] but not in noninfectious uveitis other than BS uveitis.

Retinal infiltrates, defined as retinitis or retinal exudates in earlier reports,[20, 22, 33] are the most commonly seen inflammatory lesions in uveitis attacks involving the posterior segment, and they have been recently included in the classification criteria for BS uveitis.[30] They may be in any number, size, or location in the fundus, with or without accompanying retinal hemorrhages, and typically have a tendency to resolve within days without visible chorioretinal scarring (Figure 9.2). With an increased use of high-resolution optical coherence tomography (OCT) imaging, the characteristic features of retinal infiltrates and their sequelae have been identified. A hyper-reflective retinal thickening with blurring of especially inner retinal layers and shadowing beneath the lesion without focal choroidal thickening are seen in OCT sections through these lesions. There may be subretinal fluid and disruption of outer retinal layers in large infiltrates. At the posterior pole, retinal infiltrates cause focal inner retinal atrophy, outer plexiform layer elevation, and a retinal nerve fiber layer defect extending to the optic disc (Figure 9.3).[35–37] Corresponding scotomas on visual field indicate functional significance of these infiltrates.[35] Moreover, OCT findings of such sequelae of retinal infiltrates help differentiate from intermediate uveitis and can be monitored as evidence of prior posterior uveitis attacks.[36]

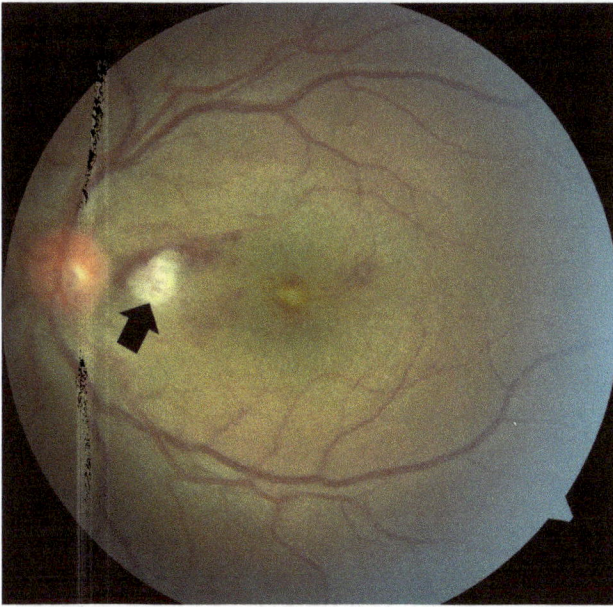

Figure 9.2 Color fundus photograph of the left eye of a patient with BS uveitis shows a white retinal infiltrate (indicated by a black arrow) and adjacent retinal hemorrhages temporal to the optic disc.

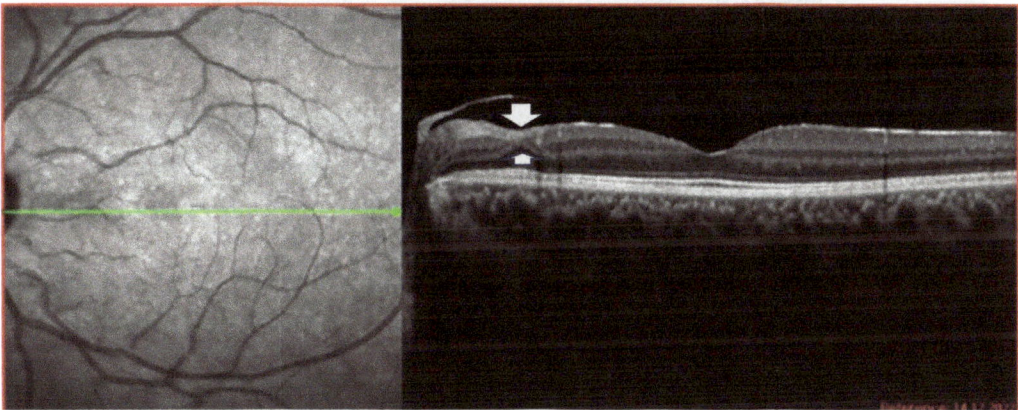

Figure 9.3 OCT scan of the same eye as in Figure 9.2 after the resolution of the retinal infiltrate shows focal retinal atrophy with inner retinal indentation (indicated by a large arrow) and outer plexiform layer elevation (indicated by a small arrow).

Inflammatory sheathing of retinal vessels may not be readily apparent due to vitreous haze at the onset of uveitis attacks. Following resolution of intraocular inflammation, diffuse gliotic sheathing of retinal veins can be seen as thin white lines along the vessel walls. Episodes of occlusive periphlebitis are characterized by fluffy sheathing of the involved vasculature, which may even have a frosted branch appearance, surrounded by retinal hemorrhages (Figure 9.4). Ghost vessels are seen following such episodes, and shunt vessels typically develop in the nonperfused retina (Figure 9.5). Branch retinal vein occlusion (BRVO) has been reported in 6% to 31% of eyes with BS uveitis.[20, 26, 31, 38, 39] Central retinal vein occlusion and retinal arteriolar occlusions are uncommon.[38, 40, 41] While Ostrovsky et al. reported that leaky type of retinal vasculitis was more frequently found in eyes with vascular occlusions,[38] suggesting the role of inflammation in the pathogenesis, Ucar et al. reported

119

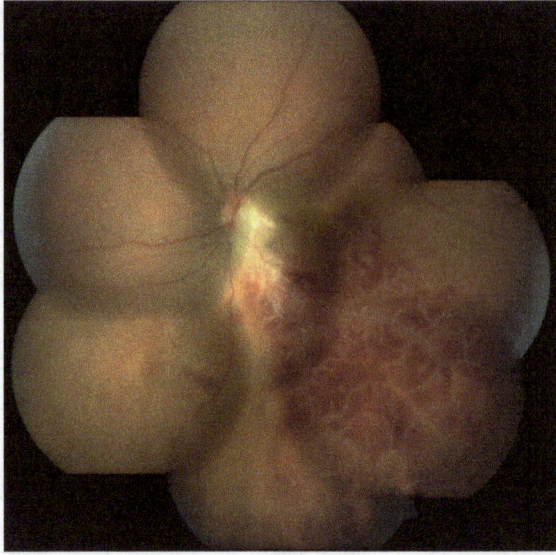

Figure 9.4 Color fundus photograph of the left eye of a patient with BS uveitis and inferior temporal branch retinal vein occlusion shows frosted branch sheathing of the occluded vein and its branches, with retinal hemorrhages surrounding the occluded vasculature.

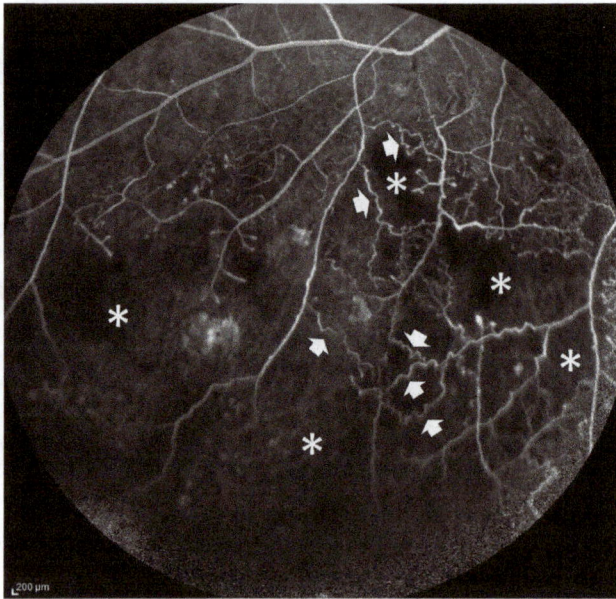

Figure 9.5 Early-phase fluorescein angiographic frame of the inferior temporal retina in the right eye of a patient with a history of inferior temporal branch retinal vein occlusion shows shunt vessels (indicated by arrows) in the nonperfused (indicated by asterisks) retinal quadrant.

that 46% of eyes with BS-associated BRVO did not have uveitis, implicating the prothrombotic state of BS patients as the underlying cause of this ocular complication.[42] Foveal ischemia is a significant cause of permanent visual loss following occlusive retinal vasculitis in BS patients.

Retinal capillaritis may manifest clinically as scattered dot hemorrhages and is revealed best by fundus fluorescein angiography (FFA). Diffuse fern-like retinal capillary leakage and staining of the

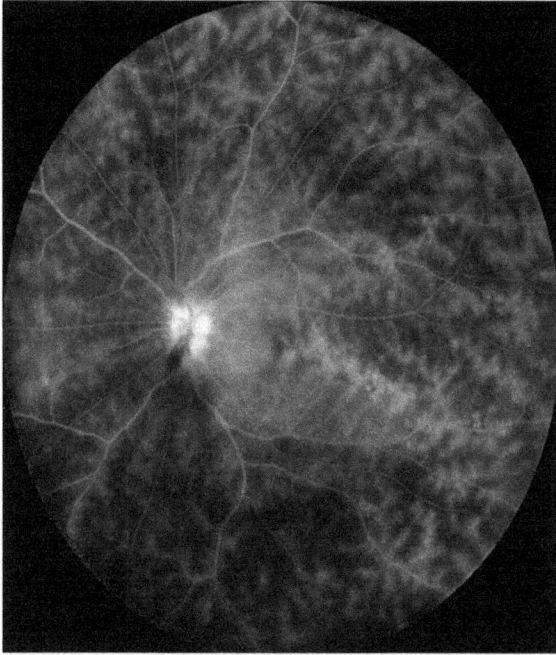

Figure 9.6 Late-phase fluorescein angiographic frame of the left eye of a patient with BS uveitis shows hyperfluorescence of the optic disc and diffuse fern-like retinal capillary leakage.

optic disc are the most common FFA findings in BS uveitis (Figure 9.6), both during acute inflammatory episodes and also during clinically quiescent periods between attacks.[33, 37, 39, 43–45] Persistent capillary leakage is a sign of uncontrolled disease and indicates a high risk of cystoid macular edema (CME), neovascularization of the optic disc (NVD), and recurrent uveitis attacks.[46, 47] Therefore, FFA is the gold standard in monitoring BS uveitis.[37, 48]

In patients with long-standing uncontrolled disease, optic atrophy, diffuse retinal atrophy with ghost vessels and pigmentary changes, and advanced macular damage constitute the end-stage fundus findings.[20] Posterior synechiae, cataract, and glaucoma are the other complications associated with recurrent anterior segment inflammation and the excessive use of corticosteroids for treatment. Both the frequency and severity of uveitis attacks and the persistent background inflammation, as evidenced by retinal capillary leakage on FFA, determine the extent of retinal damage and visual outcome.[45, 48] Table 9.2 summarizes various ocular findings in BS uveitis and their potential complications.

9.7 DIAGNOSIS OF BEHÇET SYNDROME UVEITIS

There is no specific test for the diagnosis of BS uveitis. Several sets of clinical classification criteria have been developed for BS but are widely used for the diagnosis of individual patients as well. Classification criteria are intended to ensure uniform patient populations to be included in studies of BS and require the presence of multisystemic manifestations of the disease. Uveitis is a criterion in both the International Study Group (ISG) criteria published in 1990 and the more recently developed International Criteria for Behçet's Disease (ICBD).[7, 8] In the ISG criteria, the presence of recurrent oral ulcers is an obligatory criterion, and two manifestations are required among the other four, including genital ulcers, skin lesions, uveitis, and a positive pathergy test. In the ICBD criteria, recurrent oral ulcer is not obligatory, but more weight is still given to oral ulcers (2 points) as well as to genital ulcers and uveitis (2 points each); and other manifestations, including skin lesions, neurologic, and vascular manifestations, are given 1 point each. A minimum of 4 points is required for classification of a patient as BS. Thus, a patient with uveitis and recurrent oral ulcers or genital ulcers can be classified as BS based on the ICBD criteria. An important inherent limitation of both criteria sets is the nonspecific definition of uveitis: anterior uveitis, posterior uveitis, cells in the vitreous, or retinal vasculitis.

Table 9.2 Ocular Findings in Behçet Syndrome Uveitis

	Anterior Segment of the Eye	Posterior Segment of the Eye
Acute inflammatory signs	■ Variable conjunctival hyperemia ■ Corneal endothelial dusting ■ Anterior chamber cells and flare ■ Smooth-layered hypopyon	■ Diffuse vitreous cells and haze ■ Optic disc inflammation ■ Retinal infiltrates ■ Retinal hemorrhages ■ Diffuse sheathing of retinal veins ■ Occlusive retinal periphlebitis
Sequelae of inflammatory lesions and ocular complications	■ Posterior synechiae ■ Cataract ■ Glaucoma	■ Transient inferior vitreous precipitates ■ Retinal nerve fiber layer defects ■ Diffuse gliotic sheathing of retinal veins ■ Ghost vessels ■ Cystoid macular edema ■ Neovascularization of the disc ■ Neovascularization elsewhere ■ Optic atrophy ■ Macular hole ■ Macular atrophy and scarring ■ Diffuse retinal atrophy with pigmentary changes

The Standardization of Uveitis Nomenclature (SUN) Working Group has more recently developed a new set of classification criteria for BS uveitis.[30] The first criterion is a compatible uveitic syndrome based on the presence of anterior uveitis, anterior and intermediate uveitis, and posterior or panuveitis with retinal vasculitis and/or focal retinal infiltrates. The second criterion is a diagnosis of BS based on the ISG criteria, which mandates the presence of recurrent oral ulcers and an additional manifestation of the disease. While the limitation of oral ulcer being an obligatory criterion is not avoided, the nongranulomatous feature of uveitis, occlusive nature of retinal vasculitis, or predominant involvement of retinal veins were still not specified in this new criteria set.

A diagnostic algorithm for BS uveitis has been published, which is intended to be used as a tool to guide ophthalmologists for the diagnosis of BS uveitis irrespective of the presence of extraocular manifestations of the disease.[49] In patients presenting with diffuse vitritis, the most important diagnostic clues were defined as absence of granulomatous anterior uveitis and choroiditis and the presence of retinal infiltrates or their sequelae, signs of occlusive retinal periphlebitis, and diffuse retinal capillary leakage on FFA.[49] The relapsing and remitting disease course and the spontaneous resolution of acute inflammatory lesions are also distinctive features of BS uveitis that would help distinguish it from other chronic uveitic entities. Turkish uveitis specialists correctly identified BS uveitis and non-BS uveitis in up to 81% of clinical photographs randomly presented to them in a study aiming to investigate the role of ophthalmologists in discriminating eye lesions of BS patients.[50] High levels of clinical suspicion and expertise are required for the prompt diagnosis of BS uveitis, especially in patients who develop uveitis as the initial manifestation of the disease.

9.8 TREATMENT

A standard treat-to-target strategy has not yet been established for BS.[51] The most recent European League Against Rheumatism (EULAR) recommendations published in 2018 aimed to standardize management of 10 different manifestations of BS.[52] For isolated anterior uveitis, only topical corticosteroid treatment was recommended, except in young males, who may be treated with an immunosuppressive agent because of a higher risk of developing posterior segment involvement. For patients with posterior segment involvement, the recommended treatment regimens included conventional immunosuppressive agents such as azathioprine or cyclosporine, interferon alpha, and monoclonal anti-TNF antibodies. Notably, systemic corticosteroids should be used only in combination with immunosuppressive agents. Interferon alpha has been effectively used for the treatment of refractory BS for two decades.[53–55] It has become unavailable after the publication of the EULAR recommendations.

While heterogeneity of BS patients is well recognized, cluster analyses of BS cohorts have identified the 'uveitis phenotype' as a separate cluster.[56] Therapeutic approach should be based on the severity and course of BS uveitis, which is a potentially blinding disease. Rapid suppression of severe sight-threatening acute intraocular inflammation, prevention of recurrent uveitis attacks, close monitoring and effective treatment of background chronic posterior segment inflammation, and prompt treatment of complications such as CME or NVD should be accomplished in order to preserve visual function.

While high-dose systemic corticosteroids, usually given by intravenous infusions, are widely used for the treatment of severe uveitis attacks, infliximab infusions may be used as an effective alternative treatment when corticosteroid therapy is to be avoided.[57] Intravitreal depot corticosteroid injections or implants may also be administered as an adjunct for the treatment of unilateral severe attacks or persistent CME.[58-60]

Monoclonal anti-TNF antibodies, infliximab, and adalimumab started to be used in the 2000s for the treatment of BS uveitis refractory to conventional immunosuppressive treatment.[61-64] Adalimumab has been approved for the treatment of noninfectious uveitis including BS uveitis after randomized controlled trials (VISUAL trials) proving its efficacy and safety were published in 2016.[65-66] Clinical studies have shown that both infliximab and adalimumab reduce the frequency and severity of uveitis attacks, decrease background leakage and macular thickness, have a significant corticosteroid-sparing effect, and result in favorable visual outcomes in patients with BS uveitis.[67-73] Both agents have high retention rates.[74-77] Earlier biologic treatment can provide better chances of drug-free remission.[78-80] Patients with severe BS uveitis require high doses of biologics; up to 10 mg/kg infliximab infusions may need to be given every 4 weeks following the induction doses 2 weeks apart. The standard dosing regimen for adalimumab is 80 mg initially, 40 mg 1 week later, and then 40 mg every other week. However, weekly maintenance dosing of 40 mg adalimumab is usually required in BS uveitis.

In patients who fail infliximab and adalimumab therapy, switching to other monoclonal anti-TNF antibodies, certolizumab pegol, or golimumab may be considered.[81] Favorable results have also been reported in small case series with the anti-IL6 monoclonal antibody tocilizumab and with the anti-IL1 biologics, anakinra and canakinumab.[82-84] There is very limited data on the use of Janus kinase (JAK) inhibitors in BS uveitis.[85-86] Zou et al. reported favorable results in 10 of 13 patients with BS uveitis treated with tofacitinib.[85] In the absence of randomized controlled trials and large clinical cohorts, there are no guidelines on the use of alternative immunomodulatory agents in patients who fail anti-TNF therapy. Randomized controlled trials could not prove the efficacy of daclizumab, secukinumab, or gevokizumab for the treatment of BS uveitis.[87-89]

The accumulated data suggest that biologic therapy should be started as first-line treatment in especially high-risk cases of BS uveitis, including those presenting with a severe panuveitis attack, diffuse fluorescein leakage with sight-threatening complications such as CME or NVD, or patients with irreversible damage in one or both eyes and still having active inflammation. The disease course is known to be more severe in young males; therefore, early, aggressive treatment is especially indicated in those cases. Patients with BS uveitis should be monitored by periodic FFA for subclinical background inflammation, and a complete resolution of FFA leakage should be sought in order to achieve long-term remission with preservation of potential vision.

9.9 VISUAL PROGNOSIS

The visual prognosis of BS patients used to be grim in the 1970s and the 1980s.[90, 91] An improvement in visual prognosis was reported with an earlier use of immunosuppressive agents and the availability of cyclosporine in the 1990s.[20] The estimated risk of losing useful vision (visual acuity better than 0.1; Snellen equivalent 20/200) at 7 years was significantly reduced from 30% in the 1980s to 21% in the 1990s in male patients. In the 2000s, there was further improvement with the use of interferon alpha and biologic agents in refractory cases.[68, 92, 93] A median visual acuity of 0.9 to 1.0 (Snellen equivalent 20/20) was maintained for 9 to 24 months in a large Japanese cohort of BS uveitis patients who started infliximab therapy between 2007 and 2010.[68] Taylor et al. reported that 10-year risk of severe visual loss was 13%, and anti-TNF treatment significantly reduced the risk at 5 and 10 years.[92] An expanding therapeutic armamentarium is required for the treatment of most refractory cases who have the highest risk of severe visual loss.[94]

9.10 SUMMARY

Ocular involvement in BS is typically in the form of relapsing and remitting nongranulomatous panuveitis and retinal vasculitis. Diffuse vitritis is an indication of posterior segment involvement. Transient retinal infiltrates are the most commonly seen inflammatory lesions and resolve with focal retinal atrophy that can be detected on OCT imaging. Retinal vasculitis predominantly involves the venous vasculature. Occlusive periphlebitis can cause retinal nonperfusion and foveal ischemia. Diffuse retinal capillary leakage is the most common finding on FFA and indicates uncontrolled disease, which is associated with a high risk of recurrent inflammatory attacks and cumulative damage. Visual prognosis has improved with the use of biologic agents that effectively control intra-ocular inflammation and prevent recurrences.

REFERENCES

1. Yazici H, Seyahi E, Hatemi G, et al. Behçet syndrome: a contemporary view. *Nat Rev Rheumatol.* 2018;14(2):107–119.
2. Soejima Y, Kirino Y, Takeno M, et al. Changes in the proportion of clinical clusters contribute to the phenotypic evolution of Behçet's disease in Japan. *Arthritis Res Ther.* 2021;23(1):49.
3. Yazici H, Ugurlu S, Seyahi E. Behçet syndrome: is it one condition? *Clin Rev Allergy Immunol.* 2021;43(3):275–280.
4. Yurdakul S, Gunaydin I, Tuzun Y, et al. The prevalence of Behçet's syndrome in a rural area in northern Turkey. *J Rheumatol.* 1988;15(5):820–822.
5. Kural-Seyahi E, Fresko I, Seyahi N, et al. The long-term mortality and morbidity of Behçet's syndrome: a 2-decade outcome survey of 387 patients followed at a dedicated center. *Medicine (Baltimore).* 2003;82(1):60–76.
6. Yazici Y, Adler NM. Clinical manifestations and ethnic background of patients with Behçet's syndrome in a US cohort. *Arthritis Rheum.* 2007;56(Suppl):S502.
7. International Study Group for Behçet's Disease. Criteria for diagnosis of Behçet's disease. *Lancet.* 1990;335(8697):1078–1080.
8. International Team for the Revision of the International Criteria for Behçet's Disease (ITR-ICBD). The International Criteria for Behçet's Disease (ICBD): a collaborative study of 27 countries on the sensitivity and specificity of the new criteria. *J Eur Acad Dermatol Venereol.* 2014:28(3):338–347.
9. Blake T, Pickup L, Carruthers D, et al. Birmingham Behçet's Service: classification of disease and application of the 2014 International Criteria for Behçet's Disease (ICBD) to a UK cohort. *BMC Musculoskelet Disord.* 2017;18(1):101.
10. Kobayashi T, Kishimoto M, Swearingen CJ, et al. Differences in clinical manifestations, treatment, and concordance rates with two major sets of criteria for Behçet's syndrome for patients in the US and Japan: data from a large, three-center cohort study. *Mod Rheumatol.* 2013;23(3):547–553.
11. de Menthon M, Lavalley MP, Maldini C, et al. HLA-B51/B5 and the risk of Behçet's disease: a systematic review and meta-analysis of case-control genetic association studies. *Arthritis Rheum.* 2009;61(10):1287–1296.
12. Kirino Y, Bertsias G, Ishigatsubo Y, et al. Genome-wide association analysis identifies new susceptibility loci for Behçet's disease and epistasis between HLA-B*51 and ERAP1. *Nat Genet.* 2013;45(2):202–207.
13. Hatemi G, Yazici H. Behçet's syndrome and micro-organisms. *Best Pract Res Clin Rheumatol.* 2011;25(3):389–406.
14. Seoudi N, Bergmeier LA, Drobniewski F, et al. The oral mucosal and salivary microbial community of Behçet's syndrome and recurrent aphthous stomatitis. *J Oral Microbiol.* 2015;7:27150.
15. Main DM, Chamberlain MA. Clinical differentiation of oral ulceration in Behçet's disease. *Br J Rheumatol.* 1992;31(11):767–770.
16. Mat MC, Goksugur N, Engin B, et al. The frequency of scarring after genital ulcers in Behçet's syndrome: a prospective study. *Int J Dermatol.* 2006;45(5):554–556.
17. Demirkesen C, Tuzuner N, Senocak M, et al. Clinicopathologic evaluation of nodular cutane-ous lesions of Behçet syndrome. *Am J Clin Pathol.* 2001;116(3):341–346.
18. Tascilar K, Melikoglu M, Ugurlu S, et al. Vascular involvement in Behçet's syndrome: a retrospec-tive analysis of associations and the time course. *Rheumatology (Oxford).* 2014;53(11):2018–2022.
19. Siva A, Saip S. The spectrum of nervous system involvement in Behçet's syndrome and its dif-ferential diagnosis. *J Neurol.* 2009;256(4):513–529.
20. Tugal-Tutkun I, Onal S, Altan-Yaycioglu R, et al. Uveitis in Behçet disease: an analysis of 880 patients. *Am J Ophthalmol.* 2004;138(3):373–380.
21. Tugal-Tutkun I, Gupta V, Cunningham ET. Differential diagnosis of Behçet uveitis. *Ocul Immunol Inflamm.* 2013;21(5):337–350.
22. Yang P, Fang W, Meng Q, et al. Clinical features of Chinese patients with Behçet's disease. *Ophthalmology.* 2008;115(2):312–318.

23. Kaçmaz RO, Kempen JH, Newcomb C, et al. Ocular inflammation in Behçet disease: incidence of ocular complications and of loss of visual acuity. *Am J Ophthalmol*. 2008;146(6):828–836.

24. Ostrovsky M, Rosenblatt A, Iriqat S, et al. Ocular Behçet disease–clinical manifestations, treatments and outcomes according to age at disease onset. *Biomedicines*. 2023;11(2):624.

25. Abd El Latif E, Abdel Kader Fouly Galal M, Tawfik MA, et al. Pattern of uveitis associated with Behçet's disease in an Egyptian cohort. *Clin Ophthalmol*. 2020;14:4005–4014.

26. Saleh OA, Birnbaum AD, Tessler HH, et al. Behçet uveitis in the American Midwest. *Ocul Immunol Inflamm*. 2012;20(1):12–17.

27. Posarelli C, Maglionico MN, Talarico R, et al. Behçet's syndrome and ocular involvement: changes over time. *Clin Exp Rheumatol*. 2020;38((5)Suppl 127):86–93.

28. Ksiaa I, Kechida M, Abroug N, et al. Changing pattern of clinical manifestations of Behçet's disease in Tunisia: comparison between two decades. *Reumatologia*. 2020;58(2):87–92.

29. Pathanapitoon K, Kunavisarut P, Saravuttikul FA, Rothova A. Ocular manifestations and visual outcomes of Behçet's uveitis in a Thai population. *Ocul Immunol Inflamm*. 2019; 27(1):2–6.

30. Standardization of Uveitis Nomenclature (SUN) Working Group. Classification criteria for Behçet disease uveitis. *Am J Ophthalmol*. 2021;228:80–88.

31. Khairallah M, Attia S, Yahia SB, et al. Pattern of uveitis in Behçet's disease in a referral center in Tunisia, North Africa. *Int Ophthalmol*. 2009;29(3):135–141.

32. Sachdev N, Kapali N, Singh R, et al. Spectrum of Behçet's disease in the Indian population. *Int Ophthalmol*. 2009;29(6):495–501.

33. Namba K, Goto H, Kaburaki T, et al. A major review: current aspects of ocular Behçet's disease in Japan. *Ocul Immunol Inflamm*. 2015;23(Suppl 1):S1–S23.

34. Khalsa A, Kelgaonkar A, Padhy SK, et al. Posterior subhyaloid precipitates: 'KPs' of the posterior segment. *Semin Ophthalmol*. 2021;36(8):751–756.

35. Oray M, Onal S, Bayraktar S, et al. Nonglaucomatous localized retinal nerve fiber layer defects in Behçet uveitis. *Am J Ophthalmol*. 2015;159(3):475–481.

36. Kido A, Uji A, Morooka S, et al. Outer plexiform layer elevations as a marker for prior ocular attacks in patients with Behçet's disease. *Invest Ophthalmol Vis Sci*. 2018;59(7):2828–2832.

37. Tugal-Tutkun I, Ozdal PC, Oray M, et al. Review for diagnostics of the year: multimodal imaging in Behçet uveitis. *Ocul Immunol Inflamm*. 2017;25(1):7–19.

38. Ostrovsky M, Ramon D, Iriqat S, et al. Retinal vascular occlusions in ocular Behçet disease – a comparative analysis. *Acta Ophthalmol*. 2023;101(6):619–626.

39. Ozdal PC, Ortaç S, Taşkintuna I, et al. Posterior segment involvement in ocular Behçet's disease. *Eur J Ophthalmol*. 2002;12(5):424–431.

40. Yahia SB, Kahloun R, Jelliti B, et al. Branch retinal artery occlusion associated with Behçet disease. *Ocul Immunol Inflamm*. 2011;19(4):293–295.

41. Esen E, Sizmaz S, Sariyeva A, et al. Bilateral central retinal artery occlusion in Behçet disease. *Ocul Immunol Inflamm*. 2015;23(5):416–419.

42. Ucar D, Mergen B, Gonen B, et al. Investigation of clinical profile of Behçet's syndrome-related versus idiopathic branch retinal vein occlusion. *Indian J Ophthalmol*. 2020;68(9):1876–1880.

43. Kang HM, Lee SC. Long-term progression of retinal vasculitis in Behçet patients using a fluorescein angiography scoring system. *Graefes Arch Clin Exp Ophthalmol*. 2014;252(6):1001–1008.

44. Kabaalioglu Guner M, Guner ME, et al. Correlation between widefield fundus fluorescein angiography leakage score and anterior chamber flare in Behçet uveitis. *Ocul Immunol Inflamm*. 2022:1–8.

45. Keorochana N, Homchampa N, Vongkulsiri S, et al. Fluorescein angiographic findings and Behçet's disease ocular attack score 24 (BOS24) as prognostic factors for visual outcome in patients with ocular Behçet's disease. *Int J Retina Vitreous*. 2021;7(1):48.

46. Tugal-Tutkun I, Onal S, Altan-Yaycioglu R, et al. Neovascularization of the optic disc in Behçet's disease. *Jpn J Ophthalmol*. 2006;50(3):256–265.

47. Shirahama S, Kaburaki T, Matsuda J, et al. The relationship between fluorescein angiography leakage after infliximab therapy and relapse of ocular inflammatory attacks in ocular Behçet's disease patients. *Ocul Immunol Inflamm*. 2020;28(8):1166–1170.

48. Keino H. Evaluation of disease activity in uveoretinitis associated with Behçet's disease. *Immunol Med*. 2021;44(2):86–97.

49. Tugal-Tutkun I, Onal S, Stanford M, et al. An algorithm for the diagnosis of Behçet disease uveitis in adults. *Ocul Immunol Inflamm*. 2021;29(6):1154–1163.

50. Tugal-Tutkun I, Onal S, Ozyazgan Y, et al. Validity and agreement of uveitis experts in interpretation of ocular photographs for diagnosis of Behçet uveitis. *Ocul Immunol Inflamm.* 2014;22(6):461–468.

51. Fragoulis GE, Bertsias G, Bodaghi B, et al. Treat to target in Behçet's disease: should we follow the paradigm of other systemic rheumatic diseases? *Clin Immunol.* 2023;246:109186.

52. Hatemi G, Christensen R, Bang D, et al. 2018 update of the EULAR recommendations for the management of Behçet's syndrome. *Ann Rheum Dis.* 2018;77(6):808–818.

53. Kötter I, Zierhut M, Eckstein AK, et al. Human recombinant interferon alfa-2a for the treatment of Behçet's disease with sight threatening posterior or panuveitis. *Br J Ophthalmol.* 2003;87(4):423–431.

54. Tugal-Tutkun I, Güney-Tefekli E, Urgancioglu M. Results of interferon-alfa therapy in patients with Behçet uveitis. *Graefes Arch Clin Exp Ophthalmol.* 2006;244(12):1692–1695.

55. Yang P, Huang G, Du L, et al. Long-term efficacy and safety of interferon alpha-2a in the treatment of Chinese patients with Behçet's uveitis not responding to conventional therapy. *Ocul Immunol Inflamm.* 2019;27(1):7–14.

56. Seyahi E. Phenotypes in Behçet's syndrome. *Intern Emerg Med.* 2019;14(5):677–689.

57. Markomichelakis N, Delicha E, Masselos S, et al. A single infliximab infusion vs corticosteroids for acute panuveitis attacks in Behçet's disease: a comparative 4-week study. *Rheumatology (Oxford).* 2011;50(3):593–597.

58. Tuncer S, Yilmaz S, Urgancioglu M, et al. Results of intravitreal triamcinolone acetonide (IVTA) injection for the treatment of panuveitis attacks in patients with Behçet disease. *J Ocul Pharmacol Ther.* 2007;23(4):395–401.

59. Coşkun E, Celemler P, Kimyon G, et al. Intravitreal dexamethasone implant for treatment of refractory Behçet posterior uveitis: one-year follow-up results. *Ocul Immunol Inflamm.* 2015;23(6):437–443.

60. Yalcinbayir O, Caliskan E, Ucan Gunduz G, et al. Efficacy of dexamethasone implants in uveitic macular edema in cases with Behçet disease. *Ophthalmologica.* 2019;241(4):190–194.

61. Sfikakis PP, Kaklamanis PH, Elezoglou A, et al. Infliximab for recurrent, sight-threatening ocular inflammation in Adamantiades-Behçet disease. *Ann Intern Med.* 2004;140(5):404–406.

62. Ohno S, Nakamura S, Hori S, et al. Efficacy, safety, and pharmacokinetics of multiple administration of infliximab in Behçet's disease with refractory uveoretinitis. *J Rheumatol.* 2004;31(7):1362–1368.

63. Tugal-Tutkun I, Mudun A, Urgancioglu M, et al. Efficacy of infliximab in the treatment of uveitis resistant to the combination of azathioprine, cyclosporine, and corticosteroids in Behçet's disease: an open-label trial. *Arthritis Rheum.* 2005;52(8):2478–2484.

64. Mushtaq B, Saeed T, Situnayake RD, et al. Adalimumab for sight-threatening uveitis in Behçet's disease. *Eye.* 2007;21(6):824–825.

65. Jaffe GJ, Dick AD, Brézin AP, et al. Adalimumab in patients with active noninfectious uveitis. *N Engl J Med.* 2016;375(10):932–943.

66. Nguyen QD, Merrill PT, Jaffe GJ, et al. Adalimumab for prevention of uveitic flare in patients with inactive non-infectious uveitis controlled by corticosteroids (VISUAL II): a multicentre, double-masked, randomised, placebo-controlled phase 3 trial. *Lancet.* 2016;388(10050): 1183–1192.

67. Hu Y, Huang Z, Yang S, Chen X, et al. Effectiveness and safety of anti-tumor necrosis factor-alpha agents treatment in Behçet's disease-associated uveitis: a systematic review and meta-analysis. *Front Pharmacol.* 2020;11:941.

68. Ohno S, Umebayashi I, Matsukawa M, et al. Safety and efficacy of infliximab in the treatment of refractory uveoretinitis in Behçet's disease: a large-scale, long-term postmarketing surveillance in Japan. *Arthritis Res Ther.* 2019;21(1):2.

69. Ueda S, Akahoshi M, Takeda A, et al. Long-term efficacy of infliximab treatment and the predictors of treatment outcomes in patients with refractory uveitis associated with Behçet's disease. *Eur J Rheumatol.* 2018;5(1):9–15.

70. Keino H, Okada AA, Watanabe T, et al. Long-term efficacy of infliximab on background vascular leakage in patients with Behçet's disease. *Eye.* 2014;28(9):1100–1106.

71. Sener H, Evereklioglu C, Horozoglu F, et al. Efficacy and safety of adalimumab in patients with Behçet uveitis: a systematic review and meta-analysis. *Ocul Immunol Inflamm.* 2023:1–9.

72. Yang S, Huang Z, Hu Y, et al. The efficacy of adalimumab as an initial treatment in patients with Behçet's retinal vasculitis. *Front Pharmacol.* 2021;12:609148.

73. Kim BH, Park UC, Park SW, et al. Ultra-widefield fluorescein angiography to monitor therapeutic response to adalimumab in Behçet's uveitis. *Ocul Immunol Inflamm*. 2022;30(6):1347–1353.
74. Fabiani C, Sota J, Vitale A, et al. Ten-year retention rate of infliximab in patients with Behçet's disease-related uveitis. *Ocul Immunol Inflamm*. 2019;27(1):34–39.
75. Atienza-Mateo B, Martín-Varillas JL, Calvo-Río V, et al. Comparative study of infliximab versus adalimumab in refractory uveitis due to Behçet's disease: national multicenter study of 177 cases. *Arthritis Rheumatol*. 2019;71(12):2081–2089.
76. Takeuchi M, Usui Y, Namba K, et al. Ten-year follow-up of infliximab treatment for uveitis in Behçet disease patients: a multicenter retrospective study. *Front Med (Lausanne)*. 2023;10:1095423.
77. Fabiani C, Sota J, Vitale A, et al. Cumulative retention rate of adalimumab in patients with Behçet's disease-related uveitis: a four-year follow-up study. *Br J Ophthalmol*. 2018;102(5):637–641.
78. Sfikakis PP, Arida A, Ladas DS, et al. Induction of ocular Behçet's disease remission after short-term treatment with infliximab: a case series of 11 patients with a follow-up from 4 to 16 years. *Clin Exp Rheumatol*. 2019;37((6)Suppl 121):137–141.
79. Sfikakis PP, Arida A, Panopoulos S, et al. Brief report: drug-free long-term remission in severe Behçet's disease following withdrawal of successful anti-tumor necrosis factor treatment. *Arthritis Rheumatol*. 2017;69(12):2380–2385.
80. Keino H, Watanabe T, Nakayama M, et al. Long-term efficacy of early infliximab-induced remission for refractory uveoretinitis associated with Behçet's disease. *Br J Ophthalmol*. 2021;105(11):1525–1533.
81. Tosi GM, Sota J, Vitale A, et al. Efficacy and safety of certolizumab pegol and golimumab in the treatment of non-infectious uveitis. *Clin Exp Rheumatol*. 2019;37(4):680–683.
82. Eser Ozturk H, Oray M, Tugal-Tutkun I. Tocilizumab for the treatment of Behçet uveitis that failed interferon alpha and anti-tumor necrosis factor-alpha therapy. *Ocul Immunol Inflamm*. 2018;26(7):1005–1014.
83. Arida A, Saadoun D, Sfikakis PP. IL-6 blockade for Behçet's disease: review on 31 anti-TNF naive and 45 anti-TNF experienced patients. *Clin Exp Rheumatol*. 2022;40(8):1575–1583.
84. Bettiol A, Silvestri E, Di Scala G, et al. The right place of interleukin-1 inhibitors in the treatment of Behçet's syndrome: a systematic review. *Rheumatol Int*. 2019;39(6):971–990.
85. Zou J, Lin CH, Wang Y, et al. Correspondence on 'a pilot study of tofacitinib for refractory Behçet's syndrome'. *Ann Rheum Dis*. 2023;82(4):e100.
86. Tao T, He D, Peng X, et al. Successful remission with upadacitinib in two patients with anti-TNF-refractory macular edema associated with Behçet's uveitis. *Ocul Immunol Inflamm*. 2023 Oct. 6:1–4.
87. Buggage RR, Levy-Clarke G, Sen HN, et al. A double-masked, randomized study to investigate the safety and efficacy of daclizumab to treat the ocular complications related to Behçet's disease. *Ocul Immunol Inflamm*. 2007;15(2):63–70.
88. Dick AD, Tugal-Tutkun I, Foster S, et al. Secukinumab in the treatment of noninfectious uveitis: results of three randomized, controlled clinical trials. *Ophthalmology*. 2013;120(4):777–787.
89. Tugal-Tutkun I, Pavesio C, De Cordoue A, et al. Use of gevokizumab in patients with Behçet's disease uveitis: an international, randomized, double-masked, placebo-controlled study and open-label extension study. *Ocul Immunol Inflamm*. 2018;26(7):1023–1033.
90. Mishima S, Masuda K, Izawa Y, et al. Behçet's disease in Japan: ophthalmological aspects. *Trans Am Ophthalmol Soc*. 1979;77:225–279.
91. BenEzra D, Cohen E. Treatment and visual prognosis in Behçet's disease. *Br J Ophthalmol*. 1986;70(8):589–592.
92. Taylor SR, Singh J, Menezo V, et al. Behçet disease: visual prognosis and factors influencing the development of visual loss. *Am J Ophthalmol*. 2011;152(6):1059–1066.
93. Cingu AK, Onal S, Urgancioglu M, et al. Comparison of presenting features and three-year disease course in Turkish patients with Behçet uveitis who presented in the early 1990s and the early 2000s. *Ocul Immunol Inflamm*. 2012;20(6):423–428.
94. Tugal-Tutkun I, Çakar Özdal P. Behçet's disease uveitis: is there a need for new emerging drugs? *Expert Opin Emerg Drugs*. 2020;25(4):531–547.

10 Ophthalmologic Involvement in Sjögren's Disease

Anna Flts, Esen Akpek, and Thomas Grader-Beck

10.1 INTRODUCTION: HISTORY, TERMINOLOGY, CLASSIFICATION, AND THE ROLE OF OPHTHALMOLOGY

Sjögren's is a systemic autoimmune disease that commonly presents with dry eye and dry mouth but may involve other organ manifestations in up to 50% of patients. The disease affects about 0.5% to 1% of the population.[1] However, it may be more common because of its frequent underdiagnosis. Sjögren's was first described in 1933 by Swedish ophthalmologist Dr. Henrik Sjögren in a group of 19 women with dry eye and dry mouth symptoms and suspected inflammatory arthritis.[2] The terminology was recently changed from Sjögren's syndrome to Sjögren's disease based on the efforts by the Sjögren's Foundation. The move toward this change stems from better understanding of the pathological basis and distinctiveness of the condition.[3]

Sjögren's disease was historically classified as primary and secondary. Primary Sjögren's referred to Sjögren's without any coexisting autoimmune disease, while secondary Sjögren's referred to Sjögren's in the presence of (an)other autoimmune disease(s).[4] Secondary Sjögren's is no longer recognized due to the emphasis on approaching Sjögren's disease with the same importance as any other autoimmune disease. Many have turned to terminology like "overlap Sjögren's" as a way to classify Sjögren's in the presence of another autoimmune disease, such as rheumatoid arthritis or systemic lupus erythematosus, while still maintaining the significance of the disease.

Currently, there is no single standard diagnostic criteria set that can help rule out Sjögren's. Therefore, Sjögren's remains a disease that is largely diagnosed based on clinical grounds supported by laboratory, histological, and functional testing.

Eye care providers play an important role in the diagnosis of Sjögren's disease and its appropriate management. Dry eye has been shown to precede the diagnosis of Sjögren's by a decade.[5] Therefore, we cannot overemphasize how critical it is to investigate patients with clinically significant aqueous tear deficiency for underlying autoimmune disorders like Sjögren's disease. More than 95% of patients with Sjögren's have clinically significant aqueous deficient dry eye.[6] Additionally, approximately 10% of patients with clinically significant dry eye have underlying Sjögren's disease,[5] highlighting the importance of screening for Sjögren's as a major focus in evaluating patients with dry eye.

10.2 EPIDEMIOLOGY AND RISK FACTORS

The underdiagnosis of Sjögren's disease may stem from the perception of it as a "rare" disease. However, studies have shown that Sjögren's is far from being rare. The epidemiology of Sjögren's disease showcases a varied prevalence across different populations, with estimates ranging between 0.5% to 1.0%.[1] In the United States, 400,000 to 3.1 million adults are currently living with Sjögren's disease.[1] A notable characteristic of this condition is its predominant occurrence in women, manifesting a gender disparity with a female-to-male ratio of around 9:1.[7] This ratio has been cited to be as high as 20:1 in some studies.[8] The typical dry eye and dry mouth symptoms might appear much earlier, but the formal diagnosis is made usually between the ages of 45 and 55 years old. No racial or geographic predilection has been identified.[3] Research has shown that people with a history of first-degree relative(s) with an autoimmune disease[9] are more likely to develop Sjögren's. Lastly, genetic studies have shown that DQA1*05:01, DQB1*02:01, and DRB1*03:01 alleles are risk factors.[10]

10.3 GLANDULAR AND EXTRAGLANDULAR MANIFESTATIONS

Sjögren's disease can present with a multitude of ocular, glandular, and extraglandular manifestations. Dry eye is the most common ocular manifestation of Sjögren's disease.[11] Typically, dry eye manifests as a persistent dry or gritty feeling or foreign body sensation of the eyes. Sometimes, particularly in patients with advanced dry eye, the main complaint may be fluctuating or blurry vision without significant eye discomfort. These symptoms are mainly due to a decrease in tear production by the main and accessory lacrimal glands in the setting of ocular surface inflammation. This inflammation may also lead to conjunctivitis, superficial keratitis,[11] episcleritis, or scleritis.[12] The reduced tear production increases the risk of corneal infections, epithelial defects, or ulcers due to a loss of the protective film of tears.[11, 13] Severe dryness and recurrent corneal ulcers may lead to scarring of the cornea (Figure 10.1) and decreased visual acuity.

DOI: 10.1201/9781003453710-10

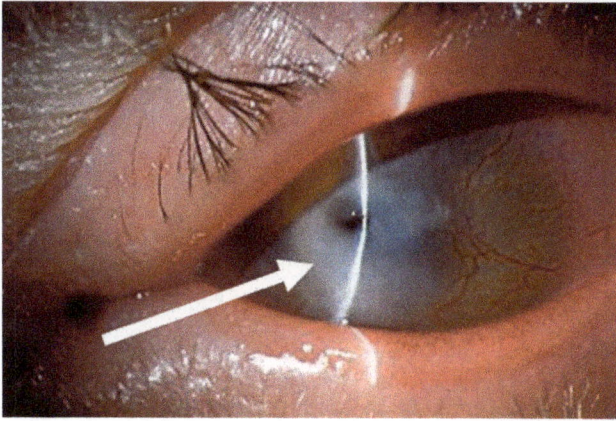

Figure 10.1 Slit lamp appearance (white arrow) of a patient with Sjögren's-related severe dry eye and corneal scarring, neovascularization, and perforation as a result of inflammation.

Although Sjögren's-related dry eye is typically known as aqueous deficient dry eye, meibomian gland dysfunction is also common and commonly overlooked. In addition, reduced corneal sensation is a prevalent finding in patients with Sjögren's disease, causing further dryness and inflammation due to impaired blink reflex and reduction in tear production.[14] Dry mouth due to decreased salivary gland production is another common glandular manifestation of the disease. Sjögren's may present with swelling of the submandibular or parotid glands, bilaterally or sometimes unilaterally. Acute swelling of the glands could also be due to bacterial sialadenitis due to overgrowth of microbial flora caused by dryness and inflammation.[13] Lack of saliva production can lead to poor oral health and the common occurrence of dental carries.[15]

Importantly, two-thirds of patients with Sjögren's disease have extraglandular systemic involvement. Clinical manifestations include inflammatory arthritis, interstitial lung disease, skin rashes and vasculitis, renal disease such as tubulointerstitial nephritis and renal tubular acidosis, peripheral and central nervous system involvement, myositis, and hematological (autoimmune cytopenia) abnormalities.[16, 17] Sjögren's disease has been associated with an increased risk of lymphoma, typically mucosa-associated lymphoid tissue (MALT) lymphoma that is most frequently found in the parotid glands.[18] The risk of lymphoma development has been documented as 43.8 times greater in Sjögren's patients compared to the normal population.[19] In addition, some patients may present with diffuse B cell lymphoma.[20] Commonly recognized risk factors for lymphoma include chronically swollen salivary glands, lymphadenopathy, cryoglobulins, C4 hypocomplementemia, monoclonal gammopathy, CD4 lymphopenia, and a high focus score on minor salivary gland biopsy.[21, 22] Recently, a scoring system has been proposed to calculate the risk of lymphoma among patients with Sjögren's disease: salivary gland enlargement, lymphadenopathy, Raynaud's phenomenon, high levels of anti-Ro/SSA autoantibodies, rheumatoid factor positivity, monoclonal gammopathy, and C4 hypocomplementemia[23] were included as the relevant factors. The risk of non-Hodgkin's lymphoma development was directly related to presence of these risk factors and ranged from a 3.8% increased risk with two or fewer risk factors to a 39.9% increased risk with the presence of three to six risk factors and 100% probability when all seven factors are present.[23]

10.4 KEY PATHOGENIC MARKERS AND MECHANISMS

Understanding the pathogenic mechanisms of Sjögren's disease is important for developing a multidisciplinary approach to treatment. First, genetic predisposition coupled with tissue damage, commonly due to viral infections or hormonal changes, may initiate early disease processes. Genome-wide association studies have revealed a number of human leukocyte antigens (HLA) and non-HLA alleles associated with Sjögren's, including HLA-DR3, HLA-DRB1, and HLA-DQB1, and variants in signal transducer and activator of transcription 4 (STAT4), CXC motif chemokine receptor 5 (CXCR5), TNF-alpha-induced protein 3 (TNFAIP3), protein tyrosine phosphatase non-receptor type 22 (PTPN22), interferon regulatory factor 5 (IRF5), and B cell activating factor (BAFF),[24] among others.[25] Early activation of the innate immune system[26, 27] is followed by the immune stimulation of the adaptive immune response and infiltration of both T and B cells into the exocrine glands.[1] This eventually leads to the dysfunction and destruction of both lacrimal and salivary gland tissues. Hyperactivity of type I interferon (IFN) and B cell activating factor (BAFF) production leads to B cell activation and hyperproliferation,[24] causing the secretion of autoantibodies, such as anti-Ro antibodies and M3 acetylcholine receptor antibodies[28] as well as the release of several cytokines, including interleukin (IL)-10 and transforming growth factor (TGF)-β, IL-2, IL-4, IL-6, IL-12, IFN-γ, and tumor necrosis factor (TNF)-α.[29] The chronic immune system activation and B cell infiltration of glandular tissues is responsible for diminished tear production by the lacrimal glands and diminished saliva production by salivary glands.[1] Typically, the clinical findings are more severe in patients with Sjögren's-related dry eye compared to non-Sjögren's with regard to tear production, tear film stability, corneal epithelial staining, and subbasal corneal nerve fiber density.[30]

Additional mechanisms also contribute to the clinical presentation. The cornea is the most densely innervated tissue supplied by the V1 branch of the trigeminal nerve.[31] A healthy nerve fiber plexus is essential for the proliferation and regeneration of corneal epithelial cells.[31] The latest research has shown a decrease in corneal sensitivity among patients with Sjögren's disease. When compared to patients with primarily evaporative dry eye in the setting of meibomian gland dysfunction, patients with Sjögren's dry eye disease have significantly reduced corneal sensitivity along with an increase in inflammatory cells density detected by in vivo confocal microscopy.[31] In addition to sicca and inflammation, the decreased corneal sensitivity due to the decreased nerve density[32] may be an additional etiological factor for the occurrence of corneal findings in Sjögren's.

10.5 CLASSIFICATION CRITERIA AND DIAGNOSTIC TOOLS IN SJÖGREN'S DISEASE

The most recent classification criteria for Sjögren's disease were published in 2016 and approved by both the European League Against Rheumatism (EULAR) and the American College of Rheumatology (ACR). The criteria are as follows:[33]

1. A patient must have at least one positive domain when screened with the EULAR Sjögren's Syndrome Disease Activity Index (ESSDAI), or they must answer "Yes" to at least one of the following questions developed by the American–European Consensus Group (AECG):[33]

    1. Have you had daily, persistent, troublesome dry eyes for more than 3 months? (Y/N)

    2. Do you have a recurrent sensation of sand or gravel in the eyes? (Y/N)

    3. Do you use tear substitutes more than 3 times a day? (Y/N)

    4. Have you had a daily feeling of dry mouth for more than 3 months? (Y/N)

    5. Do you frequently drink liquids to aid in swallowing dry food? (Y/N)

2. Next, a patient must not have any of the following: History of head and neck radiation treatment, active hepatitis C infection, AIDS, sarcoidosis, amyloidosis, graft-versus-host disease, or IgG4-related disease.

3. Last, a patient must have a total score ≥ 4 to meet the classification of Sjögren's disease, based on the weighted sum of the below 5 items (see Table 10.1).

10.5.1 Additional Diagnostic Approaches

Recently, a panel of novel auto-antibodies, namely anti-salivary protein 1 (anti-SP1), anti-carbonic anhydrase VI (anti-CA6), and anti-parotid secretory protein (anti-PSP), have been proposed as early Sjögren's antibodies.[34] Some studies suggested that these autoantibodies may identify Sjögren's patients early in their disease course and with more severe disease.[35] However, these findings were not corroborated by other studies.[36] It is important to highlight that utility of these antibodies is currently controversial and has yet to be validated in large-scale studies.

10.5.2 Ocular Testing

Although there is no pathognomonic clinical finding for Sjögren's-related dry eye, there are several tests that can be useful aids and that have been included in the 2016 classification criteria. These tests can be split into two categories: patient-reported symptoms and physician-measured signs.

Table 10.1 2016 ACR-EULAR Classification Criteria for Sjögren's Disease

Item	Criteria[33]	Weight/Score
1	Anti-SSA/Ro antibody positivity	3
2	Labial salivary gland with focal lymphocytic sialadenitis with a focus score of greater than or equal to 1 foci/4 mm^2	3
3	Ocular surface staining score of ≥5 (0–12) [or van Bijsterveld score ≥ 4 (0–9)] in one or both eyes	1
4	Schirmer's test result ≤ 5 mm/5 minutes in one or both eyes	1
5	Unstimulated whole salivary flow rate ≤ 0.1 mL/minute	1

10.5.3 Patient-Reported Symptoms

Recently, a three-question, evidence-based symptom survey was found to be useful in differentiating patients who are likely to have underlying Sjögren's, as follows:[4]

1. How often do your eyes feel dryness, discomfort, or irritation? Would you say it is often or constantly? (Y/N)

2. When you have eye dryness, discomfort, or irritation, does this impact your activities (e.g., do you stop or reduce your time doing them)? (Y/N)

3. Do you think you have dry eye? (Y/N)

A patient answering "Yes" to any of the three questions above would warrant a more comprehensive dry eye workup.

Another four-question symptom survey that is useful to screen dry eye patients for underlying Sjögren's disease is as follows:[37]

1. Is your mouth dry when eating a meal?

2. Can you eat a cracker without drinking a fluid or liquid?

3. How often do you have excessive tearing?

4. Are you able to produce tears?

Previously validated and more comprehensive questionnaires, such as the Ocular Surface Disease Index (OSDI), Standard Patient Evaluation of Eye Dryness questionnaire (SPEED), and the Symptom Assessment in Dry Eye survey (SANDE), are also available but are generally used in a clinical trial setting due to time and effort required.[38]

Lastly, the EULAR Sjögren's Syndrome Patient Reported Index (ESSPRI) is a validated tool for use in clinical trials as well as patient care.[39] It is a visual analog scale measuring pain, fatigue, and dryness (0–10). However, it should be noted that the ESSPRI has limited use for dry eye, as it only assesses overall dryness without any specific questions related to ocular dryness and does not assess vision-related symptoms.[40]

10.5.4 Physician-Measured Signs

Eye care providers can use several tests to aid in their diagnosis of Sjögren's disease, listed in the next section. These tests should be performed in the order listed here.

10.5.4.1 Measurement of Tear Quality

Tear osmolarity can be used to aid in the diagnosis of Sjögren's disease. Tear osmolarity is commonly measured with the TearLab Osmolarity System (TearLab™ Corp., San Diego, CA). Normal tear osmolarity should be ≤308 mOsm/L.[41] Research has shown that individuals with dry eye associated with Sjögren's disease may present with a higher tear osmolarity measure. There is no specific tear osmolarity cutoff in patients with Sjögren's disease; however, several studies have proposed a cutoff of 316 mOsm/L for moderate to severe aqueous deficient dry eye disease.[42] Per the Tear Film and Ocular Surface Society (TFOS) Dry Eye Workshop II, hyperosmolar tears damage the ocular surface either directly or by inducing an inflammatory cascade, which often activates genes encoding for inflammatory matrix metalloproteinases and pro-apoptotic factors. The inflammatory response leads to loss of goblet cells within the conjunctiva and dropout of corneal epithelial cells, which can manifest clinically as staining of the cornea or conjunctiva with vital dye tests.[43]

10.5.4.2 Measurement of Tear Production

Schirmer's test measures tear production within a 5-minute period by placing a strip of filter paper over the lateral section of the lower eyelid. For the testing of Sjögren's, topical anesthetics should not be administered per the 2016 classification criteria. Wetting of ≤ 5 mm in one or both eyes is an indication of an aqueous tear deficiency and can be a useful measure when considering a diagnosis of Sjögren's.[4]

10.5.4.3 Tear Film Stability

Tear breakup time (TBUT) is used to measure tear stability. TBUT is performed by using a drop of fluorescein dye to stain the tear film and measuring the time (in seconds) it takes for disruption in the tear film to occur when visualizing with the cobalt blue slit lamp light.[4] TBUT ≤ 10 seconds is considered abnormal.[44] A decrease in TBUT may be due to inadequate layer of mucin or oil in the tear film.

Meibomian gland dysfunction is frequently associated with Sjögren's, likely due to ocular surface inflammation.[11] The meibomian glands are sebaceous glands located on the upper and lower eyelid tarsal plates whose orifices are at the lid margins. These glands secrete lipids onto the ocular surface and promote tear film stability by reducing evaporation.[44] These glands can be assessed through visualization using a slit lamp, and the amount and quality of the sections are graded. Per the TFOS International Workshop on Meibomian Gland Dysfunction, meibomian gland dysfunction can be assessed using two components: meibum quality and expressibility of meibum.[45] Meibum quality is assessed by examining eight glands on the central portion of the lower lid.[45] Grading is measured from the following criteria (see Table 10.2).

10.5.4.4 Ocular Surface Damage Assessment

Ocular surface damage as measured with a vital dye staining score is another physician-measured finding that is arguably the most useful ocular element in the diagnosis of Sjögren's disease. Vital dyes can be used to visualize epithelial damage to the conjunctiva and cornea. The most common dyes used are lissamine green (Figure 10.2A) and fluorescein (Figure 10.2B), each of which has a separate scoring system.

Table 10.2 Tear Film and Ocular Surface Society Meibomian Gland Dysfunction Grading Criteria

	Meibum Quality[45]	Expressibility of Meibum[45]
Grade 0	Clear	All glands expressed
Grade 1	Cloudy	3 to 4 glands expressed
Grade 2	Cloudy with debris (granular)	1 to 2 glands expressed
Grade 3	Thick, toothpaste-like	No glands expressed

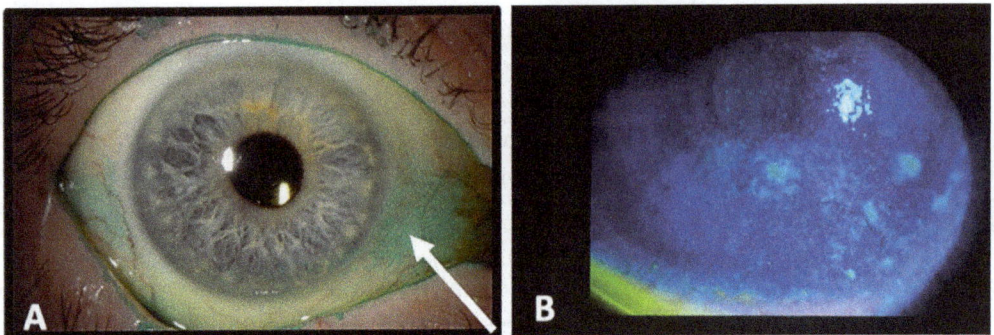

Figure 10.2 Slit lamp appearance of a patient with Sjögren's-related dry eye and (A) significant conjunctival lissamine green staining (white arrow) and (B) corneal fluorescein staining.

Table 10.3 The Sjögren's International Collaborative Clinical Alliance Ocular Staining Score: Corneal and Conjunctival Staining Criteria

	Corneal Staining Criteria[47]	Conjunctival Staining Criteria[47]
Grade 0	No staining	0 to 9 dots
Grade 1	1 to 5 dots	10 to 32 dots
Grade 2	6 to 30 dots	33 to 100 dots
Grade 3	> 30 dots	> 100 dots

The van Bijsterveld scoring system is used for rose bengal staining, albeit infrequently. The Sjögren's International Collaborative Clinical Alliance (SICCA) scoring system is the most commonly used grading system and is included in the 2016 classification criteria.[46] Based on the SICCA Ocular Staining Score (OSS), ocular surface damage can be assessed by both corneal and conjunctival staining using fluorescein and lissamine, respectively. Grading is measured for each following the criteria[47] in Table 10.3.

10.5.4.5 Other Measures

More recent research has shown that the matrix metalloproteinases, specifically MMP-9, may be elevated in the tears of patients with significant dry eye, albeit irrespective of the presence of Sjögren's. MMPs are proteolytic enzymes that can break down components of the extracellular matrix, leading to corneal epithelial cell dropout.[41] In addition, thrombospondin-1 (TSP-1) levels have been shown to be reduced among patients with dry eye in the setting of Sjögren's disease. TSP-1 is a glycoprotein that is expressed by ocular surface epithelial cells and has anti-inflammatory properties by inhibiting MMP-9.[48] Notably, the ratio of TSP-1 to MMP-9 was found to be significantly lower in dry eye with underlying Sjögren's disease compared to non-Sjögren's dry eye of similar severity.[48] These newer measures can be useful tools when assessing the presence of Sjögren's disease in patients with dry eye.

10.6 MANAGEMENT

10.6.1 Artificial Tears and Lubricants

Artificial tears and lubricants are commonly utilized to alleviate sicca symptoms regardless of underlying Sjögren's disease because they provide moisture to the ocular surface. The published literature supports the use of artificial tears to improve patient symptoms and ocular surface findings.[49–51] Hyaluronic acid, an important component of our extracellular matrix, is rich in hydroxyl groups, which allows it to attract water molecules and increase tear film stability.[52] A study of 40 patients with Sjögren's disease–related dry eye showed that both hypotonic 0.4% and isotonic 0.4% sodium hyaluronate drops used six times daily for a period of 3 months led to improved TBUT and corneal and conjunctival staining when compared to baseline.[49, 50]

Furthermore, sucralfate may act as a surface barrier, and aluminum sucrose sulfate 2% ophthalmic drops led to a significant improvement in conjunctival staining scores when used at least five times daily for 1 month in patients with Sjögren's-related dry eye.[49, 51]

10.6.2 Anti-Inflammatory Therapies

There is mounting evidence to suggest the use of topical anti-inflammatory therapy in treating patients with Sjögren's-related dry eye. Cyclosporine (CsA) works by inhibiting the expression of IL-2 and thereby preventing T cell activation and proliferation.[49, 53] Clinical trials that evaluated the use of 2% topical cyclosporine on Sjögren's disease–related dry eye showed significant improvement in TBUT scores and conjunctival staining after 2 months of use when compared to placebo (olive oil), but there was no significant change in Schirmer's test results.[49, 54] A study that looked at the use of 0.05% CsA drops in patients with Sjögren's disease–associated dry eye showed a significant improvement in TBUT and Schirmer's scores after both 1 week and 1 month.[55]

Although topical steroids have several well-known side effects over long-term use, short-term topical preservative-free methylprednisolone therapy has been shown to improve corneal staining scores, TBUT scores, and Schirmer test results in several previous studies.[49, 56]

Lastly, lifitegrast is a topical integrin antagonist and blocks the binding of intercellular adhesion molecule 1 (ICAM-1) to lymphocyte function-associated antigen 1 (LFA-1), interrupting the T cell–mediated inflammatory cascade and release of cytokines.[57] The efficacy of lifitegrast 5% ophthalmic solution has been studied in four randomized controlled studies that showed an improvement in symptoms among patients with dry eye, including improved corneal staining scores and OSDI scores.[58–62] However, research regarding the efficacy of lifitegrast in patients with Sjögren's disease dry eye is limited; further investigation is needed.

10.6.3 Other Therapies

Varenicline nasal spray is the first FDA-approved nasal spray for dry eye disease. Varenicline has a high affinity for the nicotinic acetylcholine receptor and can act as an agonist.[57] Varenicline nasal spray activates the nasolacrimal reflex, which increases tear production.[57] The ONSET-2 phase 3 randomized trial assessed the efficacy of varenicline nasal spray on dry eye disease over 6 months and showed statistically significant improvement in eye dryness scores and Schirmer's test scores compared to baseline.[63] The most common side effects are coughing and sneezing due to the route of administration.[63] However, there is no current research on the efficacy of varenicline nasal spray among Sjögren's patients.

Autologous serum eye drops can also be considered for the treatment of Sjögren's disease–related dry eye. Unlike artificial tears and lubricants, autologous serum contains many of the same components found in tears, including vitamin A, nerve growth factor, and epidermal growth factor,[49, 64] which can be advantageous in the treatment of dry eye. Platelet-rich plasma also has been considered as an effective treatment for dry eye associated with Sjögren's disease. Research suggests that the use of eye drops that contain platelet-rich plasma can improve ocular surface damage because platelets play an important role in wound healing.[64] A randomized clinical trial studied the efficacy of autologous serum and platelet-rich plasma in patients with Sjögren's disease and assessed various ocular parameters at baseline, 4 weeks, and 12 weeks.[64] Results showed a significant improvement in TBUT and ocular staining scores among both groups compared to baseline but no significant change in Schirmer's test or OSDI scores in either group.[64]

An amniotic membrane device (Prokera; BioTissue Inc, Doral, FL) may also be considered as a treatment for patients with Sjögren's disease dry eye. A small-scale case study showed an improvement in corneal and conjunctival staining; however, in all (six) patients, a relapse of symptoms was noted after removal of the membrane.[65] Given the limited studies on the efficacy of amniotic membrane implants in patients with Sjögren's disease, further research is needed.

10.6.4 In-Office Treatments and Procedures

Punctal plugs and tear duct cauterization are commonly used to conserve tears and improve tear volume. Patients with Sjögren's disease who had punctal plug insertion were followed for 1 year and showed a significant improvement in TBUT and Schirmer test scores.[49, 66] Similarly, another study that looked at short-term (6 weeks) efficacy of punctal occlusion among patients with Sjögren's disease and severe dry eye showed an improvement in eye discomfort and corneal punctate epithelial keratitis score determined using vital dye staining.[49, 67] The most common side effect following punctal plug occlusion is the loss of plugs, which occurs in about one-third of patients. The formation of pyogenic granulomas is another risk associated with punctal plug use. The granulomas can lead to partial or complete extrusion of the plug and cause discomfort.[68] Typically, the granulomas resolve a few weeks after removal of the plugs.[68]

Prosthetic Replacement of the Ocular Surface Ecosystem (PROSE) therapy is a custom scleral contact lens device that is filled with sterile preservative-free saline or other therapeutics and helps to provide constant lubrication to the ocular surface.[69] PROSE has been shown to improve visual acuity and dry eye symptoms among Sjögren's patients[69] and may be an ideal option for patients who have previously failed plugs.

Lastly, for patients with meibomian gland dysfunction, various in-office procedures to improve meibum and hence tear stability can be recommended. LipiFlow (Johnson & Johnson, Jacksonville, FL, USA),[70] a thermodynamic pulsatile therapeutic procedure, has been shown to improve meibomian gland scores, dry eye symptoms (measured via a SPEED score), and TBUT among patients with Sjögren's disease.[70]

10.6.5 Systemic Therapies

Systemic therapies may be considered in the management of Sjögren's disease in the setting of severe dry eye not responding to topical or local therapies. In addition, systemic immunosuppressive drugs may be appropriate for patients experiencing extraglandular and ocular manifestations of Sjögren's disease; although many of the drugs studied have shown some benefits, it is important to note that all large phase 3 trials[71] up until now have not shown any benefit for dry eye.

Systemic secretagogues, including pilocarpine (Salagen, Novartis Pharmaceuticals, Basel, Switzerland) and cevimeline (Evoxac, Daiichi Pharmaceutical Corp, Montvale, NJ), have been FDA approved to treat dry mouth. Both drugs are muscarinic cholinergic agonists that act on M3 receptors to stimulate exocrine glands.[49] Evidence suggests a significant relief of dry mouth symptoms, along with modest improvement in dry eye symptoms with both drugs,[49, 72, 73] with patients reporting a reduced need for artificial tear usage while on pilocarpine.[49, 72] Although these medications are generally considered safe, side effects such as sweating, flushing, and urinary frequency are not uncommon.[49, 13]

Hydroxychloroquine, a disease-modifying anti-rheumatic drug, is often used to treat various autoimmune diseases. Although the exact mechanism of action is not known, it is thought that the hydroxychloroquine interferes with macrophage antigen processing and T cell activation.[49, 74] With regard to Sjögren's disease, the use of hydroxychloroquine has not been found to improve sicca symptoms, although some studies have shown worsening TBUT, corneal staining, conjunctival staining, and dry eye symptoms after withdrawal of treatment.[49, 75] The pivotal JOQUER trial did not demonstrate any significant benefit for salivary flow or tear production.[76] Typically, hydroxychloroquine is used at a dose of ≤ 5 mg/kg to limit its toxicity.[77]

Other immunosuppressive medications, such as mycophenolic acid and methotrexate, are commonly used to treat the extraglandular ocular or systemic manifestations of Sjögren's disease. Mycophenolic acid works as a selective inhibitor of inosine monophosphate dehydrogenase, which inhibits nucleotide synthesis in T and B cells, inhibiting their proliferation.[49, 78, 79] Research that examined the efficacy of mycophenolic acid in treating patients with Sjögren's disease over a period of 6 months showed an improvement of subjective ocular dryness and reduced the need for artificial tears.[49, 78] Similarly, methotrexate, which works by inhibiting dihydrofolate reductase, has been tried in the treatment of Sjögren's disease. A 1-year pilot study examining the efficacy of methotrexate among patients with Sjögren's disease showed an improvement in the patient-reported measure of dry eyes and dry mouth but no significant improvement in the objective parameters.[49, 80] Immunosuppressive medications should not be used during times of active infection due to their potential to weaken the immune system's ability to fight off disease.

Systemic corticosteroids such as prednisone are often used to treat autoimmune disorders, including Sjögren's disease. Prednisone and other corticosteroids work by blocking phospholipase A2, which decreases the production of inflammatory mediators and suppresses the immune system.[81] A 6-month randomized controlled study examined the efficacy of prednisone among patients with Sjögren's disease; outcomes showed an improvement in salivary flow compared to baseline, but no significant improvement in dry eye measures was noted.[49, 82] However, corticosteroids are not without their effects, including immunosuppression, weight gain, anxiety, worsening diabetes, osteoporosis, elevated intraocular pressure, and cataracts.[83] Therefore, a careful consideration of a patient's individual health needs and circumstances is essential when determining the appropriateness of treatment.

10.6.6 Biologics and Additional Systemic Therapies

Rituximab, which targets CD20 molecules on B cells and leads to B cell depletion, may be beneficial in patients with Sjögren's disease due to the overactive B cells that commonly present with the disease.[49] An open-label phase 2 study that looked at the efficacy of rituximab treatment among patients with Sjögren's disease showed an improvement in TBUT and corneal staining score at 5 weeks and 12 weeks of follow-up compared to baseline, but no significant improvement in Schirmer's test scores was found.[49, 84]

Interferon alpha-2 can also be considered in the treatment of Sjögren's disease by modulating the immune system and exerting a suppressive effect. An open pilot study compared the effects of interferon alpha-2 to hydroxychloroquine in 20 patients with Sjögren's disease over an 11-month period. Results showed a statistically significant improvement in salivary and lacrimal function by 67% and 61% compared to 15% and 18%, respectively.[85]

Another pilot study investigated the efficacy of D-penicillamine in treating patients with Sjögren's disease.[86] Nineteen patients where followed, and results showed a statistically significant increase in salivary flow after 3 months of treatment compared to baseline. No statistically significant findings were observed with Schirmer's test and parotid salivary flow.[86] Eight patients had to stop treatment due to various side effects, with the most common side effect being loss of taste.[86]

Given the limited studies and small sample sizes, more research is needed to assess the efficacy of interferon alpha-2 and D-penicillamine among patients with Sjögren's disease.

Per the 2020 EULAR recommendations for the treatment of Sjögren's disease, corticosteroids should be considered a first-line option in patients with active systemic disease and should be used at the lowest effective dose. Immunosuppressive agents can be used as a second-line treatment, while biologics are considered as a third-line option.[87] However, careful systemic evaluation is needed before starting any immunosuppressive therapies to prevent side effects.[87]

10.7 DISEASE COURSE AND PROGNOSIS

Sjögren's is a slowly progressing disease that often presents with sicca symptoms but frequently causes extraglandular ocular and systemic manifestations, including keratitis, scleritis, uveitis, joint inflammation, lung involvement, decreased renal function, and increased risk for MALT and diffuse B cell lymphoma. The glandular and extraglandular manifestations, along with the chronic nature of Sjögren's disease, can take a negative toll on the patient's quality of life and cause significant morbidity and increased risk of mortality.[88]

An international study using the Sjögren's Registry data from 27 countries analyzed 11,372 primary Sjögren's disease patients over an average of 8.6 years, recording 876 (7.7%) deaths.[88] Information was available for 640 of the deaths, showing that 14% were due to systemic manifestations of Sjögren's disease.[88] The study showed that patients with a high systemic activity score on the ESSDAI and positive cryoglobulins had twice as high a risk of Sjögren's disease–related death.[88] Additionally, Sjögren's disease is recognized as a cause of disability by many social security systems. Research has showed an increased work disability status in patients with Sjögren's when compared to the general public in both Swedish[89] and Dutch[90] populations. Given the nature of the disease, it is very possible that there are similar trends among other populations.

Furthermore, looking at the outcomes of the "Living with Sjögren's" survey designed by the Sjögren's Foundation in conjunction with Harris Poll in 2016,[91] there are many burdens that patients living with Sjögren's disease face daily. Patients reported a high prevalence of symptoms including dry mouth (94%), dry eye (93%), and fatigue (82%).[91] Additionally, treatment burden was assessed, and results showed that 97% of participants used nonprescription eye drops, 88% used health food supplements, and 87% took vitamin D.[91] Therefore, the cost burden for patients with Sjögren's disease is also an important aspect to consider. Patients spent the most on dental coverage, at an average of $2026 yearly, which is, on average, higher than the general population,[92] along with prescription medications, over-the-counter medications, and the need for numerous healthcare appointments to manage their chronic illness.[53] Most importantly, almost all participants agreed that there is desire for new therapies to address dryness, fatigue, and the risk of lymphoma.[91]

Although the results have not yet been published in peer-reviewed journals, we can see many similar trends in the 2021 "Living with Sjögren's"[93] survey (https://sjogrens.org/sites/default/files/inline-files/LivingwithSjogrens-8.5x11-2022-Mar31_7pm.pdf), which highlights the need for prioritizing Sjögren's disease diagnosis and management in order to provide patients with a better quality of life.

10.8 SUMMARY

Sjögren's disease is a common autoimmune disorder, particularly among women, that is both underdiagnosed and underappreciated. Given the complex nature of the disease, its chronic and relentless clinical course, and vast array of symptoms, understanding the early presentation of the disease is key to timely diagnosis. Dry eye precedes the diagnosis of Sjögren's disease by a decade.[5] Improving education regarding signs and symptoms of the disease and heightening the awareness among eye care providers can help improve early detection. Along the same lines, educating patients regarding the dry eye and dry mouth symptoms potentially associated with Sjögren's can help reduce delays in seeking medical care. Dryness, fatigue, and joint pain decrease the quality of life of the afflicted patients considerably. Sjögren's-related dry eye has a significant impact on activities that require sustained gaze such as reading, driving, or computer work due to blurred vision and eye discomfort. More importantly, Sjögren's is not just dryness of the eyes and mouth. Two-thirds of patients may have serious extraglandular systemic or ocular manifestations, leading to significant morbidity and even mortality. Management of Sjögren's requires a multidisciplinary approach involving a team of healthcare professionals specialized in treating autoimmune diseases. Use of systemic medications specifically for ocular findings, whether severe dry eye or extraglandular ocular findings, requires a close collaboration between rheumatologists and ophthalmologists.

REFERENCES

1. Carsons SE, Patel BC. Sjogren syndrome. In: *StatPearls [Internet]*. Treasure Island, FL: StatPearls Publishing, 2023 Jan. Updated 2023 Jul. 31. https://www.ncbi.nlm.nih.gov/books/NBK431049/.
2. Sjögren H. On knowledge of keratoconjunctivitis sicca: keratitis filiformis due to lacrimal gland hypofunction. *Acta Ophthalmol*. 1933;1:1–151.
3. Baer AN, Hammitt KM. Sjögren's disease, not syndrome. *Arthritis Rheumatol*. 2021;73(7):1347–1348. doi:10.1002/art.41676.
4. Beckman KA, Luchs J, Milner MS. Making the diagnosis of Sjögren's syndrome in patients with dry eye. *Clin Ophthalmol*. 2015;10:43–53. Published 2015 Dec. 24. doi:10.2147/OPTH.S80043.
5. Akpek EK, Bunya VY, Saldanha IJ. Sjögren's syndrome: more than just dry eye. *Cornea*. 2019;38(5):658–661. doi:10.1097/ICO.0000000000001865.
6. Fernandez Castro M, Sánchez-Piedra C, Andreu JL, et al. Factors associated with severe dry eye in primary Sjögren's syndrome diagnosed patients. *Rheumatol Int*. 2018;38(6):1075–1082. doi:10.1007/s00296-018-4013-5.
7. Kassan SS, Moutsopoulos HM. Clinical manifestations and early diagnosis of Sjögren syndrome. *Arch Intern Med*. 2004;164(12):1275–1284. doi:10.1001/archinte.164.12.1275.
8. Alamanos Y, Tsifetaki N, Voulgari PV, et al. Epidemiology of primary Sjögren's syndrome in North-West Greece, 1982–2003. *Rheumatol Oxf Engl*. 2006;45:187–191.
9. Priori R, Medda E, Conti F, et al. Risk factors for Sjögren's syndrome: a case-control study. *Clin Exp Rheumatol*. 2007;25(3):378–384.
10. Cruz-Tapias P, Rojas-Villarraga A, Maier-Moore S, et al. HLA and Sjögren's syndrome susceptibility: a meta-analysis of worldwide studies. *Autoimmun Rev*. 2012 Feb.;11(4):281–287. doi:10.1016/j.autrev.2011.10.002. Epub 2011 Oct. 7. PMID:22001416.
11. Roszkowska AM, Oliverio GW, Aragona E, et al. Ophthalmologic manifestations of primary Sjögren's syndrome. *Genes (Basel)*. 2021;12(3):365. Published 2021 Mar. 4. doi:10.3390/genes12030365.
12. McGavin DD, Williamson J, Forrester JV, et al. Episcleritis and scleritis: a study of their clinical manifestations and association with rheumatoid arthritis. *Br J Ophthalmol*. 1976;60(3):192–226. doi:10.1136/bjo.60.3.192.
13. Vivino FB, Bunya VY, Massaro-Giordano G, et al. Sjogren's syndrome: an update on disease pathogenesis, clinical manifestations and treatment. *Clin Immunol*. 2019 June;203:81–121. doi:10.1016/j.clim.2019.04.009. Epub 2019 Apr. 29. PMID:31022578.
14. Adatia FA, Michaeli-Cohen A, Naor J, et al. Correlation between corneal sensitivity, subjective dry eye symptoms and corneal staining in Sjögren's syndrome. *Can J Ophthalmol*. 2004;39(7):767–771. doi:10.1016/s0008-4182(04)80071-1.
15. Mathews SA, Kurien BT, Scofield RH. Oral manifestations of Sjögren's syndrome. *J Dent Res*. 2008 Apr.;87(4):308–318. doi:10.1177/154405910808700411. PMID:18362310.
16. Fox RI. Extraglandular manifestations of Sjögren's syndrome (SS): dermatologic, arthritic, endocrine, pulmonary, cardiovascular, gastroenterology, renal, urology, and gynecologic manifestations. *Sjögren's Syndrome*. 2011;285–316. Published 2011 Apr. 12. doi:10.1007/978-1-60327-957-4_17.
17. Mihai A, Caruntu C, Jurcut C, et al. The spectrum of extraglandular manifestations in primary Sjögren's syndrome. *J Pers Med*. 2023 June 7;13(6):961. doi:10.3390/jpm13060961. PMID:37373950; PMCID:PMC10305413.
18. Yachoui R, Leon C, Sitwala K, et al. Pulmonary MALT lymphoma in patients with Sjögren's syndrome. *Clin Med Res*. 2017 June;15(1–2):6–12. doi:10.3121/cmr.2017.1341. Epub 2017 May 9. PMID:28487450; PMCID:PMC5573524.
19. Kassan SS, Thomas TL, Moutsopoulos HM, et al. Increased risk of lymphoma in sicca syndrome. *Ann Intern Med*. 1978 Dec.;89(6):888–892. doi 10.7326/0003-4819-89-6-888. PMID:102228.
20. Gorodetskiy VR, Probatova NA, Vasilyev VI. Characteristics of diffuse large B-cell lymphoma in patients with primary Sjögren's syndrome. *Int J Rheum Dis*. 2020;23(4):540–548. doi:10.1111/1756-185X.13800.
21. Solans-Laqué R, López-Hernandez A, Bosch-Gil JA, et al. Risk, predictors, and clinical characteristics of lymphoma development in primary Sjögren's syndrome. *Semin Arthritis Rheum*. 2011;41(3):415–423. doi:10.1016/j.semarthrit.2011.04.006.
22. Risselada AP, Kruize AA, Goldschmeding R, et al. The prognostic value of routinely performed minor salivary gland assessments in primary Sjögren's syndrome. *Ann Rheum Dis*. 2014;73(8):1537–1540. doi:10.1136/annrheumdis-2013-204634.

23. Fragkioudaki S, Mavragani CP, Moutsopoulos HM. Predicting the risk for lymphoma development in Sjogren syndrome: an easy tool for clinical use. *Medicine (Baltimore)*. 2016 June;95(25):e3766. doi:10.1097/MD.0000000000003766. PMID:27336863; PMCID:PMC4998301.

24. Li H, Ice JA, Lessard CJ, et al. Interferons in Sjögren's syndrome: genes, mechanisms, and effects. *Front Immunol*. 2013 Sept. 20;4:290. doi:10.3389/fimmu.2013.00290. PMID:24062752; PMCID:PMC3778845.

25. Yura Y, Hamada M. Outline of salivary gland pathogenesis of Sjögren's syndrome and current therapeutic approaches. *Int J Mol Sci*. 2023;24(13):11179. Published 2023 Jul. 6. doi:10.3390/ijms241311179.

26. Nguyen CQ, Peck AB. Unraveling the pathophysiology of Sjogren syndrome-associated dry eye disease. *Ocul Surf*. 2009 Jan.;7(1):11–27. doi:10.1016/s1542-0124(12)70289-6. PMID:19214349; PMCID:PMC2861866.

27. Wu KY, Kulbay M, Tanasescu C, et al. An overview of the dry eye disease in Sjögren's syndrome using our current molecular understanding. *Int J Mol Sci*. 2023 Jan. 13;24(2):1580. doi:10.3390/ijms24021580. PMID:36675090; PMCID:PMC9866656.

28. Abe S, Tsuboi H, Kudo H, et al. M3 muscarinic acetylcholine receptor-reactive Th17 cells in primary Sjögren's syndrome. *JCI Insight*. 2020;5(15):e135982. Published 2020 Aug. 6. doi:10.1172/jci.insight.135982.

29. Kroese FG, Abdulahad WH, Haacke E, et al. B-cell hyperactivity in primary Sjögren's syndrome. *Expert Rev Clin Immunol*. 2014;10(4):483–499. doi:10.1586/1744666X.2014.891439.

30. Zhao S, Le Q. Analysis of the first tear film break-up point in Sjögren's syndrome and non-Sjögren's syndrome dry eye patients. *BMC Ophthalmol*. 2022;22(1). doi:10.1186/s12886-021-02233-6.

31. Luzu J, Labbé A, Réaux-Le Goazigo A, et al. In vivo confocal microscopic study of corneal innervation in Sjögren's Syndrome with or without small fiber neuropathy. *Ocul Surf*. 2022 Jul.;25:155–162. doi:10.1016/j.jtos.2022.07.003. Epub 2022 Jul. 22. PMID:35872076.

32. Tuisku IS, Konttinen YT, Konttinen LM, et al. Alterations in corneal sensitivity and nerve morphology in patients with primary Sjögren's syndrome. *Exp Eye Res*. 2008 June;86(6):879–885. doi:10.1016/j.exer.2008.03.002. Epub 2008 Mar. 12. PMID:18436208.

33. Shiboski CH, Shiboski SC, Seror R, et al. 2016 American College of Rheumatology/European League Against Rheumatism classification criteria for primary Sjögren's syndrome: a consensus and data-driven methodology involving three international patient cohorts. *Arthritis Rheumatol*. 2017 Jan.;69(1):35–45. doi:10.1002/art.39859. Epub 2016 Oct. 26. PMID:27785888; PMCID:PMC5650478.

34. Karakus S, Baer AN, Agrawal D, et al. Utility of novel autoantibodies in the diagnosis of Sjögren's syndrome among patients with dry eye. *Cornea*. 2018;37(4):405–411. doi:10.1097/ICO.0000000000001471.

35. Veenbergen S, Kozmar A, van Daele PLA, et al. Autoantibodies in Sjögren's syndrome and its classification criteria. *J Transl Autoimmun*. 2021;5:100138. Published 2021 Dec. 27. doi:10.1016/j.jtauto.2021.100138.

36. Thatayatikom A, Jun I, Bhattacharyya I, et al. The diagnostic performance of early Sjögren's syndrome autoantibodies in juvenile Sjögren's syndrome: the University of Florida pediatric cohort study. *Front Immunol*. 2021;12:704193. Published 2021 June 25. doi:10.3389/fimmu.2021.704193.

37. Bunya VY, Maguire MG, Akpek EK, et al. A new screening questionnaire to identify patients with dry eye with a high likelihood of having Sjögren syndrome. *Cornea*. 2021;40(2):179–187. doi:10.1097/ICO.0000000000002515.

38. Foulks GN, Forstot SL, Donshik PC, et al. Clinical guidelines for management of dry eye associated with Sjögren disease. *Ocul Surf*. 2015;13(2):118–132. doi:10.1016/j.jtos.2014.12.001.

39. Seror R, Ravaud P, Mariette X, et al. EULAR Sjogren's syndrome patient reported index (ESSPRI): development of a consensus patient index for primary Sjogren's syndrome. *Ann Rheum Dis*. 2011;70(6):968–972. PubMed:21345815.

40. Saldanha IJ, Bunya VY, McCoy SS, et al. Ocular manifestations and burden related to Sjögren syndrome: results of a patient survey. *Am J Ophthalmol*. 2020;219:40–48. doi:10.1016/j.ajo.2020.05.043.

41. Lemp MA, Bron AJ, Baudouin C, et al. Tear osmolarity in the diagnosis and management of dry eye disease. *Am J Ophthalmol*. 2011;151(5):792–798.e1. doi:10.1016/j.ajo.2010.10.032.

42. Bunya VY, Langelier N, Chen S, et al. Tear osmolarity in Sjögren syndrome. *Cornea.* 2013;32(7):922–927. doi:10.1097/ICO.0b013e31827e2a5e.
43. Bron AJ, de Paiva CS, Chauhan SK, et al. TFOS DEWS II pathophysiology report [published correction appears in *Ocul Surf.* 2019 Oct.;17(4):842; *Ocul Surf.* 2017;15(3):438–510. doi:10.1016/j.jtos.2017.05.011.
44. Chan TCY, Chow SSW, Wan KHN, et al. Update on the association between dry eye disease and meibomian gland dysfunction. *Hong Kong Med J.* 2019;25(1):38–47. doi:10.12809/hkmj187331.
45. Nichols JJ, Berntsen DA, Mitchell GL, et al. An assessment of grading scales for meibography images. *Cornea.* 2005;24:382–388.
46. Shiboski SC, Shiboski CH, Criswell L, et al. American College of Rheumatology classification criteria for Sjögren's syndrome: a data-driven, expert consensus approach in the Sjögren's International Collaborative Clinical Alliance cohort. *Arthritis Care Res (Hoboken).* 2012;64(4):475–487. doi:10.1002/acr.21591.
47. Whitcher JP, Shiboski CH, Shiboski SC, et al. A simplified quantitative method for assessing keratoconjunctivitis sicca from the Sjögren's syndrome international registry. *Am J Ophthalmol.* 2010;149(3):405–415. doi:10.1016/j.ajo.2009.09.013.
48. Masli S, Akpek EK. Reduced tear thrombospondin-1/matrix metalloproteinase-9 ratio can aid in detecting Sjögren's syndrome etiology in patients with dry eye. *Clin Transl Sci.* 2022 Aug.;15(8):1999–2009. doi:10.1111/cts.13316. Epub 2022 June 8. PMID:35610740; PMCID:PMC9372415.
49. Akpek EK, Lindsley KB, Adyanthaya RS, et al. Treatment of Sjögren's syndrome-associated dry eye an evidence-based review. *Ophthalmology.* 2011 Jul.;118(7):1242–1252. doi:10.1016/j.ophtha.2010.12.016. Epub 2011 Apr. 3. PMID:21459453.
50. Aragona P, Di Stefano G, Ferreri F, et al. Sodium hyaluronate eye drops of different osmolarity for the treatment of dry eye in Sjögren's syndrome patients. *Br J Ophthalmol.* 2002;86(8):879–884. doi:10.1136/bjo.86.8.879.
51. Prause JU, Bjerrum K, Johansen S. Effects of sodium sucrose-sulfate on the ocular surface of patients with keratoconjunctivitis sicca in Sjögren's syndrome. *Adv Exp Med Biol.* 1994;350:691–696.
52. Hynnekleiv L, Magno M, Vernhardsdottir RR, et al. Hyaluronic acid in the treatment of dry eye disease. *Acta Ophthalmol.* 2022;100(8):844–860. doi:10.1111/aos.15159.
53. Hess AD, Colombani PM, Esa AH. Cyclosporine and the immune response: basic aspects. *Crit Rev Immunol.* 1986;6:123–149.
54. Gündüz K, Ozdemir O. Topical cyclosporin treatment of keratoconjunctivitis sicca in secondary Sjögren's syndrome. *Acta Ophthalmol (Copenh).* 1994;72:438–442.
55. Devecı H, Kobak S. The efficacy of topical 0.05% cyclosporine A in patients with dry eye disease associated with Sjögren's syndrome. *Int Ophthalmol.* 2014;34(5):1043–1048. doi:10.1007/s10792-014-9901-4.
56. Hong S, Kim T, Chung SH, et al. Recurrence after topical nonpreserved methylprednisolone therapy for keratoconjunctivitis sicca in Sjögren's syndrome. *J Ocul Pharmacol Ther.* 2007;23:78–82.
57. Wu KY, Chen WT, Chu-Bédard YK, et al. Management of Sjogren's dry eye disease-advances in ocular drug delivery offering a new hope. *Pharmaceutics.* 2022 Dec. 31;15(1):147. doi:10.3390/pharmaceutics15010147. PMID:36678777; PMCID:PMC9861012.
58. Lollett IV, Galor A. Dry eye syndrome: developments and lifitegrast in perspective. *Clin Ophthalmol.* 2018;12:125–139. Published 2018 Jan. 15. doi:10.2147/OPTH.S126668.
59. Semba CP, Torkildsen GL, Lonsdale JD, et al. A phase 2 randomized, double-masked, placebo-controlled study of a novel integrin antagonist (SAR 1118) for the treatment of dry eye. *Am J Ophthalmol.* 2012;153(6):1050.e1–1060.e1.
60. Sheppard JD, Torkildsen GL, Lonsdale JD, et al. Lifitegrast ophthalmic solution 5.0% for treatment of dry eye disease: results of the OPUS-1 phase 3 study. *Ophthalmology.* 2014;121(2):475–483.
61. Tauber J, Karpecki P, Latkany R, et al. Lifitegrast ophthalmic solution 5.0% vs placebo for treatment of dry eye disease: results of the randomized phase III OPUS-2 study. *Ophthalmology.* 2015;122(12):2423–2431.
62. Holland EJ, Luchs J, Karpecki PM, et al. Lifitegrast for the treatment of dry eye disease: results of a phase III, randomized, double-masked, placebo-controlled trial (OPUS-3). *Ophthalmology.* 2017;124(1):53–60.

63. Wirta D, Vollmer P, Paauw J, et al. Efficacy and safety of OC-01 (varenicline solution) nasal spray on signs and symptoms of dry eye disease: the ONSET-2 phase 3 randomized trial. *Ophthalmology.* 2022;129(4):379–387. doi:10.1016/j.ophtha.2021.11.004.

64. Kang MJ, Lee JH, Hwang J, et al. Efficacy and safety of platelet-rich plasma and autologous-serum eye drops for dry eye in primary Sjögren's syndrome: a randomized trial. *Sci Rep.* 2023;13:19279. doi:10.1038/s41598-023-46671-2.

65. Shafer B, Fuerst NM, Massaro-Giordano M, et al. The use of self-retained, cryopreserved amniotic membrane for the treatment of Sjögren syndrome: a case series. *Digit J Ophthalmol.* 2019;25(2):21–25. Published 2019 June 8. doi:10.5693/djo.01.2019.02.005.

66. Egrilmez S, Aslan F, Karabulut G, et al. Clinical efficacy of the Smartplug in the treatment of primary Sjögren's syndrome with keratoconjunctivitis sicca: one-year follow-up study. *Rheumatol Int.* 2010 May 21;31. [Epub ahead of print].

67. Mansour K, Leonhardt CJ, Kalk WW, et al. Lacrimal punctum occlusion in the treatment of severe keratoconjunctivitis sicca caused by Sjögren syndrome: a uniocular evaluation. *Cornea.* 2007;26:147–150.

68. Kim BM, Osmanovic SS, Edward DP. Pyogenic granulomas after silicone punctal plugs: a clinical and histopathologic study. *Am J Ophthalmol.* 2005 Apr.;139(4):678–684. doi:10.1016/j.ajo.2004.11.059. PMID:15808164.

69. Pan BX, Chiu GB, Heur M. Prosthetic replacement of the ocular surface ecosystem therapy for Sjogren's syndrome patients. *Invest Ophthalmol Vis Sci.* 2016;57(12):3890.

70. Epitropoulos AT, Goslin K, Bedi R, et al. Meibomian gland dysfunction patients with novel Sjögren's syndrome biomarkers benefit significantly from a single vectored thermal pulsation procedure: a retrospective analysis. *Clin Ophthalmol.* 2017 Apr. 13;11:701–706. doi:10.2147/OPTH.S119926. PMID:28458508; PMCID:PMC5402721.

71. Baer AN, Gottenberg J, St Clair EW, et al. Efficacy and safety of abatacept in active primary Sjögren's syndrome: results of a phase III, randomised, placebo-controlled trial. *Ann Rheum Dis.* 2021;80:339–348.

72. Papas AS, Sherrer YS, Charney M, et al. Successful treatment of dry mouth and dry eye symptoms in Sjögren's syndrome patients with oral pilocarpine: a randomized, placebo-controlled, dose-adjustment study. *J Clin Rheumatol.* 2004;10:169–177.

73. Petrone D, Condemi JJ, Fife R, et al. A double-blind, randomized, placebo-controlled study of cevimeline in Sjögren's syndrome patients with xerostomia and keratoconjunctivitis sicca. *Arthritis Rheum.* 2002;46:748–754.

74. Fox RI, Kang HI. Mechanism of action of antimalarial drugs: inhibition of antigen processing and presentation. *Lupus.* 1993;2(Suppl):S9–S12.

75. Yavuz S, Asfurogˆlu E, Bicakcigil M, et al. Hydroxychloroquine improves dry eye symptoms of patients with primary Sjögren's syndrome. *Rheumatol Int.* 2010 Mar. 23;31. [Epub ahead of print].

76. Gottenberg JE, Ravaud P, Puéchal X, et al. Effects of hydroxychloroquine on symptomatic improvement in primary Sjögren syndrome: the JOQUER randomized clinical trial. *JAMA.* 2014;312(3):249–258. doi:10.1001/jama.2014.7682.

77. Stokkermans TJ, Falkowitz DM, Trichonas G. Chloroquine and hydroxychloroquine toxicity. In: *StatPearls [Internet].* Treasure Island, FL: StatPearls Publishing, 2023 Jan. Updated 2023 Aug. 18. https://www.ncbi.nlm.nih.gov/books/NBK537086/#.

78. Willeke P, Schlüter B, Becker H, et al. Mycophenolate sodium treatment in patients with primary Sjögren syndrome: a pilot trial. *Arthritis Res Ther.* 2007;9(6):R115. doi:10.1186/ar2322. PMID:17986340; PMCID:PMC2246233.

79. Allison AC, Eugui EM. Mycophenolate mofetil and its mechanisms of action. *Immunopharmacology.* 2000;47:85–118.

80. Skopouli FN, Jagiello P, Tsifetaki N, et al. Methotrexate in primary Sjögren's syndrome. *Clin Exp Rheumatol.* 1996;14:555–558.

81. Sorenson DK, Kelly TM, Murray DK, et al. Corticosteroids stimulate an increase in phospholipase A2 inhibitor in human serum. *J Steroid Biochem.* 1988;29(2):271–273. doi:10.1016/0022-4731(88)90276-2.

82. Fox PC, Datiles M, Atkinson JC, et al. Prednisone and piroxicam for treatment of primary Sjögren's syndrome. *Clin Exp Rheumatol.* 1993;11:149–156.

83. Liu D, Ahmet A, Ward L, et al. A practical guide to the monitoring and management of the complications of systemic corticosteroid therapy. *Allergy Asthma Clin Immunol*. 2013;9(1):30. Published 2013 Aug. 15. doi:10.1186/1710-1492-9-30.

84. Pijpe J, van Imhoff GW, Spijkervet FK, et al. Rituximab treatment in patients with primary Sjögren's syndrome: an open-label phase II study. *Arthritis Rheum*. 2005;52:2740–2750.

85. Ferraccioli GF, Salaffi F, De Vita S, et al. Interferon alpha-2 (IFN alpha 2) increases lacrimal and salivary function in Sjögren's syndrome patients: preliminary results of an open pilot trial versus OH-chloroquine. *Clin Exp Rheumatol*. 1996;14(4):367–371.

86. ter Borg EJ, Haanen HC, Haas FJ, et al. Treatment of primary Sjögren's syndrome with D-penicillamine: a pilot study. *Neth J Med*. 2002;60(10):402–406.

87. Ramos-Casals M, Brito-Zerón P, Bombardieri S, et al. EULAR recommendations for the management of Sjögren's syndrome with topical and systemic therapies. *Ann Rheum Dis*. 2020;79(1):3–18. doi:10.1136/annrheumdis-2019-216114.

88. Brito-Zerón P, Flores-Chávez A, Horváth IF, et al. Mortality risk factors in primary Sjögren syndrome: a real-world, retrospective, cohort study. *EClinicalMedicine*. 2023;61:102062. Published 2023 Jul. 4. doi:10.1016/j.eclinm.2023.102062.

89. Mandl T, Jørgensen TS, Skougaard M, et al. Work disability in newly diagnosed patients with primary Sjögren syndrome. *J Rheumatol*. 2017 Feb.;44(2):209–215. doi:10.3899/jrheum.160932. Epub 2016 Nov. 15. PMID:28148755.

90. Meijer JM, Meiners PM, Huddleston Slater JJ, et al. Health-related quality of life, employment and disability in patients with Sjogren's syndrome. *Rheumatology (Oxford)*. 2009;48(9):1077–1082. doi:10.1093/rheumatology/kep141.

91. McCoy SS, Woodham M, Bunya VY, et al. A comprehensive overview of living with Sjögren's: results of a national Sjögren's Foundation survey. *Clin Rheumatol*. 2022 Jul.;41(7):2071–2078. doi:10.1007/s10067-022-06119-w. Epub 2022 Mar. 8. PMID:35257256; PMCID:PMC9610846.

92. Hung M, Lipsky MS, Moffat R, et al. Health and dental care expenditures in the United States from 1996 to 2016. *PLoS One*. 2020;15(6):e0234459. Published 2020 June 11. doi:10.1371/journal.pone.0234459.

93. Sjögren's Foundation. *Living with Sjögren's* [PDF document]. 2022. https://sjogrens.org/sites/default/files/inline-files/LivingwithSjogrens-8.5x11-2022-Mar31_7pm.pdf.

11 Ophthalmologic Disease in IgG4-Related Disease

Curtis E. Margo, Norberto Mancera, and Zachary S. Wallace

11.1 INTRODUCTION

The subclasses of IgG immunoglobulins had been discovered and largely characterized by the 1960s, but only in the last few decades have their roles in the context of human disease been widely recognized. One of the most recent disorders associated with a single subclass immunoglobulin is *IgG4-related disease (-RD)*, a multisystem fibroinflammatory condition with wide-ranging clinical manifestations. IgG4-positive plasma cells at the center of this disease were first observed among dense inflammatory infiltrates of the pancreas and hepatobiliary tract before they were associated with elevated serum IgG4.[1] The inflamed pancreatic disease, commonly referred to as type 1 auto-immune pancreatitis, is now recognized as a common manifestation of IgG4-RD.[2] The key histopathologic features in these cases were scrutinized and expanded beyond the IgG4-plasma cell–rich infiltrate to include fibrosis – often described as "storiform" – and obliterative phlebitis.

The association of elevated serum IgG4 with the histopathologic triad described already would soon be recognized in other organs and tissues, like the salivary gland, kidney, aorta, thyroid, and mediastinum.[3] As this knowledge diffused through the medical community, retrospective studies confirmed that many cases of IgG4-RD had previously gone unrecognized. For example, a retrospective study of thoracic aortitis found as many as 10% displayed IgG4 plasma cell–rich fibrous inflammation.[4,5] In another series, over 50% of cases previously reported to be "idiopathic" retroperitoneal fibrosis were found to be IgG4-RD.[6] The birth of this novel multisystem inflammatory disease got off to an explosive start, with cases reported from around the world across racial and ethnic groups. The flood of case reports and series forced clinicians to reexamine dozens of entrenched eponyms (e.g., Ormond's disease, Riedel's thyroiditis, Küttner's tumor, etc.) and replaced them with IgG4-RD. The same process took place for many purely descriptive diagnoses (e.g., multifocal fibro-sclerosis, periaortitis, sclerosing mesenteritis, etc.) that had been entrenched in the medical vernacu-lar. The effort in finding a single suitable term for these antiquated diagnoses likely helped speed the acceptance of the new entity.[7]

Seldom has such a seemingly diverse assortment of disorders of unknown etiology been placed under an umbrella of presumed shared pathogenesis. This chapter will review those components of IgG4-RD that affect the eye and ocular adnexa, the latter term referring to the conjunctiva, eyelids, and tissues contained within the orbit, including the lacrimal gland and optic nerve.

11.2 DIAGNOSIS

The gold standard for IgG4-RD was initially defined by histopathologic and immunohistochemical criteria. Typical morphologic features include a dense polyclonal (and T cell–rich) lymphoplasma-cytic infiltrate in which the number of IgG4-positive plasma cells is greater than 10/high-power microscopic field, and the ratio of IgG4-positive plasma cells to IgG-plasma cells is usually greater than 40%.[8] Since the distribution of plasma cells is not uniform throughout any involved tissue, this leaves the pathologist some flexibility in finding the most appropriate area to count cells. Other key findings are fibrosis, which can be highly variable depending on the stage of the disease (and the tis-sue involved) (Figure 11.1). The characteristic arrangement of fibrous tissue is described as storiform, which, according to Stedman's Medical Dictionary, means "having a cartwheel pattern." A third key feature is obliterative phlebitis, although it may be the least consistently reported finding in the early literature. The distinction between obliterative and non-obliterative venous inflammation is a matter of judgement. Inflammation of small venous channels must also be distinguished from small-vessel vasculitis characterized by vessel wall necrosis. Eosinophils are often encountered in IgG4-RD in mild to moderate numbers, but prominent neutrophilic infiltrates are distinctly uncom-mon. Obliterative arteritis may also be encountered, particularly in affected lung tissue. Certain pathology findings help exclude IgG4-RD, including granulomas, granulomatous inflammation, vasculitis, and prominent necrosis.

It is important to recognize that this combination of histopathologic features, and any of them individually, are not specific to IgG4-RD, including the high density of IgG4-plasma cells. They can be encountered in certain malignancies, inflammatory myofibroblastic proliferation, several rheu-matologic diseases, several types of vasculitis, and certain macrophage/histiocytic disorders.[9, 10] Other conditions with dense collections of lymphocytes – like indolent lymphomas (e.g., extranodal marginal zone lymphoma, etc.), Castleman's disease, and Kimura's disease – present challenging

DOI: 10.1201/9781003453710-11

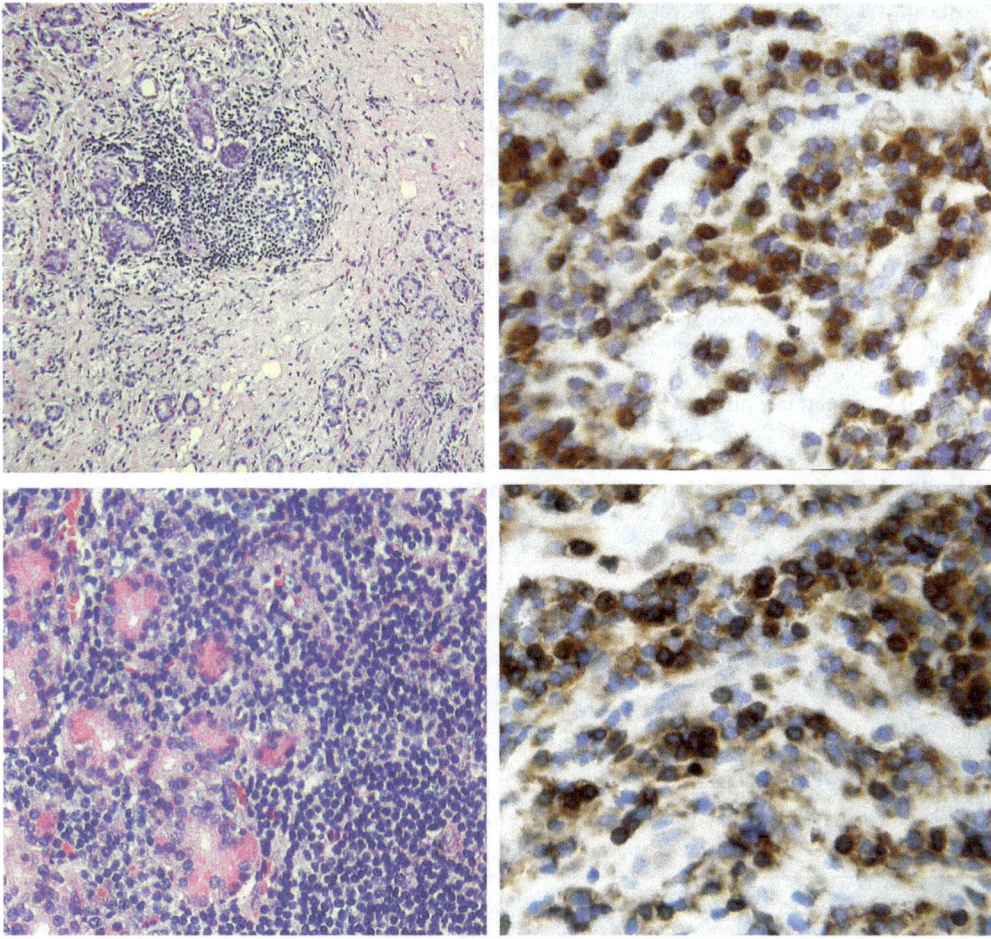

Figure 11.1 Biopsy of lacrimal gland showing near-total replacement of glandular tissue with fibrous tissue (upper left). Only interlobular ducts are visible. Under higher magnification from another part of the biopsy (lower left), remaining acinar cells are surrounded by a dense collection of lymphocytes. Immunohistochemical studies for IgG (upper right) reveals that most lymphoplasmacytic cells stain positive. That same general region, when stained for IgG4 (lower right), shows almost all cells (> 90%) express the immunoglobulin subclass.

histopathologic diagnoses, particularly in small biopsies. Because of these issues, there was an early attempt to assess the diagnostic utility of elevated serum IgG4.[11]

The serum concentration of IgG4 is normally the lowest among the four IgG subclasses, but the range varies by age, sex, race, ethnicity, and other demographic features.[12] Among normal individuals concentration may also range nearly 100-fold (0.01 to 1.4 mg/mL).[13, 14] Approximately 20% to 30% of patients with established IgG4-related disease have normal IgG4 serum concentrations.[15] Nonetheless, concentrations above the upper limit of normal should raise suspicion of IgG4-RD in the proper clinical setting. In addition to their poor sensitivity, serum IgG4 concentrations also lack high specificity. Roughly a quarter of cases with very high-serum IgG4 concentration (greater than fivefold) end up having an alternative diagnosis, including allergic conditions, autoimmune diseases, malignancy, infections, and other conditions.[13–16] Serum concentrations, however, may serve a function in monitoring responses to therapy.[8]

Given the limitations of pathology findings and serum IgG4 concentration testing, the diagnosis of IgG4-RD is established by clinicopathologic correlation. This is particularly relevant in the eye and ocular adnexa, where biopsy may not always be feasible, or doing so could cause significant morbidity. This contemporary approach is illustrated in the recently defined 2019 ACR/EULAR

Classification Criteria for IgG4-RD, where a combination of clinical findings, laboratory abnormalities, pathology findings, and imaging results are used to classify patients as having or not having IgG4-RD.[17, 18] These criteria were developed using a data-driven approach and are meant to be used for research to enroll somewhat homogenous populations. However, they provide a useful framework for approaching the diagnostic evaluation of a patient suspected of having IgG4-RD. There are three steps to assessing someone's classification as having IgG4-RD. First, one must fulfill entry criteria, meaning that they have a typical manifestation of IgG4-RD (e.g., orbital disease, salivary gland, hepatobiliary, retroperitoneal) or a biopsy at one of these sites with a dense lymphoplasmacytic infiltrate. Second, anyone satisfying an exclusion criterion is ineligible for classification as having IgG4-RD; exclusion criteria refer to clinical, pathologic, radiologic, or laboratory findings that are most suggestive of an alternative diagnosis (Table 11.1). Third, inclusion criteria are tallied. These include common features of IgG4-RD, including the serum IgG4 concentration, manifestations (e.g., symmetric lacrimal gland enlargement), histopathologic findings (e.g., IgG4+ plasma cell infiltrate), and radiographic features (e.g., diffuse pancreatic enlargement). Each criterion is assigned points so that a total score can be summed and, if at least 20, the patient can be classified as having IgG4-RD.

Table 11.1 Exclusion Criteria Definition*

Clinical

Fever: Documented, recurrent temperature > 38°C, with fever being a prominent part of the patient's overall presentation with the underlying disease, in the absence of any clinical features of infection.

No objective response to glucocorticoids: If the patient has been treated with prednisone at a minimum of 40 mg/day (~0.6 mg/kg/day) for a period of 4 weeks, the patient has not demonstrated an objective clinical response. An objective response includes unequivocal improvement of the clinical lesions, biochemical abnormalities, or radiological findings. There are two additional points to consider with regard to glucocorticoid response: Improvement only in the serum IgG4 concentration should not be regarded as a clinical response without improvement in other aspects of the disease. Some forms of IgG4-related disease (IgG4-RD) associated with advanced fibrosis, for example, some cases of retroperitoneal fibrosis, or sclerosing mesenteritis, may not demonstrate obvious radiological responses to glucocorticoids.

Serological

Leukopenia and thrombocytopenia without alternative explanation: Reduction in the total white cell count and platelet count to levels below those normal for the reference laboratory, having no apparent explanation except for the underlying disease. Reductions in both the white cell count and platelet count are unusual in IgG4-RD but are typical of, for example, myelodysplastic syndromes, haematopoietic malignancies, and autoimmune conditions within the systemic lupus erythematosus spectrum.

Peripheral eosinophilia: To a concentration of > 3000 mm³.

Positive antineutrophil cytoplasmic antibody (ANCA): ELISA results positive for ANCA targeted against proteinase three or myeloperoxidase.

Positive antibodies: Ro, La, double-stranded DNA, RNP, or Sm antibodies positive in titers greater than normal suggest an alternative diagnosis. Other autoantibody associated with high specificity for another immune-mediated condition is a reasonable explanation for the patient's presentation. Such specific autoantibodies include antisynthetase antibodies (e.g., anti-Jo-1), anti-topoisomerase III (Scl-70), and antiphospholipase A2 receptor antibodies. This does not include autoantibodies of low specificity, such as rheumatoid factor, antinuclear antibodies, anti-mitochondrial antibodies, anti–smooth muscle antibodies, and antiphospholipid antibodies.

Cryoglobulinemia: Cryoglobulinemia (type I, II, or III) occurring in a clinical context that provides a reasonable explanation for the patient's presentation.

Radiological

Known radiological findings suspicious for malignancy or infection that have not been investigated sufficiently: Such radiological findings include mass lesions that have not been evaluated thoroughly, necrosis, cavitation, hypervascular or exophytic mass, bulky or matted lymphadenopathy, or loculated abdominopelvic fluid collection, among others.

Rapid radiological progression: Defined as significant worsening within a 4- to 6-week interval.

Long bone abnormalities consistent with Erdheim–Chester disease: Multifocal osteosclerotic lesions of the long bones, usually associated with bilateral diaphyseal involvement.

Splenomegaly: > 14 cm in the absence of alternative explanation (e.g., portal hypertension).

Table 11.1 (*Continued*)

Pathological

Cellular infiltrates suspicious for malignancy that have not been investigated sufficiently: A high likelihood of malignancy may be suggested by cellular atypia, a monotypic nature of immunohistochemistry findings, or light chain restriction on in situ hybridization studies. If malignancy is suspected, this must be excluded by appropriate studies before inclusion.

Markers consistent with inflammatory myofibroblastic tumor: Known positivity for a marker suggestive of inflammatory myofibroblastic tumor, for example, anaplastic lymphoma kinase one or ROS, a receptor tyrosine kinase that is encoded by the gene ROS1. Prominent neutrophilic inflammation: Neutrophilic infiltrates are unusual in IgG4-RD, with the exception of occasional examples in the lung or near mucosal sites. Extensive neutrophilic infiltrates or neutrophilic abscesses strongly indicate the possibility of a non-IgG4-RD diagnosis.

Necrotizing vasculitis: Although vascular injury (e.g., obliterative phlebitis or arteritis) is a hallmark of IgG4-RD, the presence of fibrinoid necrosis within blood vessel walls provides strong evidence against IgG4-RD.

Prominent necrosis: Small foci of necrosis may rarely be present around the luminal surface of ductal organs, but zonal necrosis with no alternative explanation (e.g., stenting) provides strong evidence against IgG4-RD.

Primary granulomatous inflammation: Inflammation rich in epithelioid histiocytes, including multinucleated giant cell formation and granuloma formation, is highly atypical of IgG4-RD.

Pathological features of a macrophage/histiocytic disorder: For example: known S100-positive macrophages demonstrating emperipolesis, a pathological feature of Rosai Dorfman disease.

Specific Disease Exclusions

Known diagnoses of the following diseases are exclusion criteria: Multicentric Castleman's disease, Crohn's disease (if pancreatobiliary disease is present), ulcerative colitis (if pancreatobiliary disease is present), Hashimoto thyroiditis (if the thyroid is the only proposed disease manifestation). Patients with IgG4-RD can certainly have Hashimoto thyroiditis separately from IgG4-RD, but Hashimoto thyroiditis is part of the IgG4-RD spectrum.

* From the 2019 American College of Rheumatology/European League Against Rheumatism Classification Criteria for IgG4-Related Disease.[19] (With permission and courtesy of BJM Publishing Group Ltd.)

It is important to note that these criteria are imperfect. Some patients with atypical manifestations of the disease (e.g., breast mass, prostate disease) or unusual features (e.g., prominent peripheral eosinophilia) may certainly have IgG4-RD but not fulfill these classification criteria. Thus, they may be excluded from a clinical trial but may still be managed clinically as IgG4-RD based on the treating clinician's overall judgement. The sensitivity of the 2019 ACR/EULAR classification criteria has been tested in a European cohort.[18] Among the group of 79 patients in the 2020 study, overall sensitivity was 91%.[18]

The untreated, natural history of IgG4-related disease is poorly understood but likely variable.[19–21] In many cases of unrecognized or untreated disease, patients sustain progressive tissue injury and new organ involvement. Additionally, it is likely that the nature of the lesion may shift with time from a more inflammatory phenotype toward one characterized by greater fibrosis. This is difficult to prove, and in some manifestations like retroperitoneal fibrosis, impressive fibrosis with less of an inflammatory infiltrate may be present early in the process. At least one case of early-onset fibrosis involving the orbit has been described.[22] It may be difficult to establish a diagnosis from pathology specimens characterized by predominant fibrosis because the IgG plasma cells may be minimal, a dilemma encountered in many retrospective studies of mostly fibrotic tumors including so-called brawny scleritis.[23, 24]

11.3 THE IgG4 SUBCLASS

IgG4 makes up just 4% of IgG serum concentration and 3% less than the next-lowest subclass (IgG3). It is normally produced only after repeated or sustained exposure to antigens, has a half-life of 21 days, and is the only subclass that poorly activates complement.[25, 26] Although its heavy chains have 95% amino acid homology with other IgG subclasses, its indifference towards complement is explained by variances in a portion of the constant domain of the heavy chain that causes negligible binding to both C1q and Fcγ receptors.[27]

Another unique property of IgG4 is known as *Fab-arm exchange*, a process in which different half-molecules of IgG4 can recombine with one another, forming bi-specific and monovalent antibodies.

Since a majority of circulating IgG4 has this divided (dual) specificity, it can bind to unrelated antigens. Being monovalent also eliminates its ability to cross-link antigens, further distinguishing IgG4 from its immunoglobulin cousins.[25] Any relationship between the molecular features of IgG4 and the pathogenesis of IgG4-RD is highly speculative at this time.

11.4 GENERAL CLINICAL MANIFESTATIONS OF IgG4-RELATED DISEASE

One explanation for the belated awareness of IgG4-RD has been attributed to its diverse clinical presentations. There were simply too few clues to make connections before immunohistochemistry for immunoglobulin subclasses was available. Much like sarcoidosis, clinical manifestations depend on the organ and tissue involved. For many organs and sites of disease activity, the first clinical manifestation may be due to the mass effect caused by the lesions (e.g., obstructive uropathy from retroperitoneal fibrosis, proptosis from a retro-orbital mass). In other cases, patients present as a result of organ insufficiency (e.g., exocrine pancreatic insufficiency) or incidentally when lab abnormalities are detected (e.g., chronic kidney disease from tubulointerstitial nephritis). Pain is uncommon but may occur at certain sites like the retroperitoneum, where nerves may be encased. Why intense inflammation of lacrimal gland, orbital connective tissue, and recti muscles causes no pain in IgG4-RD is unclear, since comparable degrees of chronic inflammation from other causes consistently result in discomfort and pain.[28, 29] With such an assortment of clinical manifestations, the early diagnosis can be easily overlooked without a high index of suspicion.

Few generalizations can be made about presentation of ocular adnexal IgG4-RD other than it is usually symmetric and painless.

11.5 OCULAR IgG4-RELATED DISEASE

The general principles and approach to diagnosing IgG4-related disease of the eye and ocular adnexal are the same as those applied elsewhere in the body. The relative rarity of IgG4-RD of the eye and periocular tissues prevents most single institutions from accumulating much experience dealing with the disorder.

11.6 LACRIMAL GLAND

As knowledge of IgG4-RD spread throughout specialties, it was inevitable that reports of involvement of the eye and ocular adnexa would follow. The most commonly affected ocular adnexal structure is the lacrimal gland.[30, 31] The lacrimal gland is similar in structure to salivary glands with fewer mucin-bearing acinar cells. Residing partially in the orbit and eyelid, the gland is accessible to biopsy (preferably the orbital lobe in order to limit scarring of secretary ducts) but approached cautiously due to concern of permanent impairment of tear production. Its larger orbital lobe, which represents two-thirds the volume of the gland, is separated from the palpebral portion by the levator aponeurosis. Much of the orbital lobe is behind the equator of the eye, so any enlargement will produce outward, medial, and downward displacement of the globe.

These reports also clarified the distinction between IgG4-RD disease of lacrimal gland and primary Sjögren's syndrome, the former of which lacks serum antibodies against SSA (Ro) and SSB (La) as well as anti-nuclear antibodies and rheumatoid factor. The salivary glands in persons with Sjögren's syndrome classically display localized proliferations of myoepithelial cells. While these collections of myoepithelial cells are uncommonly found in lacrimal glands of persons with primary Sjögren's syndrome, they have not been reported in IgG4-RD.[29] A number of other systemic immune-mediated diseases can involve the lacrimal gland, including granulomatosis with polyangiitis, Churg–Strauss syndrome, and microscopic polyangiitis. However, the single most common tissue diagnosis of noninfectious dacryoadenitis remains idiopathic.[29, 32–34]

Most patients with lacrimal gland involvement by IgG4-RD have symmetric disease.[35–37] Though enlarged, the inflammatory process in the lacrimal gland is typically painless and lacks overt signs of inflammation (e.g., tenderness, erythema, chemosis, etc.). Concomitant enlargement of salivary glands is common, and many patients have disease, often asymptomatic, elsewhere (e.g., kidney, retroperitoneum, pancreas). Although imaging studies will confirm lacrimal gland pathology of some sort, they cannot reliably distinguish such conditions as lymphoma, sarcoidosis, or infection (e.g., mumps, etc.) from IgG4-RD (Figure 11.3). Painless enlargement of the gland usually requires exclusion of an epithelial neoplasm, but both benign and malignant neoplasms arise unilaterally. Lymphoma can present as either unilateral or bilateral disease. While elevated serum IgG4 levels may heighten the suspicion of IgG4-RD, clinicopathologic correlation is needed. When the lacrimal gland is the only site of disease activity, a biopsy is needed to establish the diagnosis.

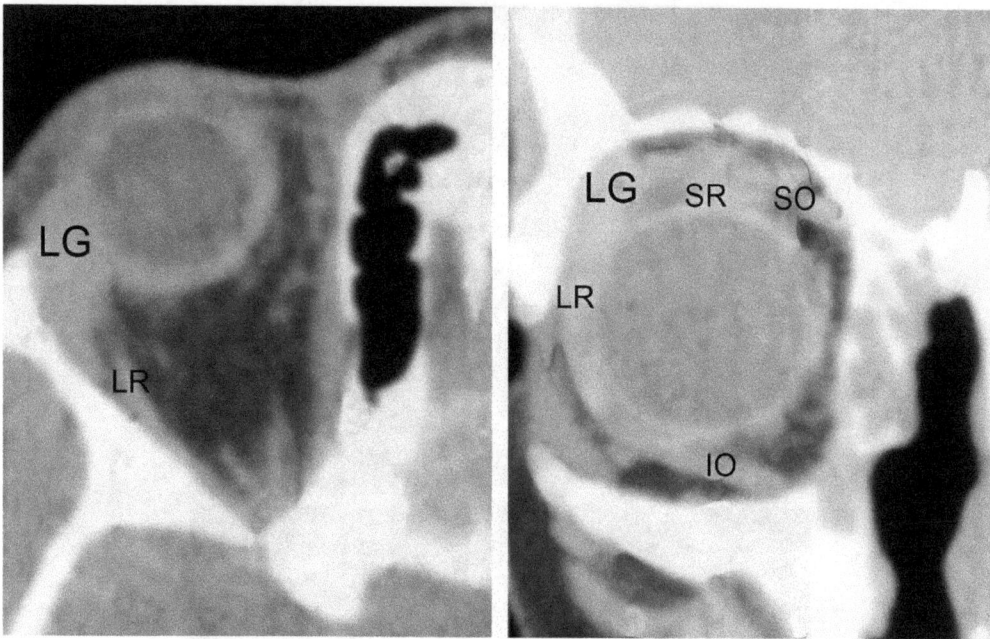

Figure 11.2 Computed tomogram (CT) of normal right lacrimal gland (LG). The LG consists of two portions, the larger orbital segment that makes up two-thirds of the gland and the smaller palpebral portions. The normal gland in adults is roughly 2 cm in length and 12 mm in maximum girth. The orbital gland rests in the bony lacrimal fossa and is separated from the palpebral portion by the levator aponeurosis. The anterior edge of the palpebral lobe ends at the superior conjunctival cul-de-sac and can be visualized when the lid is elevated. The inferior edge of the orbital lobe ends at the superior margin of the lateral rectus (LR) muscle. Its medial border is separated from the superior rectus muscle (SR). The presence of a space-occupying mass of the LG will cause different symptoms and signs depending on whether all or portions of the tissue are affected. Since much of the gland is behind the equator of the eye, enlargement typically displaces the eye downward, outward (proptosis), and medial. A space-occupying lesion of the palpebral lobe will result in an upper lateral eyelid mass without proptosis. The coronal CT also shows locations of the superior and inferior oblique (SO, IO) muscles.

The importance of biopsy when there is no other evidence of systemic IgG4-RD other than ocular adnexal is self-evident, since a host of neoplastic and other diseases can present as a painless mass. Even when IgG4-RD is documented elsewhere, a tissue sample is needed to exclude such conditions as marginal-zone B cell lymphoma and other indolent lymphomas known to rarely arise within IgG4-related disease.[38, 39] As familiarity with IgG4-RD increases, so too have reports of other conditions that are mistaken for it, including in the lacrimal gland.[40, 41]

Given the rapidity with which histopathologic criteria for IgG4-RD were drafted and diffused into the medical community, it may have biased reporting in the literature. How should cases of reactive lymphoid hyperplasia with high ratios and absolute concentrations of IgG4-plasma cells but lacking storiform fibrosis or obliterative phlebitis, for example, be classified?[42] Such ambiguities encourage investigation into new criteria and diagnostic strategies.[43] Under the ACR/EULAR classification criteria, storiform fibrosis is not necessary for diagnosis.[17]

11.7 THE ORBIT

The pear-shaped orbit is confined laterally and posteriorly by seven bones and anteriorly by the eye. The curtain-like anterior orbital septum completes the partitioning of orbit from eyelid. The orbit contains an array of connective tissues, lacrimal gland (already discussed), and optic nerve (a white track of the brain). Numerous vessels and nerves pass through the orbit. All tissues of the orbit appear vulnerable to IgG4-RD.[44] Most cases reported in the literature are found in retrospective clinical series, with individual case reports making up a minority.[45–48] The goal of many

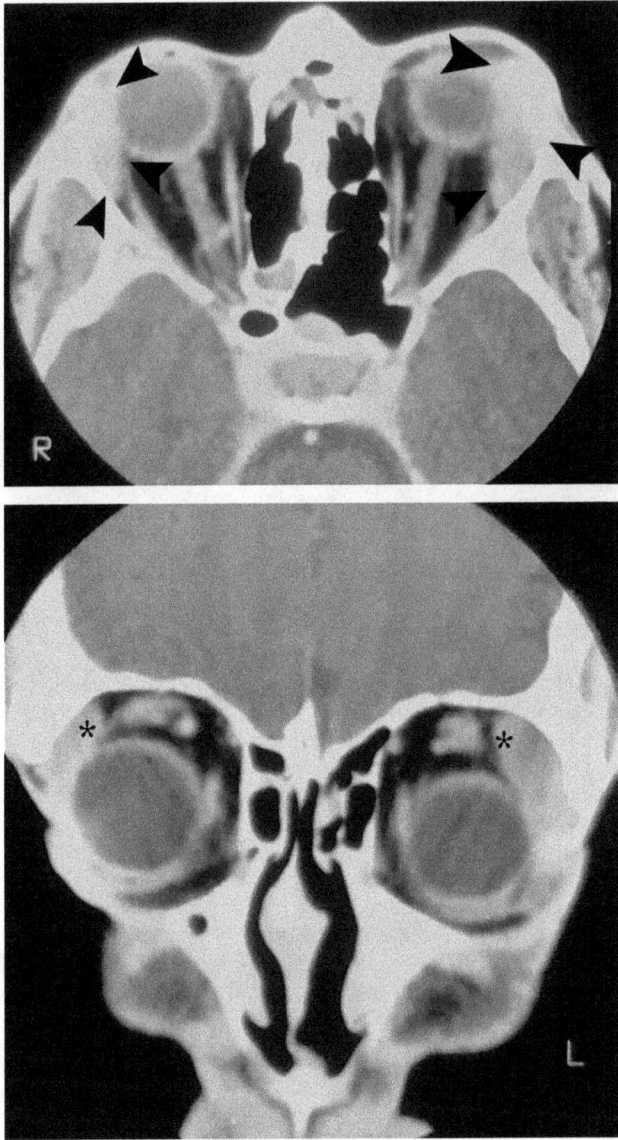

Figure 11.3 Computed tomograms showing bilateral enlargement of lacrimal glands, left larger than right. The axial view (upper) reveals relatively homogeneous, electron-dense masses with their epicenters in the lacrimal glands (arrowheads). Most of the masses are behind the equator of the globes. They obscure the distal lateral recti muscles. The coronal section (lower) at the equator of the eyes shows the lacrimal glands (*) occupying the space between the globes and the superior lateral orbital walls. Both enlarged glands approach the superior recti muscles but do not touch them.

retrospective clinical series has been to determine if past diagnoses of idiopathic orbital inflammation, orbital pseudotumor, lymphoid hyperplasia, and idiopathic sclerosing inflammation can be re-classified as IgG4-RD. Most studies have succeeded in documenting that IgG4-RD existed in the past under a variety of diagnoses ranging from idiopathic inflammatory pseudotumor, reactive lymphoid hyperplasia, and pseudolymphoma to sclerosing pseudotumor. A national prospective study involving 87 patients came to a similar conclusion, finding more than a third of patients with "biopsy-proven" idiopathic orbital inflammation satisfied the criteria for IgG4-RD.[49] Though most patients with IgG4-RD have bilateral orbital involvement, roughly 30% do not.[50, 51]

Table 11.2 Typical Orbital Manifestations of IgG4-Related Disease

Structure	Symptoms	Clinical Findings
Lacrimal gland (most common orbital manifestation)	▪ Swelling around eye ▪ May experience dry eye symptoms, but this is not common	▪ Enlarged gland, often symmetric, on physical exam ▪ Proptosis ▪ Painless
Extraocular muscle	▪ Pain with eye movement ▪ Double vision ▪ Protuberant eye	▪ Proptosis ▪ Abnormal ocular motility
Orbit	▪ Orbital pain (retrobulbar), headache ▪ Change in vision ▪ Double vision ▪ Drooping eyelid ▪ Protuberant eye	▪ Effects of space-occupying lesion (e.g., abnormal position of globe, abnormal retropulsion of the globe, etc.) ▪ Proptosis (manifestation of space-occupying lesion) ▪ Ptosis ▪ Diminished vision ▪ Abnormal ocular motility

The large number of patients with IgG4-RD orbital disease that are reported in the literature confirm that essentially any tissue in the orbit is susceptible, that bone destruction is distinctly uncommon, and that the orbit may or may not be associated with disease elsewhere in the body. Depending on the specific tissue involved, patients may experience pain, decreased vision, or double vision. Others may notice a protruding eye (proptosis) or droopy eyelid. On examination, there is evidence of an orbital mass (space-occupying lesion) and possibly a disturbance in ocular motility when diplopia is present (Table 11.2). In nearly all early cases reported in the literature, diagnoses were established through histopathologic interpretation with immunohistochemical studies. Practical findings have emerged from these clinical series, as illustrated by the observation that the infraorbital canal is often expanded on imaging studies from patients with chronic orbital inflammation, including IgG4-RD.[52] These retrospective clinical series also reflect the reality that a substantial number of cases could not be re-classified, highlighting the fact that the category "idiopathic" inflammation continues to exist, albeit a bit less often.

11.8 OCULAR IgG4-RELATED DISEASE

Verifying ocular (eyeball) involvement with IgG4-RD presents several problems, foremost of which is validating the diagnosis with biopsy. Most diagnoses to date have been made presumptively without ocular biopsy, relying on biopsies from extraocular tissues. The more convincing cases reported have dealt with presumptive IgG4-related scleritis. Less persuasive accounts of ocular involvement are related to IgG4-related uveitis.

Sclera is a common target of immune-mediated disease and autoimmune disease, so that the association with IgG4-RD is feasible.[52–55] Cases of so-called brawny scleritis reported in the past literature display marked thickening of posterior sclera, which can mimic uveal melanoma.[52] In the few cases of brawny scleritis studied, however, so few inflammatory cells remained in the sclera that it precluded interpretation of immunohistochemical studies.[52] At least one case of IgG4-related scleritis has been associated with meningeal involvement.[54] Another case has been associated with periaortitis.[56]

The literature on IgG4-related uveitis is more difficult to interpret because ocular tissue is rarely biopsied, and many patients have other disorders that can be associated with uveitis. Take, for example, a 69-year-old man with fibroinflammatory liver nodules that contained IgG4-positive plasma cells and who also developed granulomatous anterior uveitis.[57] His intraocular inflammation was attributed to IgG4-related disease, but other comorbidities could have explained his granulomatous uveitis. Another patient of the same age with IgG4-plasma cell interstitial nephritis also suffered from granulomatous anterior uveitis.[58] But this patient also had cutaneous leukocytoclastic vasculitis. Neither granulomatous inflammation nor vasculitis are features of IgG4-RD. In another case report, a 79-year-old with Lewy body dementia was found to have periaortitis, scleritis, and uveitis. An elevated serum IgG4 level led to the diagnosis of IgG4-related disease.[56] Without a tissue biopsy, the validity of these diagnoses is challengeable. IgG4-related uveitis may exist, but its prevalence appears exceptionally low, and evidence supporting a causal association with IgG4-RD could be coincidental.

IgG4-related optic neuropathy is an exceptionally rare diagnosis.[54, 58] Historical cases reported before the era of IgG immunohistochemistry subtyping called sclerosing pseudotumor (pachymeningitis) of the optic nerve sheath may have represented IgG4-related optic neuropathy.[59]

11.9 EPIDEMIOLOGY

How much insight might be gained from examining the epidemiology of multiorgan systemic disease, which was virtually unknown at the turn of the 21st century? A meta-analysis of orbital cases from 2013 found a male-to-female ratio of 1.3 to 1 for all definite and probable cases in the literature.[20] This male predominance is consistent with early surveys examining IgG4-related disease in general.[8] The male predominance is particularly high in Japan, where a 2.8-to-1 ratio has been reported for IgG4-related pancreatic disease.[60] In a more recent US study using a claims-based administrative data set, investigators found 58% of patients with IgG4-related disease were women.[61] That same study reported the incidence of IgG4-related disease was similar to that of systemic rheumatic diseases like ANCA-associated vasculitis. The average age of persons with IgG4-related disease in general as well as those with orbital involvement is the mid-50s.[8, 20, 60] Demographic findings must be interpreted cautiously, however, given the inherent biases associated with clinical series coming from tertiary care facilities and the limitations of claims-based analyses. A majority of cases found in the literature have come from Japan and other Asian countries, which has led to studies examining genetic predispositions.[8] Although genetic factors may influence some aspects of susceptibility and clinical course, to date, the impact remains uncertain.

11.10 MANAGEMENT AND THERAPY

This section appraises management and therapy from the context of initial diagnosis of "ocular" IgG4-related disease, which translates in practical terms to involvement of orbit connective tissues and/or lacrimal gland. The fraction of cases arising in conjunctiva or optic nerve and intraocularly are vanishingly small. Assuming accurate diagnosis, patients should undergo an expeditious systemic evaluation to identify or exclude disease elsewhere. This usually entails a combination of laboratory studies and cross-sectional imaging, most often with computed tomography or magnetic resonance imaging. The role of positron emission tomography is less well defined. Cross-sectional imaging may identify other features common to IgG4-RD as well as sites that may be more amenable to biopsy to support a diagnosis.

Glucocorticoids of varying doses and preparations have been first-line agents used to treat the many obsolete-named disorders that now fall under the IgG4-related disease umbrella.[8, 62, 63] Oral glucocorticoids in dosage appropriate for the clinical situation is favored for its rapid response. Most courses begin with 40 to 60 mg/d of prednisone, which is tapered over the subsequent 8 to 12 weeks. The response to glucocorticoids is typically swift, but relapses are common as the dose is tapered and, especially, after discontinuation. Because prolonged monotherapy with corticosteroids is usually untenable due to treatment toxicities, other immunosuppressive agents have been explored.[64–69] One study gave 20 patients with solitary lacrimal gland IgG4-RD the option of "watchful waiting" and found that 18 had lesions that remained stable over a median follow-up of 27 months.[51]

Informed decision-making for alternatives to corticosteroids is hampered by lack of randomized controlled trials, small size of studies, varying clinical endpoints, scarcity of long-term follow-up, absence of standardized data collection, and the heterogeneous nature of IgG4-RD. Studies reporting outcomes with conventional disease-modifying antirheumatic drugs like azathioprine, methotrexate, mycophenolate, and cyclophosphamide suggest efficacy but have been typically studied in combination with glucocorticoids.[45] When available, one of the most commonly used steroid-sparing agents is the anti-CD20 antibody rituximab.[45, 65, 66] There are currently two phase 3 clinical trials evaluating the efficacy and safety of B cell–targeted therapies in comparison with a three month glucocorticoid taper. These trials are expected to address some of the ongoing major knowledge gaps.

There are no specific therapeutic guidelines for the management of intraocular inflammation attributed to IgG4-related disease, including scleritis. The goal of therapy in this situation is to suppress and eliminate inflammation through the stepwise implementation of anti-inflammatory and immune-modulating agents. Such execution is optimally achieved through the combined efforts of ophthalmologic and medical specialists. The escalated employment of local and systemic agents to achieve lasting remission should generally follow the basic algorithm for IgG4-RD when intraocular pharmacokinetics properties are known and deemed appropriate. If not, treatment of IgG4-related intraocular inflammation can follow practice guidelines for uveitis.[70]

11.11 SUMMARY

IgG4-RD was not recognized until the start of the 21st century. As research into its pathogenesis continues, so does the development of therapies that can induce a lasting remission. The lacrimal gland and orbit make up a majority of all cases of ophthalmic IgG4-RD. Successful long-term management will likely include targeted immune-modulating therapy coordinated with medical and surgical expertise to alleviate local complications caused by an inflammatory, space-occupying mass around the eye.

REFERENCES

1. Hamano H, Kawa S, Horiuchi A, et al. High serum IgG4 concentrations in patients with sclerosing pancreatitis. *N Engl J Med.* 2001 Mar. 8;344(10):732–738. doi:10.1056/NEJM200103083441005.
2. Kamisawa T, Funata N, Hayaski Y, et al. A new clinicopathological entity of IgG4-related autoimmune disease. *J Gastoenterol.* 2003;38:982–984. doi:10.1007/s00535-003-1175-y.
3. Khosroshaki A, Stone JH. IgG4-related systemic disease: the age of discovery. *Curr Opin Rheumatol.* 2011;23:72–73. doi:10.1097/BOR.0b013e328341a229.
4. Stone JH, Khosroshahi A, Hilgenberg A, et al. IgG4-related systemic disease and lymphoplasmacytic aortitis. *Arthritis Rheum.* 2009;60:3139–3145. doi:10.1002/art.24798.
5. Stone JH, Khosroshahi A, Deshpande V, et al. IgG4-related systemic disease accounts for a significant proportion of thoracic lymphoplasmacytic aortitis cases. *Arthrit Care Res.* 2010;62:316–322.
6. Khosroshahi A, Carruthers MN, Stone JH, et al. Rethinking Ormond's disease: "idiopathic" retroperitoneal fibrosis in the era of IgG4-related disease. *Medicine (Baltimore)* 2013;92(2):82–91.
7. Stone JH, Khosroshahi A, Deshpanda V, et al. Recommendations for the nomenclature of IgG4-related disease and its individual organ system manifestations. *Arthritis Rheum.* 2012;64(10):3061–3067.
8. Stone JH, Zen Y, Deshpande V. IgG4-related disease. *N Engl J Med.* 2012;366:539–551.
9. Carruthers MN, Khosroshahi A, Augustin T, et al. The diagnostic utility of serum IgG4 concentrations in IgG4-related disease. *Ann Rheum.* 2015;74(1):14–18.
10. Varghese JL, Fung AW, Mattman A, et al. Clinical utility of serum IgG4 measurements. *Clin Chim Acta.* 2020;506:228–235.
11. Chang S, Lee C-C, Chang M-L, et al. Comparison of clinical manifestations and pathology between Kimura disease and IgG4-related disease: a report of two cases and literature review. *J Clin Med.* 2022 Dec.;11(23):6887. doi:10.3390/jcm11236887.
12. Harkness T, Fu X, Zhang Y, et al. Immunoglobulin G and immunoglobulin G subclass concentrations differ according to sex and race. *Ann Allergy Asthma Immunol.* 2020;125(2):190–195.
13. Nirula A, Glaser SM, Kalled SL, et al. What is IgG4? A review of the biology of a unique immunoglobulin subtype. *Curr Opin Rheumatol.* 2001;23:119–124.
14. Aucouturier P, Danon F, Daveau M, et al. Measurement of serum IgG4 levels by a competitive immunoenzymatic assay with monoclonal antibodies. *J Immunol Methods.* 1984;74:151–162.
15. Kamisawa T, Zen Y, Pillai S, et al. IgG4-related disease. *Lancet.* 2015;385:1460–1471.
16. Baker WC, Cook C, Fu Z, et al. The positive predictive value of a very high serum IgG4 concentration for the diagnosis of IgG4-related disease. *J Rheumatol.* 2023;50:408–412.
17. Wallace ZS, Naden RP, Chari S, et al. The 2019 American College of Rheumatology/European League Against Rheumatism classification criteria for IgG4-related disease. *Ann Rheum Dis.* 2020;79(1):77–87.
18. Vikse J, Midtvedt Ø, Fevang BT, et al. Differential sensitivity of the 2020 revised comprehensive diagnostic criteria and the 2019 ACR/EULAR classification criteria across IgG4-related disease phenotypes: results from a Norwegian cohort. *Arthritis Res Ther.* 2023;25:16374.
19. Ren H, Mori N, Sato S, et al. American College of Rheumatology and the European League Against Rheumatism classification criteria of IgG4-related disease: an update for radiologists. *Jpn J Radiol.* 2022;40:876–893.
20. Andrew NH, Sladden N, Kearney DJ, et al. An analysis of IgG4-related disease (IgG4-RD) among idiopathic orbital inflammations and benign lymphoid hyperplasia using two consensus-based diagnostic criteria for IgG4-RD. *Br J Ophthalmol.* 2015;99:376–381.
21. Umehera H, Okazaki K, Masaki Y, et al. Comprehensive diagnostic criteria for IgG4-related disease (IgG4-RD), 2011. *Mod Rheumatol.* 2012;22:21–30.
22. Mehta M, Jakobiec F, Fay A. Idiopathic fibroinflammatory disease of the face, eyelids, and periocular membrane with immunoglobulin IgG4-positive plasma cells. *Arch Pathol Lab Med.* 2009;133:1251–1255.

23. Margo CE, Espana EM, Harman LE. Scleritis. In: Margo CE, ed, *Ophthalmic pathology: the evolution of modern concepts*, chapter 22. London: Academic Press, 2023:134–137.

24. Butterfield SD, Silkiss R. Idiopathic sclerosing dacryoadenitis. *J Ophthalmic Inflamm Infect*. 2023;13:43–48.

25. Rispens T, Huijbers MG. The unique properties of IgG4 and its role in health and disease. *Nat Rev Immunol*. 2023;24:1–16. doi:10.1038/x41577-023-00871z.

26. Sigal LH. Basic science for the clinician 58. IgG subclasses. *J Clin Rheumatol*. 2012;18:316–318.

27. Vidarsson G, Dekkers G, Rispens T. IgG subclasses and allotypes: from structure to effector functions. *Front Immunol*. 2014 Oct. 20. doi:103389/fimmu.2014.00520.

28. Kennerdell JS, Dresner SC. The nonspecific orbital inflammatory syndromes. *Surv Ophthalmol*. 1984;29:93–103.

29. Singh S, Selva D. Non-infectious dacryoadenitis. *Surv Ophthalmol*. 2022;67:353–368.

30. Andrew NH, Sladden N, Kearney DJ, et al. An analysis of IgG4-related disease (IgG4-RD) among idiopathic orbital inflammations and benign lymphoid hyperplasia using two consensus-based diagnostic criteria for IgG4-RD. *Br J Ophthalmol*. 2015;99(3):76–81.

31. Abad S, Margin A, Heéran F, et al. IgG4-related disease in patients with idiopathic orbital inflammation syndrome: data from the French SIOI prospective cohort. *Acta Ophthalmol*. 2019;97(4):e648–e656.

32. Teo L, Seah LL, Choo CT, et al. A survey of the histopathology of lacrimal gland lesion in a tertiary referral centre. *Orbit*. 2013;32:1–7.

33. Ahn C, Kang S, Sa HS. Clinicopathologic features of biopsied lacrimal gland masses in 95 Korean patients. *Graefes Arch Clin Exp Ophthalmol*. 2019;257:1527–1533.

34. Andrew NH, McNab AA, Selva D. Review of 268 lacrimal gland biopsies in an Australian cohort. *Clin Exp Ophthalmol*. 2015;43:5–11, 35.

35. Salama OH, Ibrahim EN, Hussein MO, et al. IgG4-related dacryoadenitis in Egyptian patients: a retrospective study. *Clin Ophthalmol*. 2022;16:2765–2773.

36. Takahira M, Kawano M, Zen Y, et al. IgG4-related chronic sclerosing dacryoadenitis. *Arch Ophthalmol*. 2007;125:1575–1578.

37. Cheuk W, Yuen HK, Chank JK. Chronic sclerosing dacryoadenitis: part of the spectrum of IgG4-related sclerosing disease? *Am J Surg Pathol*. 2007;31:643–645.

38. Ochoa ER, Harris NL, Pilch BZ. Marginal zone B-cell lymphoma of the salivary gland arising in chronic sclerosing sialadenitis (Kuttner tumor). *Am J Surg Pathol*. 2001;25:1546–1550.

39. Ferry JA, Klepeis V, Sohani AR, et al. IgG4-related orbital disease and its mimics in a western population. *Am J Surg Pathol*. 2015;39:1688–1700.

40. Strehl JD, Hartmann A, Sgaimy A. Numerous IgG4-positive plasma cells are ubiquitous in diverse localized chronic inflammatory conditions and need to be distinguished from IgG4-related systemic disorders. *J Clin Pathol*. 2011;64:237–243.

41. Asano N, Sato Y. Rheumatoid lymphadenopathy with abundant IgG4+ plasma cells: a case mimicking IgG4-related disease. *J Clin Exp Hematopath*. 2012;52:57–61.

42. Mancera N, Bajric J, Margo CE. IgG4-rich reactive lymphoid hyperplasia of the lacrimal gland. *Orbit*. 2020;39:285–288.

43. Chan AS, Mudhar H, Shen SY, et al. Serum IgG2 and tissue IgG2 plasma cell elevation in orbital IgG4-related disease (IgG4-RD): potential use in IgG4-RD assessment. *Br J Ophthalmol*. 2017;101:1576–1582.

44. Wallace ZS, Khosroshahi A, Jakobiec FA, et al. IgG4-related systemic disease as a cause of "idiopathic" orbital inflammation, including orbital myositis, and trigeminal nerve involvement. *Surv Ophthalmol*. 2012;57:26–33.

45. Andrew N, Kearney D, Selva D. IgG4-related orbital disease: a meta-analysis and review. *Acta Ophthalmol*. 2013;91:694–700.

46. Mulay K, Aggarwal E, Honavar SG. Clinicopathologic features of orbital immunoglobulin G4-related disease (IgG4-RD): a case series and literature review. *Graefes Arch Clin Exp Ophthalmol*. 2015;253:803–809.

47. Sa H-S, Lee J-H, Woo KI, et al. IgG4-related disease in idiopathic sclerosing orbital inflammation. *Br J Ophthalmol*. 2015;99:1493–1497.

48. Andron A, Hostovsky A, Nair AG, et al. The impact of IgG4-ROD on the diagnosis of orbital tumors: a retrospective analysis. *Orbit*. 2017;35:359–364.

49. Abad S, Margin A, Heéran F, et al. IgG4-related disease in patients with idiopathic orbital inflammation syndrome: data from the French SIOI prospective cohort. *Acta Ophthalmol*. 2019;97(4):e648–e656.

50. Wallace ZS, Deshpande V, Stone JH. Ophthalmic manifestations of IgG4-related disease: single-center experience and literature review. *Semin Arthritis Rheum.* 2014;43(6):806–817.

51. Kubota T, Kayayama M, Nishimura R, et al. Long-term outcomes of ocular adnexal lesions in IgG4-related ophthalmic disease. *Br J Ophthalmol.* 2020;104:345–349.

52. Hardy TG, McNab AA, Rose GE. Enlargement of the infraorbital nerve: an important sign associated with orbit reactive lymphoid hyperplasia or IgG4-R inflammation. *Ophthalmology.* 2014;121:1297–1303.

53. Hankins M, Margo CE. Histopathological evaluation of scleritis. *J Clin Pathol.* 2019;72:386–390.

54. Kim EC, Lee SJ, Hwang HS, et al. Bilateral diffuse scleritis as a first manifestation of immunoglobulin G4-related sclerosing pachymeningitis. *Can J Ophthalmol.* 2013;48:e31–e33.

55. Ohno K, Sato Y, Ohshima K, et al. IgG4-related disease involving the sclera. *Mod Rheumatol.* 2014;24:195–198.

56. Mase Y, Kubo A, Matsumoto A, et al. Posterior scleritis with choroidal detachments and periaortitis associated with IgG4-related disease: a case report. *Medicine (Baltimore).* 2022;101:e29611.

57. Chen JL, Men M, Naini BV, et al. IgG4-related hypertensive granulomatous anterior uveitis. *Am J Ophthalmol Case Rep.* 2022;26:101465.

58. Katz E, Harvey L, Stone JH. Granulomatous uveitis secondary to IgG4-related disease. *Rheumatol Adv Prac.* 2021;1:1–2.

59. Margo CE, Levy MH, Beck RW. Bilateral idiopathic inflammation of the optic nerve sheaths: light and electron microscopic findings. *Ophthalmology.* 1989;96:200–206.

60. Nishimori I, Tamakoski A, Otsuki M. Prevalence of autoimmune pancreatitis in Japan from a nationwide survey in 2002. *J Gastroenterol.* 2007;42(Suppl 18):6–8.

61. Wallace ZS, Miles G, Smolkina E, et al. Incidence, prevalence, and mortality of IgG4-related disease in the USA: a claims-based analysis of commercially insured adults. *Ann Rheum Dis.* 2023;82:957–962.

62. Khosroshahi A, Wallace WS, Crowe JL, et al. International consensus guidance statement on the management and treatment of IgG4-related disease. *Arthritis Rheumatol.* 2015;67:1688–1699.

63. Kamisawa T, Okazaki K. Diagnosis and treatment of IgG4-related disease. *Curr Top Microbiol Immunol.* 2017;401:19–33.

64. Yoshifuji H, Umehara H. Glucocorticoids in the treatment of IgG4-related disease – prospects for new international treatment guidelines. *Mod Rheumatol.* 2022:roac097.

65. Ebbo M, Grados A, Samson M, et al. Long-term efficacy and safety of rituximab in IgG4-related disease: data from a French nationwide study of thirty-three patients. *PLoS One.* 2017 Sept. 15;12(9):e0183844. doi:10.1371/journal.pone. 0183844.

66. Carruthers MN, Topazian MD, Khosroshahi A, et al. Rituximab for IgG4-related disease: a prospective, open-label trial. *Ann Rheum Dis.* 2015;74:1171–1177.

67. Kanda M, Kamekura R, Sugawara M, et al. IgG4-related disease administered dupliumab: case series and review of the literature. *RMD Open.* 2023:9e003026. doi:10.1136/rmdopen-2023-003026.

68. Nakayamada S, Tanaka Y. Development of targeted therapies in IgG4-related disease. *Mod Rheumatol.* 2023;3:266–270.

69. Lanzillotta M, Fernandez-Codina A, Culver E, et al. Emerging therapy options for IgG4-related disease. *Expert Rev Clin Immunol.* 2021;17:471–483.

70. Levy-Clarke G, Margo CE. Uveitis. In: Kellerman RD, Rakel DP, eds, *Conn's current therapy 2023*, Section 7. Philadelphia, PA: Elsevier Inc., 2023:535–539.

12 Ophthalmologic Disease in Cogan's Syndrome, Relapsing Polychondritis, VEXAS Syndrome, and Other Disorders

Kirby Taylor, Eric Crowell, and Veena Patel

12.1 COGAN'S SYNDROME

12.1.1 Introduction

Cogan's syndrome (CS) was first delineated in the medical literature in 1945 by ophthalmologist David G. Cogan in a five-case series. It is a rare, enigmatic multisystemic disease thought to be an immune-mediated vasculitis typified by ocular and audio-vestibular symptoms and has associations with systemic vasculitis.[1, 2] The syndrome often presents in young, Caucasian adults with interstitial keratitis, leading to symptoms of eye redness, pain, and light sensitivity, coupled with neurosensory hearing loss, dizziness, tinnitus, nausea, and vomiting. In 1980, Haynes et al. introduced a classification for CS, distinguishing between 'typical' CS, which adheres to the initial description by Cogan, and 'atypical' CS, which encompasses a spectrum of symptoms including persistent conjunctivitis, scleritis, uveitis, optic disc edema, and retinal vasculitis.[3, 4]

12.1.2 Epidemiology

Usually, CS, in both its typical and atypical forms, manifests within the first three decades of life, predominantly affecting Caucasians and occurring in males and females equally. A comprehensive retrospective case series studying 62 patients with CS reported a median onset age of 37 years, including an even distribution of 31 females and 31 males.[4] In another case series examining 32 patients with CS, 90% were identified as Caucasian, with the remaining 10% being Black.[4]

12.1.3 Etiology and Pathogenesis

12.1.3.1 Etiology

Since 1945, there have been approximately 250 reported cases of CS, which is presumed to have an autoimmune basis. Nonetheless, the precise cause of CS remains a subject of debate. There is a theory proposing an infectious etiology, potentially linked to viral involvement that may initiate a molecular mimicry response. Recent interest has centered on the role of autoimmunity in CS pathogenesis. Evidence of autoantibodies targeting antigens in the cornea, inner ear, and endothelial tissues in some CS patients lends weight to the theory of an autoimmune mechanism driving the disease. Some research has indicated a possible cell-mediated reaction.[3, 5]

12.1.3.2 Pathogenesis

The autoimmune hypothesis of CS was substantiated in the 1980s by the identification of numerous autoantibodies targeting corneal, inner ear, and endothelial antigens, some of which are now considered to be specific indicators for diagnosis. Additionally, other autoantibodies, such as anti-neutrophilic cytoplasmic antibody (ANCA) and rheumatoid factor (RF), although nonspecific, have been linked to CS. Histopathological findings from this era, which revealed infiltration by lymphocytes and plasma cells in the cornea and cochlea, have further corroborated the immune-mediated nature of CS.[5]

Immunofluorescent staining has revealed the presence of IgG and IgA antibodies against human corneal tissue and IgG antibodies against inner ear tissue in CS patient serum. There has also been documentation of anti-corneal IgM binding to the non-keratinizing squamous epithelium within corneal tissue. Moreover, CS patient serum has shown IgM and IgG reactivity with fresh cryosections of rat labyrinth and cornea. IgG immunoglobulins in CS patient serum have been identified, reacting against peptides that are like known antigens such as SSA/Ro and the reovirus III core protein lambda 1. These peptides also show homology to the cell-density-enhanced protein tyrosine phosphatase-1 (DEP-1/CD 148) expressed in the sensory epithelia of the inner ear and endothelial cells. IgG antibodies purified from a patient's serum have been found to recognize and bind to autoantigens and the DEP-1/CD 148 protein, inhibiting the proliferation of cells that express DEP-1/CD 148.[5] The "Cogan antigen" is an antigen that shares specific sequence homology with CD148 and connexin 26, which are expressed in inner-ear endothelial cells. Connexin 26 shares similarity with other connexin proteins in corneal fibroblasts. It is important to understand that immune-mediated processes play a role in the pathogenesis of CS, with the Cogan antigen being present in many of the sera of CS patients.[1]

DOI: 10.1201/9781003453710-12

While these autoantibodies are highly specific for CS diagnosis, they have also been detected in other patients without CS but with neurosensory hearing loss. In addition, these specific antibodies are not readily available for clinicians to use to aid in their diagnosis.[5]

Upper respiratory tract infections precede the onset of disease in 50% of cases, suggesting a possible infectious origin to the immune-mediated process. Chlamydial infections have received much attention for their ability to evade host immune defenses and cause chronic infection. However, there has not been a proven link between any chlamydial species and Cogan's syndrome. The IgG and IgM autoantibodies against Cogan peptide have been shown to cross-react with a structural protein of reovirus type III, suggesting that it could be viral involvement that elicits the immune-mediated response.[1]

12.1.4 Clinical Presentation

Cogan syndrome unfolds gradually, with patients taking an average of 12 months from initial symptom onset to secure a definitive diagnosis. This delay in diagnosis is often due to the staggered appearance of the syndrome's hallmark vestibulo-auditory and ocular symptoms. In many cases, auditory symptoms emerge first, followed by ocular manifestations within a median interval of 2 months. However, instances of simultaneous development of these symptoms are also noted.[3] In a 32-patient case series of CS patients, vestibulo-auditory symptoms were present in approximately 98% of the cases, with 41% experiencing bilateral hearing loss and 31% suffering from deafness. Ocular symptoms were noted in 92% of these patients, with interstitial keratitis, an immune-mediated stromal corneal lesion, being the primary ocular manifestation (51%).[4] An intriguing aspect of CS is its potential link to preceding events, observed in 31% of patients within a specific study group. These precursor conditions include rhinitis, pharyngitis, otitis, chlamydia pneumonia, and flu-like illnesses.[4]

Further complicating the clinical picture, a comprehensive meta-analysis encompassing over 222 patients identified that 58% presented with symptoms typical of CS, whereas the remaining 42% demonstrated atypical characteristics. Remarkably, CS can coexist with a myriad of other systemic conditions, extending beyond the auditory and visual symptoms. These include but are not limited to weight loss, joint and muscle pain, aortic insufficiency, arteritis in areas like the iliac and renal arteries, peripheral neuropathy, skin rashes, mouth ulcers, pericarditis, abdominal pain, esophagitis, encephalitis, facial nerve palsy, fever, splenomegaly, Raynaud's phenomenon, hepatic steatosis, chondritis, headache, aortitis, and coronary arteritis.[4]

12.1.4.1 Typical Cogan's Syndrome

Typical Cogan's syndrome involves:

- Ocular symptoms, primarily non-syphilitic interstitial keratitis

- Ménière's syndrome-like audio-vestibular symptoms, such as sudden tinnitus, vertigo, and hearing loss

- A gap of less than 2 years between the onset of ocular and audio-vestibular symptoms[5]

12.1.4.2 Atypical Cogan's Syndrome

Atypical Cogan's syndrome features:

- Various inflammatory ocular issues, which may include interstitial keratitis

- Audio-vestibular symptoms differing from those in Ménière's syndrome

- A delay of more than 2 years between the appearance of ocular and audio-vestibular symptoms

Systemic manifestations occur more frequently (30% to 50%) in atypical CS, aiding in differentiation between the two types.[5] Some patients with atypical CS have presented with rheumatoid arthritis, idiopathic juvenile arthritis, and ankylosing spondylitis.[4] The other ocular symptoms in the atypical form include conjunctivitis, anterior or posterior scleritis, uveitis, optic disc edema, closed-angle glaucoma, papillitis, central vein occlusion, vasculitis optic neuropathy, and retinal vasculitis.[6] Table 12.1 lists the criteria for both typical and atypical Cogan's syndrome.

12.1.4.3 Ophthalmic Manifestations

Ocular involvement in Cogan syndrome varies widely. Interstitial keratitis is the most prevalent manifestation, affecting 80% of cases. Other potential ocular issues include scleritis, episcleritis,

Table 12.1 Features of Typical and Atypical Cogan's Syndrome

Feature	Typical Cogan's Syndrome	Atypical Cogan's Syndrome
Ocular Symptoms	Primary: Non-syphilitic interstitial keratitis	Various inflammatory issues: May include interstitial keratitis, conjunctivitis, scleritis, uveitis, optic disc edema, papillitis, central vein occlusion, optic neuropathy, retinal vasculitis
Audio-Vestibular Symptoms	Ménière's syndrome-like: Sudden tinnitus, vertigo, hearing loss	Differing from Ménière's syndrome
Time Gap between Ocular and Audio-Vestibular Symptoms	Gap of less than 2 years between onset	Delay of more than 2 years between appearance
Systemic Manifestations	Not common	Occurs more frequently (30–50%): Rheumatoid arthritis, juvenile arthritis, ankylosing spondylitis

angle-closure glaucoma, retinal vascular disease, uveitis, conjunctivitis, optic disc edema, exoph-thalmos, vasculitic optic neuropathy, and extraocular muscle tendonitis. Common clinical symptoms include ocular redness (74%), light sensitivity with tearing (50%), eye pain (50%), and decreased visual acuity (42%). Slit lamp examination may reveal ciliary injection and small opacities in the cornea's posterior stroma near the limbus. Inflammatory signs like cells and flare are also visible in the anterior chamber. The earliest corneal signs are subepithelial infiltrates, resembling those in viral epidemic keratoconjunctivitis. Typically, both eyes are affected, though symptoms and findings can be markedly asymmetric, with the more affected eye varying over time.[1]

12.1.4.4 Audio-Vestibular Manifestations

The most frequent symptoms include hearing loss, vertigo, ataxia, nausea, vomiting, and oscillopsia, which can appear anytime during the disease. Typically, the vestibular system is affected first, followed by the cochlear system within days to weeks. Vestibular symptoms tend to recede once auditory symptoms emerge. Hearing loss in CS, both unilateral and bilateral, often resembles sensorineural hearing loss and may progress to complete deafness in 1 to 3 months, occurring in about 50% of patients. Permanent hearing loss is noted in 20% of patients. CS-induced vasculitis can lead to degeneration in the organ of Corti and fibrosis and osteogenesis in the perilymphatic space, which may represent one of the mechanisms causing permanent hearing loss. Notably, at least 20% of patients exhibit spontaneous or gaze-induced nystagmus.[1, 5]

12.1.4.5 Systemic Manifestations

Systemic manifestations tend to present within the first 2 months of onset. In a retrospective case series of 32 patients, 78% of CS patients presented with systemic findings. They presented as a total of 65 different systemic manifestations that could be grouped into nine separate groups.[4]

1. *Constitutional features*: Fever, fatigue, weight loss

2. *Musculoskeletal manifestations*: Arthralgia/myalgia

3. *Cardiovascular manifestations*: Aortitis, aortic insufficiency, iliac, coronary, and renal artery stenosis, pericarditis, Raynaud's phenomenon

4. *Gastrointestinal manifestations*: Abdominal pain, splenomegaly, hepatitis, esophagitis, liver steatosis

5. *Neurological manifestations*: Headache, lymphocytic meningitis, encephalitis, peripheral neuropathy, facial nerve palsy

6. *Skin and/or mucous membrane signs or chondritis*: Mouth ulcers, skin rashes, vitiligo, photosensitivity, chondritis

7. *Urogenital manifestations*: Peyronie disease, orchitis

8. *Renal manifestations*: Membranoproliferative glomerulonephritis

9. *Lymphadenopathy*

Table 12.2 Diagnostic Criteria for Cogan's Syndrome

Criteria	Clinical Finding
Mandatory Criteria	Sensorineural hearing loss, inflammatory ocular disease, exclusion of alternative causes
Prevalent and Additional Criteria	Vertigo, tinnitus, ataxia, dizziness, fever, weight loss, fatigue, lymphadenopathy, headache
Suggested Additional Diagnostic Criterion	Large-, medium-, or small-vessel vasculitis; positive inflammatory laboratory biomarkers

The most common systemic vasculitis associated with CS is aortitis and is present in 10% of CS patients. CS has been found to be associated with systemic autoimmune diseases in 8% to 10% of cases including Takayasu arteritis, polyarteritis nodosa, granulomatosis with polyangiitis, relapsing polychondritis, rheumatoid arthritis, renal amyloidosis associated with monoclonal gammopathy, and tubulointerstitial nephritis and uveitis (TINU syndrome).[7] Although atypical CS tends to present with more systemic manifestations, other case series report similar incidence of systemic features between typical and atypical CS.[4]

12.1.5 Diagnosis

CS is a clinical diagnosis that involves a multidisciplinary approach. Clinical diagnostic criteria of CS include mandatory, prevalent, and additional criteria with exclusion of other causes of the patient's clinical finding. Mandatory criteria are needed for the diagnosis and include sensorineural hearing loss, inflammatory ocular disease, and exclusion of alternative causes of inflammation or infection.[1] Prevalent and additional criteria aid in the diagnosis but are not mandatory and include vertigo, tinnitus, ataxia, dizziness, fever, weight loss, fatigue, lymphadenopathy, and headache. Some have suggested additional diagnostic criterion such as evidence of large-, medium-, or small-vessel vasculitis and positive inflammatory laboratory biomarkers.[1] Table 12.2 displays the diagnostic criteria for Cogan's syndrome.

There is no specific marker to diagnose Cogan's syndrome, but workup should include a complete blood count (CBC), erythrocyte sedimentation rate (ESR), C-reactive protein (CRP), and potentially magnetic resonance imaging (MRI) to show high signals in the cochlear and vestibular structures and to exclude acoustic neuromas. Nonspecific inflammatory markers such as CRP and ESR are often elevated. An infectious workup should be undergone for various organisms such as *Treponema pallidum*, chlamydia, *Borrelia burgdorferi*, brucellosis, toxoplasmosis, tularaemia, *Coxiella rickettsia*, *Bartonella*, Epstein–Barr virus, cytomegalovirus, HIV, herpes virus, hepatitis A, B, and C, mumps, Coxsackie virus, and parvovirus B19.[1]

Some studies have evaluated that the rate of CS patients positive for Hsp70 is 45% to 50%. Typical CS has higher rates of positivity to Hsp70 than atypical.[1] Other antibodies such as ANCA, myeloperoxidase (MPO), and proteinase3 (PR3) have been identified in sera of patients with CS. Additionally, some patients have a mildly positive antinuclear antibody (ANA). Few have shown a positive RF and anticardiolipin antibodies. However, these are all highly nonspecific for CS.[4] Cogan's syndrome is diagnosed based on clinical criteria, and while certain antibodies have been associated with the condition, their presence is not definitive for diagnosis. MPO and PR3 testing can be considered to rule out other vasculitic causes of a patients inflammatory symptoms as opposed to a diagnosis of CS. It is important to remember that CS patients can also have a positive MPO or PR3, so a positive test does not rule out CS. No antibody is specific for CS; however, antibody testing can be considered to rule out other causes of inflammation.

12.1.6 Differential Diagnosis

Cogan's syndrome, with its combination of ophthalmic and audio-vestibular symptoms, can be confused with several diseases. These include congenital syphilis, which is a key exclusion criterion in diagnosing Cogan's syndrome, Susac syndrome (retinocochleocerebral vasculopathy), Vogt–Koyanagi–Harada syndrome (VKH), and various systemic vasculitides like granulomatosis with polyangiitis, polyarteritis nodosa, and Takayasu's arteritis. VKH is particularly distinguishable from Cogan's syndrome due to the presence of poliosis (white patches of hair) and alopecia (hair loss), which are not seen in Cogan's syndrome. Susac syndrome is characterized by unique neuroimaging findings in the corpus callosum, a feature not present in Cogan's syndrome.[1] Systemic vasculitis, such as granulomatosis with polyangiitis, Behçet's disease, and systemic lupus erythematosus with secondary vasculitis, tend to not have both ocular and audio-vestibular findings at the time of diagnosis and can be distinguished from CS in that way.

12.1.7 Treatment

The therapeutic landscape for Cogan's syndrome encompasses a spectrum of interventions tailored to mitigate its multifaceted manifestations. Treatment strategies are devised with a dual focus: to promptly alleviate the acute symptoms and to prevent long-term sequelae. The cornerstone of CS management is the judicious use of corticosteroids, which, despite the paucity of double-blind controlled studies, have demonstrated substantial clinical benefit, particularly in the early stages of the disease. The response of ocular symptoms to corticosteroid therapy is typically more pronounced than that of the audio-vestibular symptoms, guiding the choice between topical versus systemic immunosuppressive treatment modalities. The selection of the initial therapy, the adjustment of dosages, and the transition to maintenance therapy or second-line agents are guided by the severity and progression of the disease as well as by the patient's response to treatment. A clinician has an arsenal of therapeutics to employ – from the frontline use of corticosteroids to the implementation of additional immunosuppressive agents like cyclophosphamide, methotrexate, azathioprine, and cyclosporine A, each with its distinct therapeutic profiles and side effect spectra. Furthermore, biological therapies offer novel mechanisms of action, and the judicious timing of surgical interventions may offer the promise of restored hearing.

12.1.7.1 Corticosteroids

Corticosteroids remain the primary treatment for CS, showing positive outcomes, though there's a lack of double-blind controlled studies affirming their efficacy in CS management. Ocular symptoms often respond better to corticosteroids than audio-vestibular symptoms. Topical corticosteroids and local atropine may suffice for ocular issues, but systemic immunosuppression is usually necessary. A poor response to steroids might indicate a misdiagnosis rather than a resistant strain of CS. Since CS-induced vasculitis can lead to degeneration in the organ of Corti and fibrosis and osteogenesis in the perilymphatic space, improvement in audio-vestibular symptoms with steroids is not always expected. Early high-dose corticosteroids (1 to 1.5 mg/kg of prednisone equivalent daily) are advised for audio-vestibular dysfunction, with beneficial effects typically seen within 2 to 3 weeks. Pure-tone audiometry is recommended for monitoring hearing improvements. Once improvement is observed, steroids should be gradually tapered over 2 to 6 months. Haynes et al. noted that 95% of untreated CS patients suffered permanent hearing loss, compared to 55% who received systemic steroids within 2 weeks of initial hearing loss. However, corticosteroids come with short- and long-term side effects. Due to these potential long-term effects, other immunosuppressive treatments are being explored.[1, 2]

12.1.7.2 Immunomodulatory Therapy

In the management of CS, the use of immunomodulatory therapy (IMT) is essential, with each subclass offering unique benefits. Cyclophosphamide (Cys), an alkylating agent, when combined with oral glucocorticoids, has been effective in achieving clinical stabilization in most patients, as revealed in a retrospective multicenter study. However, its usage is often limited by severe side effects, including hemorrhagic cystitis and bone marrow suppression, leading to discontinuation in some cases.[1] Similarly, methotrexate (MTX), a dihydrofolate reductase inhibitor, acts as a second-line, steroid-sparing therapy. It has demonstrated effectiveness in refractory autoimmune inner ear disease associated with CS in two small prospective studies and is also suitable for pediatric patients.[1]

In contrast, azathioprine (AZA), an immunosuppressant, is primarily used in the maintenance phase of CS treatment. Its efficacy is mainly supported by several case reports.[1] Cyclosporine A (CyA), known for inhibiting T-lymphocyte maturation and production, has been used in conjunction with corticosteroids in various studies. While CyA shows good responses for ocular and systemic vascular involvement in CS, it is less effective for auditory and vestibular symptoms.[1] Together, these DMARDs provide a comprehensive approach to CS treatment, allowing for tailored therapies based on individual patient needs and the specific manifestations of the disease.

12.1.7.3 Biological Therapy

Biological therapies used in CS include anti-TNF alpha agents, rituximab (RTX), and tocilizumab (TCZ). All current anti-TNF alpha agents – etanercept, adalimumab, golimumab, certolizumab pegol, and infliximab (IFX) – have been used to treat CS in various case series and case reports.

Conventional synthetic disease-modifying anti-rheumatic drugs (cs-DMARDS) like MTX and AZA may prevent serum anti-drug antibody production that can occur with anti-TNF alpha agents and may be added as adjunct therapy. Infliximab has been effective in cs-DMARD and steroid-refractory CS, particularly for vestibulo-auditory response.[3] Etanercept does not improve hearing loss. Rituximab has demonstrated utility in CS by potentially preventing deafness or the need for cochlear implants in severe cases, reducing the number of medications needed for systemic control and showing improvement in symptoms of hearing loss.[2,7] Adalimumab and tocilizumab have shown varied efficacy in preventing long-term hearing loss but may help stabilize the disease for maintenance.[1]

12.1.7.4 Surgical Treatment

Surgery is recommended only after the disease is inactive and controlled with long-term medication. Surgical interventions mainly focus on treating hearing loss with cochlear implants. Postoperative hearing outcomes have generally been good to excellent, lasting up to 5 years.[1]

12.2 RELAPSING POLYCHONDRITIS

12.2.1 Introduction

Relapsing polychondritis (RPC) is a rare, chronic, multisystem inflammatory disorder characterized by relapsing and remitting episodes. The disease is believed to be autoimmune in nature. It predominantly affects cartilaginous, hyaline, elastic, and fibrous tissues. The most involved structures are the cartilaginous portions of the ears, nose, and tracheobronchial tree.[8–10] RPC can also impact other cartilaginous and proteoglycan-rich structures, such as the inner ear, eyes, and cardiovascular system.[10] Initially described by Jaksch-Wartenhorst in 1923, the condition gained broader recognition in the 1960s when Pearson and colleagues coined the term 'relapsing polychondritis.' The identification of RPC is challenging due to its nonspecific signs and the relapsing-remitting pattern of the disease.[9,10]

12.2.2 Epidemiology

The epidemiological understanding of RPC is still evolving, with limited data available due to the low prevalence of disease. In the United States, the incidence of RPC is estimated at approximately 3.5 cases per million people per year. A cohort study conducted in the United Kingdom from 1990 to 2012 reported an incidence rate of 0.71 cases per million people per year.[8]

A detailed retrospective analysis involving 68 RPC patients in the United Kingdom revealed a female predominance, accounting for 68% of the cases. Other larger meta-analyses have shown equal predominance for the genders.[9] The median age at which symptoms first appeared was 44 years. However, a notable diagnostic delay averaging 55 weeks resulted in the median age at diagnosis being approximately 48 years. Demographically, of these 68 patients, a majority of 55 patients (81%) were Caucasian, followed by 8 Afro-Caribbean, 4 Asian, and 1 of mixed ethnicity.

Regarding clinical criteria, 82% of the patients in this study met the Michet criteria for RPC (see Table 12.3). A commonality among these patients was the involvement of two or more organs, with pulmonary involvement being the most frequently observed.[11]

12.2.3 Etiology and Pathogenesis

RPC affects a wide range of tissues, not limited to cartilaginous structures like the ears, nose, respiratory tract, and joints, but also extending to non-cartilaginous tissues such as the eyes, skin, heart, and central nervous system.[8] RPC is an autoimmune process, as evidenced by (1) its frequent association with other autoimmune disorders; (2) the effectiveness of glucocorticoids and immunosuppressive therapy; (3) infiltration of cartilaginous structures by CD4+ T lymphocytes; (4) the presence of immunoglobulins and plasma cells in lesions; and (5) the presence of autoantibodies against types II, IX, and XI collagen.[12]

The exact pathogenesis of RPC remains unclear, but autoimmune reactions against type II collagen are believed to play a crucial role. Evidence suggests involvement of both humoral and cellular immunity, with cartilaginous tissue biopsies often showing infiltration by CD4+ T cells. Stabler et al. and colleagues highlighted the role of other cell-mediated immune responses, particularly the activation of monocyte and macrophage lineages in RPC's development.[12]

RPC is predominantly considered an immune-mediated disease and is known to have significant overlap with other autoimmune disorders. A notable genetic link is its strong association with the human leukocyte antigen (HLA) allele DR4. Various immune responses directed against cartilage components have been documented in RPC. Autoantibodies targeting multiple collagen types (II, IX,

Table 12.3 Relapsing Polychondritis Diagnostic Criterion Overview

Michet's Criteria	McAdam's Criteria with Damiani/Levine Modification

1. Chondritis at 2 sites:
  ▪ Auricular, nasal, laryngotracheal
2. One site of chondritis + 2 other of the following signs:
  ▪ Ocular inflammation
  ▪ Vestibular dysfunction
  ▪ Hearing loss
  ▪ Seronegative inflammatory arthritis
	1. 3 of the following 6 features:
	  ▪ Bilateral auricular chondritis
	  ▪ Nasal chondritis
	  ▪ Respiratory tract chondritis
	  ▪ Ocular inflammation
	  ▪ Non-erosive seronegative inflammatory arthritis
	  ▪ Cochlear/Vestibular dysfunction
	2. One of the above + histological confirmation
	3. Chondritis at 2 or more sites + response to steroids or dapsone

Source: Modified from Figure 12.1 in Gallagher et al.[9]

and XI), as well as cartilage matrix proteins like matrilin-1 and cartilage oligomeric matrix protein (COMP), have been identified in studies.[12]

Triggering factors for RPC include mechanical stimuli such as trauma or piercings, which might expose hidden antigens within the cartilaginous matrix, initiating the autoimmune process. Additionally, RPC occurrences have been linked to glucosamine chondroitin supplementation, intravenous drug use, and post-TNF-alpha inhibition with medications like etanercept. Intriguingly, RPC can also manifest during pregnancy, suggesting a hormonal influence on its pathogenesis. Cross-reactivity with structural homologs of cartilaginous autoantigens found in *Mycobacterium tuberculosis* and myxoma virus may also trigger the autoimmune cascade in RPC.[12]

12.2.4 Diagnostic Criterion

Relapsing polychondritis is a clinical diagnosis based on established criteria sets, primarily those developed by Michet and McAdam, with the latter being later modified by Damiani and Levine.[9] Historically, RPC diagnosis was characterized by chondritis at multiple sites (such as the nose, ears, laryngotracheal region), vestibulo-auditory dysfunction, seronegative inflammatory arthritis, and ocular inflammation.[9]

The revised criteria, as modified by Damiani and Levine, require the presence of three of the following features for diagnosis: bilateral auricular chondritis, nasal chondritis, respiratory tract chondritis, ocular inflammation, non-erosive seronegative inflammatory arthritis, and cochlear/vestibular dysfunction. A diagnosis can be established if one of these features is present alongside histological confirmation or if the patient exhibits chondritis at two or more sites and responds favorably to steroids or dapsone treatment.

Table 12.3 provides a detailed comparison of the original McAdam criteria alongside the modified Damiani and Levine criteria, as well as the Michet criteria, to facilitate a comprehensive understanding of the diagnostic process for RPC.[9]

12.2.5 Clinical Presentation

The diagnosis of RPC is mostly clinical and may be informed by laboratory data, imaging techniques, and occasionally cartilage biopsies. As mentioned earlier, there are established diagnostic criteria such as the Michet, McAdam, and Daminani and Levine to help clinicians establish a diagnosis of RPC. RPC has a wide spectrum of presentations and tissues that can be affected. RPC mimickers such as granulomatosis with polyangiitis (GPA), T cell lymphoma, and sarcoidosis must be distinguished from RPC. In addition, other immune-mediated disease, such as systemic lupus erythematosus, Sjögren's syndrome, systemic vasculitis, antiphospholipid syndrome, rheumatoid arthritis, spondylarthritis, inflammatory bowel disease, and thyroiditis, are associated with RPC in up to 30% of cases and should be searched for systematically.[10]

12.2.5.1 Ocular Manifestations in Patients with RPC

Table 12.4 displays the ocular manifestations of RPC. Large case series have reportedly observed a range of 20% to 61% prevalence of ocular symptoms of patients with RPC. The most common ocular manifestations include scleritis (41%), uveitis (26%), conjunctivitis (35%), and keratitis (7%). The most common ocular symptoms include eye redness, blurred vision, and eye pain.[8]

Table 12.4 Ocular Manifestations of Relapsing Polychondritis

Orbit	Orbital inflammation, proptosis and exophthalmos
Eyelids	Lid edema, ptosis, Horner's syndrome, tarsitis
Conjunctiva	Conjunctivitis, keratoconjunctivitis sicca
Cornea	Keratitis, ulceration, peripheral thinning, infiltrates, perforation
Sclera	Anterior and posterior scleritis, episcleritis, scleromalacia
Lens	Cataracts (posterior subcapsular)
Uvea	Anterior, intermediate, posterior and panuveitis
Retina	Retinopathy, CRVO/BRVO, CRAO/BRAO, retinal detachment, retinal vasculitis, retinal pigment epithelium defects, cystoid macular edema, choroiditis
Optic Nerve	Optic neuritis, optic perineuritis, ischemic optic neuropathy, optic disc edema
Ocular Adenxa	Dacryocystitis, ophthalmoplegia due to extraocular muscle palsy

Source: Modified from Table 1 of Fukuda et al.[8]
Abbreviations: CRVO: central retinal vein occlusion, BRVO: branch retinal vein occlusion, CRAO: central retinal artery occlusion, BRAO: branch retinal artery occlusion.

12.2.5.2 Scleritis

Scleritis/episcleritis is the most common ocular complication associated with RPC. Most cases of scleritis are bilateral, and the most common subtype of scleritis is diffuse anterior scleritis. However, nodular, necrotizing, and posterior scleritis have all been observed. The scleritis in RPC is accompanied by more visual disturbances, rates of recurrence, rates of necrotization, and bilaterality when compared to other immune-mediated scleritis.[8]

12.2.5.3 Uveitis

Uveitis ranks among the more prevalent ophthalmic manifestations of RPC, accounting for 12% to 20% of patients who are diagnosed with RPC presenting with uveitis.[8] Typically presenting as chronic and anterior uveitis, it frequently involves a hypopyon. Notably, RPC can also manifest as panuveitis, which may include retinitis, and can be accompanied by retinal vasculitis, retinal hemorrhages, and cystoid macular edema.

12.2.5.4 Conjunctivitis

In RPC, conjunctivitis typically manifests as nonspecific conjunctival injection, often described as painful or itchy by patients. Clinical examination may reveal subconjunctival hemorrhages and significant chemosis. Prolonged conjunctival inflammation in RPC can lead to the development of salmon patch lesions, characterized by reactive lymphoid hyperplasia. This condition is frequently bilateral, and excisional biopsy of these lesions typically shows granulomatous obliterative microangiopathy. The biopsy reveals an array of inflammatory cells in the substantia fascia, including eosinophils, plasma cells, lymphocytes, and epithelioid cells.[8] Immunofluorescence staining in RPC patients often indicates deposition of complement (C3) and immunoglobulins IgM and IgG on the walls of conjunctival vessels.

12.2.5.5 Cornea

Peripheral ulcerative keratitis (PUK) is identified as a common type of keratitis in RPC, sharing similarities with other connective tissue disorders such as rheumatoid arthritis.[8] PUK in RPC can progress rapidly, potentially leading to corneal melting and perforation. Histological examinations of enucleated eyes affected by corneal melt in RPC have revealed necrotic corneal stroma infiltrated with polymorphonuclear leukocytes and plasma cells, particularly in the peripheral stroma. Additionally, corneal infiltrates often occur alongside scleritis in cases of RPC.[8]

12.2.5.6 Eyelid

Lid edema is observed in 8% of patients with RPC and occurs in association with orbital inflammation or independently. Both retraction and ptosis have been observed in RPC.[8]

12.2.5.7 Lens

In cases of RPC, the development of posterior subcapsular cataracts is a frequent observation. This occurrence is presumably linked to prolonged intraocular inflammation or as a consequence of systemic corticosteroid therapy, which is often employed in the management of RPC.[8]

12.2.5.8 Retina

Isaak and colleagues observed that approximately 8% of patients with RPC exhibit some form of retinopathy. This retinopathy can manifest as cotton-wool spots, retinal hemorrhage, and microaneurysms. In RPC, retinal vascular occlusions, including both vein and artery occlusions, are often associated with the vasculitis characteristic of the condition. Additionally, occurrences of exudative retinal detachments and defects in the retinal pigment epithelium (RPE) have been reported. Furthermore, cystoid macular edema is a common observation in RPC patients who have uveitis.[8]

12.2.5.9 Optic Nerve and Other Cranial Nerves

Although uncommon, optic neuropathy is recognized as the most prevalent cranial nerve disorder associated with RPC. The term 'optic neuropathy' in RPC encompasses a range of conditions including optic neuritis, papilledema, ischemic optic neuropathy, and optic nerve perineuritis. There have been instances in which optic perineuritis emerged as the initial complication of RPC despite its rarity.

Apart from the optic nerve, RPC can also affect other cranial nerves, notably the oculomotor and abducens nerves, inducing palsies and potentially diplopia.[8]

12.2.5.10 Orbit and Miscellaneous

In patients with RPC, a rare but notable complication is orbital inflammation. Orbital inflammation in RPC can manifest as proptosis, periorbital lid edema, eye pain, and restricted movement of the extraocular muscles. Additionally, orbital inflammation has the potential to induce cranial nerve palsies and optic perineuritis.

In cases where orbital inflammation in RPC leads to the formation of orbital masses, biopsies have revealed them to often be reactive lymphoid hyperplasia or mucosa-associated lymphoid tissue B cell lymphoma. It's important to note that patients with RPC are at an increased risk of hematological malignancies, including leukemia, multiple myeloma, and lymphoma. Therefore, when an orbital mass is identified in an RPC patient, a biopsy is strongly recommended to determine the nature of the mass and guide appropriate treatment.[8]

12.2.5.11 Systemic Manifestations of RPC

The spectrum of systemic manifestations of RPC is vast. In principle, RPC symptomatically affects any tissue containing specific types of collagen, proteoglycans, cartilaginous connective proteins, elastin, fibrin, and other various connective tissues. That, in turn, produces pathologic disease in many organ systems. However, it is important to remember that chondritis is the hallmark manifestation of the disease entity. Auricular chondritis is the most common chondritis and occurs in almost 60% to 90% of cases.[8] This presents as unilateral or bilateral ear pain, redness, or swelling. Prolonged or repeated inflammation of the ear can produce floppy pinna or cauliflower ear.[8] Other common symptoms include nasal chondritis, hearing loss, vestibular dysfunction, and dyspnea due to laryngotracheal involvement. Arthritis is also a very common presenting symptom. Table 12.5 describes the systemic manifestations of RPC based on organ system.

12.2.6 Diagnostics

Diagnosis of RPC is based on clinical manifestations and pathologic examination, adhering to established diagnostic criteria. Currently, there are no validated diagnostic biomarkers specifically for RPC. Laboratory analysis does not reveal any characteristic findings unique to RPC. However, nonspecific inflammatory markers such as ESR, CRP, and other acute-phase reactants are present in about 60% of cases. Elevated antinuclear antibodies and ANCA levels, without a preference for PR3 or MPO, may be observed but are nonspecific. Common baseline laboratory tests like ESR, CRP, CBC, and a comprehensive metabolic panel (CMP) are utilized, but none provide findings specific to RPC.[8, 10]

Imaging techniques, including computed tomography (CT), MRI, ^{18}F-fluorodeoxyglucose-positron emission tomography/CT (FDG-PET/CT), and color Doppler ultrasonography, are valuable for assessing local inflammation and aiding in the diagnosis of RPC. CT is particularly useful for evaluating the larynx to the subsegmental bronchi. Chest CT scans in RPC patients often show airway thickening and narrowing due to cartilaginous destruction but without involvement of the posterior membranous wall. FDG-PET/CT is effective in detecting a range of RPC lesions across various sites, including the auricular, nasal, and bronchial regions, as well as laryngeal, tracheal, costal, and joint chondritis.[8] MRI and ultrasonography are particularly useful in evaluating articular and ear

Table 12.5 Clinical Systemic Manifestations of Relapsing Polychondritis

System	Manifestation
Ear	Auricular chondritis, hearing loss, tinnitus, serous otitis media, vertigo, nausea, vomiting, ataxia
Nose	Nasal chondritis, saddle nose deformity, rhinorrhea, epistaxis
Respiratory	Hoarseness, cough, aphonia, dyspnea, wheezing, inspiratory stridor, laryngotracheal stricture and collapse
Renal	Creatinine elevation, microhematuria, proteinuria, necrotizing glomerulonephritis, glomerulosclerosis, IgA nephropathy, tubulointerstitial nephritis
Musculoskeletal	Arthritis, costochondral cartilage tenderness, flail chest, dislocation
Cardiovascular	Valvular heart disease, aneurysm, pericarditis, vasculitis, coronary heart disease, atrioventricular block, tachycardia
Skin	Urticaria, purpura, oral aphthosis, angioedema, erythema multiforme, erythema nodosum, livedo reticularis, panniculitis, superficial phlebitis, dermatomyositis like lesions
Neurologic	Headache, cranial neuropathy, encephalopathy, seizure, hemiplegia, ataxia
General	Fatigue, malaise, weight loss, night sweats, lymphadenopathy

Source: Table modified from Table 5 of Fukuda et al.[8]

involvement of RPC. In atypical cases, deep cartilage biopsy in affected cartilage may be necessary to help aid in diagnosis.

To measure disease activity, 27 experts developed the Relapsing Polychondritis Disease Activity Index (RPDAI), which identifies 27 items with individual weights ranging from 1 to 24, culminating in a maximum theoretical score of 265. The RPDAI considers the patient's condition over a 28-day period preceding the medical examination.[12]

Monitoring disease activity and predicting progression in RPC is crucial for optimizing management. Various biomarkers have been studied for this purpose. Anti–type II collagen antibodies are present in approximately 50% of RPC patients. Serum cartilage oligomeric matrix protein levels have been proposed as a marker, but their reliability in distinguishing active from non-active disease is inconclusive. The soluble triggering receptor expressed on myeloid cells-1 (sTREM-1) has shown promise in predicting disease activity, but its utility is limited due to elevation in other autoimmune diseases like systemic lupus erythematosus and rheumatoid arthritis. Increases in interferon-gamma and interleukin-2 have been observed during RPC flares, yet these markers are not exclusive to RPC and have variable clinical utility.[10, 12]

12.2.7 Treatment and Management

12.2.7.1 A Focus on Ocular Treatment and Management

Due to its rarity, there are no randomized trials or evidence-based guidelines for treating RPC. Ocular inflammation in RPC typically requires systemic treatment under a rheumatologist's guidance, as topical treatments alone are often insufficient. The choice of therapy depends on the disease's severity and organ systems involved, ranging from non-steroidal anti-inflammatory drugs (NSAIDs), dapsone, and colchicine for mild cases to systemic glucocorticoids for severe cases, including those with ocular inflammation. Long-term immunosuppression is often necessary to prevent relapse.

For patients intolerant to steroids or in need of steroid-sparing options, immunosuppressants such as cyclophosphamide, methotrexate, azathioprine, and cyclosporine are second-line treatments. Additionally, biologics like infliximab, etanercept, adalimumab, rituximab, anakinra, tocilizumab, and abatacept have been employed with varying success. Specifically, refractory scleritis in RPC has been effectively managed with immunosuppressants (cyclosporine, azathioprine, cyclophosphamide), infliximab, or tocilizumab, alongside corticosteroids. Surgical interventions may be necessary for complications from ocular inflammation, including cataract, secondary glaucoma, or corneal perforation.[8]

12.2.7.2 Management for Specific Clinical Manifestations

A systemic review by Petitdemange et al. looked to find the most efficacious therapeutics for RPC. As stated earlier, corticosteroids are commonly used for their anti-inflammatory effects, particularly

Table 12.6 Main Clinical Features of Relapsing Polychondritis and Proposed Management

Clinical Manifestation	Typical Therapeutic Management
Nasal, Auricular, Parasternal Chondritis	NSAIDs, glucocorticoids (GCs). For relapses, consider colchicine, dapsone, methotrexate.
Tracheal Chondritis	GC (oral or intravenous), conventional synthetic DMARDs (csDMARDs), other immunosuppressives (e.g., cyclophosphamide), or biologics.
Articular Manifestations	NSAIDs, GCs, csDMARDs, conventional immunosuppressives (e.g., methotrexate), or biologics.
Cutaneous Involvement	GCs, colchicine, dapsone (particularly for neutrophilic dermatitis), methotrexate.
Cardiac or Valvular Involvement	GCs, csDMARDs, conventional immunosuppressives (e.g., methotrexate), or biologics.
Ocular Involvement	Referral to an ophthalmologist is essential. Topical GCs, cycloplegics. csDMARDs, conventional immunosuppressives, or biologics may be required.
Audio-Vestibular Involvement	GCs, methylprednisolone infusion, csDMARDs, conventional immunosuppressives or biologics.
Neurological Manifestations	GCs, methylprednisolone infusion, csDMARDs, conventional immunosuppressives (e.g., cyclophosphamide), or biologics.
Renal Involvement	Uncommon manifestation. Often indicates differential diagnoses like ANCA-associated vasculitis.

Source: Table adapted from Rednic et al.[10]
Abbreviations: ANCA: antineutrophil cytoplasmic autoantibodies, GCs: glucocorticoids, NSAIDs: non-steroidal anti-inflammatory drugs, csDMARDs: conventional synthetic disease-modifying antirheumatic drugs.

in severe cases of RPC, and are often paired with other immunosuppressants or biologic therapies to enhance treatment efficacy and reduce steroid dependence. The review found that treatments such as TNF-alpha inhibitors (TNFi), methotrexate, tocilizumab (TCZ), and abatacept (ABT) were associated with the best outcomes. ABT showed a pooled response rate of 72%, TCZ 66%, and TNFi 64%, with MTX slightly less at 56%.[13] The evidence suggests ABT, IFX, ADA, TCZ, and MTX are most effective, but the choice of therapy should be tailored to the patient's specific needs, including the severity of disease and potential side effects, and patient comorbidities.[13]

Table 12.6 lists a wide array of clinical manifestations of RPC and typical therapeutics and management based on experts' opinion and literature.

12.3 VACUOLES, E1 ENZYME, X-LINKED, AUTOINFLAMMATORY, SOMATIC (VEXAS) SYNDROME

12.3.1 Introduction

Vacuoles, E1 enzyme, X-linked, autoinflammatory, somatic (VEXAS) syndrome was initially identified in 2020 by Beck et al. through a case series of 25 men who exhibited multisystem autoinflammation and hematological disorders. These manifestations were attributed to a somatic mutation in the E1 ubiquitin-conjugating enzyme encoded by the UBA1 gene on the X chromosome.[14, 15] Patients with VEXAS have been found to exhibit elevated levels of inflammatory cytokines, including interferon-gamma, interleukin-8, and interferon-inducible protein 10. These pro-inflammatory mediators trigger an inflammatory cascade that activates the innate immune system, resulting in the diverse symptoms observed. Ophthalmic symptoms in VEXAS patients, as reported in the original case series by Beck et al., include orbital inflammation, orbital myositis, dacryoadenitis, orbital cellulitis, ophthalmoplegia due to cranial neuritis, optic neuritis, scleritis, various forms of uveitis (anterior, intermediate, posterior), and retinal vasculitis.[15]

12.3.2 Epidemiology

Most patients with VEXAS syndrome are older men, reflective of the X-linked nature of the mutation, with a median age of 74 years at diagnosis.[16] The estimated prevalence of VEXAS is roughly 1 in 14,000 individuals, with the prevalence increasing to 1 in 4000 if one is male and above the age of 50 years. A case series by Georgin-Lavialle et al., involving patients with VEXAS syndrome, revealed a male predominance of 96%. The median age at symptom onset was 67 years, while the age at diagnosis was 71 years.

12.3.3 Etiology and Pathogenesis

In VEXAS syndrome, an acquired inactivating mutation affects the X-linked UBA1 gene. UBA1 is responsible for encoding the E1 activating enzyme, which plays a crucial role in activating ubiquitin in roughly 90% of cases. The process of ubiquitination, facilitated by the E1 activating enzyme, leads to the ubiquitylation-dependent degradation of intracellular proteins, essential for maintaining cellular homeostasis.[17] UBA1 has two isoforms: UBA1a, a nuclear form initiated at p.Met1, and UBA1b, a shorter cytoplasmic form beginning at p.Met41. Pathogenic mutations in VEXAS syndrome predominantly occur at the methionine-41 position. About half of all documented VEXAS cases involve a c.122 T > C, p.Met41Thr mutation; mutations at c.121A > G, Met41Val, and c.121A > C, Met41Leu, are also common.[17] These mutations lead to either a complete loss of UBA1b protein function or the production of a novel isoform, UBA1c, with significantly reduced catalytic activity.[17]

The mutation that occurs in VEXAS syndrome originates in multipotent hematopoietic progenitors. It has been observed that a selection pressure develops, which influences the mutated allele to express predominantly in certain cell lines, specifically neutrophils, monocytes, and megakaryocytes, while sparing B and T lymphocytes.[17] The selective expression leads to impaired activity of cytoplasmic UBA1 in these immune cells, triggering an overproduction of interferon gamma, interleukin-8, and interferon-inducible proteins. These molecular alterations contribute to the autoinflammatory pathologies seen in individuals with VEXAS syndrome.

12.3.4 Clinical Features

12.3.4.1 Systemic Manifestations

Patients with VEXAS syndrome experience an array of symptoms due to inflammation. Two extensive case series from France and the United States revealed that skin lesions are the most frequent clinical feature, present in 82% to 83% of patients.[17] Skin manifestations include neutrophilic dermatoses, vasculitic rashes, erythema nodosum, urticaria, erythematous papules, periorbital edema, and injection-site reactions. The most common vasculitic rash present is leukocytoclastic vasculitis. Other systemic features include noninfectious fevers (64% to 83%), weight loss (62%), lung involvement (50% to 57%), arthralgia/arthritis (27% to 58%), relapsing chondritis (36% to 52%), ocular manifestations (24% to 40%), venous thrombosis (35% to 41%), and lymphadenopathy (34%). Less common symptoms are pericarditis, myocarditis, and orchitis.[17] Most VEXAS patients exhibit elevated CRP levels, neutropenia, thrombocytopenia, and macrocytic anemia. Many other clinical inflammatory phenotypes have been diagnosed in patients with VEXAS, including relapsing polychondritis, polyarteritis nodosa, Sweet's syndrome, and large- and small-vessel vasculitis.[17]

12.3.4.2 Ocular Manifestations

Ocular symptom prevalence in VEXAS syndrome varies, ranging from 16% to 39%. Recent case studies suggest a prevalence closer to 30% to 35% (Abumanhal). Since the discovery of VEXAS syndrome in 2020, the list of ocular manifestations has expanded. These include orbital inflammation, orbital myositis, dacryoadenitis, ophthalmoplegia, optic neuritis, scleritis, uveitis, and retinal vasculitis.[15]

Orbital inflammatory syndrome, encompassing dacryoadenitis, posterior scleritis, and extraocular muscle orbital myositis, appears to be the most common ocular manifestation. Notably, the Met41Val mutation is more frequently associated with ocular symptoms compared to other common mutations.[15]

Georgin-Lavialle et al.'s study of patients identified uveitis, scleritis, and episcleritis as the three most common ocular manifestations outside of an orbital inflammatory syndrome. Myint et al.'s literature review found anterior uveitis to be the most prevalent type of uveitis. Table 12.7 compiles data from 21 case reports and series, detailing their most common ocular manifestations. Note, not all cases had associated documentation of ocular manifestations, so the percentile does not add up to 100%.

12.3.4.3 Hematological Manifestations

The hematologic manifestations of the syndrome include macrocytic anemia and various cytopenias, such as neutropenia and thrombocytopenia, which may be accompanied by myelodysplasia or present as myelodysplastic syndrome.[15] VEXAS syndrome establishes a genetic connection between

Table 12.7 Prevalence of Ocular Manifestations in Documented Cases of VEXAS

Ocular Manifestation	Sample Size of 216 patients (%)
Episcleritis	35 (16)
Scleritis (anterior/posterior)	49 (22)
Orbital Inflammation	12 (5)
Uveitis (anterior/intermediate/posterior/panuveitis)	29 (13)
Orbital Myositis	4 (2)

Source: Table modified from Table 2 of Myint et al.[16]

autoinflammation and myelodysplastic syndromes (MDS). MDS is diagnosed in approximately 25% to 55% of patients with VEXAS syndrome. While the UBA1 protein plays a crucial role in cellular protein degradation, the UBA1 gene is not yet recognized as a gene associated with MDS. Current research is exploring whether this represents a novel gene mutation contributing to MDS development or if the UBA1 protein mutation creates a chronic inflammatory environment that promotes the clonal expansion of myeloid neoplasms.[18] Additionally, it's significant to note that patients with VEXAS syndrome have an increased risk of developing multiple myeloma, suggesting that mutations in UBA1 may predispose individuals to this condition.[18] Patients with VEXAS-MDS had more frequent recurrent fevers, gastrointestinal tract involvement, pulmonary infiltrates, and arthralgias when compared to VEXAS patients without MDS.[14]

12.3.5 Diagnosis

VEXAS can be suspected based on clinical features, but definitive diagnosis requires genetic testing for the UBA1 gene mutation. Additional laboratory indicators, beyond the abnormal hematological markers, can assist in diagnosing VEXAS syndrome. Markedly elevated CRP levels are a notable finding in many VEXAS patients, with some case series reporting values as high as 133.0 mg/dL.[14] Elevated RF, increased IgG4 levels, ANA, and ANCA positivity are also seen but nonspecific. There is some evidence suggesting that patients with VEXAS might also have elevated factor VIII activity and a positive lupus anticoagulant. DNA analysis from bone marrow biopsies is crucial for identifying the UBA1 mutation and should be strongly considered in patients suspected of having VEXAS.[17] Additionally, if orbital symptoms are present, magnetic resonance imaging (MRI) of the orbits can be valuable for diagnostic purposes.

12.3.6 Treatment and Management

There are two primary therapeutic strategies for treating VEXAS syndrome: (1) targeting and eradicating the UBA1-mutated hematopoietic population and (2) inhibiting the disease's pro-inflammatory state. Managing inflammatory symptoms can be challenging, often necessitating prolonged high-dose steroids or immunosuppression, which carries associated risks of toxicity.[17] Currently, the only curative treatment is allogeneic hematopoietic stem cell transplantation (AHSCT), but this approach entails significant risks.[17] Risk stratification of VEXAS patients is crucial, especially as clinical predictors of increased mortality are identified. For instance, patients with the Met41Leu mutation generally have a better prognosis, whereas those with Met41Thr and Met41Val mutations have poorer 5-year survival rates.[14] The presence of MDS has not been shown to significantly impact the survival rate of VEXAS patients.[14] Factors associated with mortality include gastrointestinal involvement (OR 3.7), lung infiltrate (OR 3.3), and mediastinal lymph node enlargement (OR 7.73).

Therapeutic management includes glucocorticoids, conventional disease-modifying anti-rheumatic drugs (DMARDs), and biological targeted therapies. Steroid-sparing therapies are selected based on severity of disease, specific organ involvement, and patient comorbidities. Common conventional DMARDs used for VEXAS include methotrexate, cyclophosphamide, and mycophenolate. Biological therapies used include anti-IL-6R (tocilizumab), IL-1 receptor antagonists (anakinra and canakinumab), TNF-alpha inhibitors, and rituximab. JAK inhibitors (baricitinib and ruxolitinib) and azacytidine are also used, though less frequently. There is insufficient data for a head-to-head comparison of these therapeutic agents. More than half of VEXAS patients are glucocorticoid dependent, with a median daily dose of 20 mg.[14, 17]

It's also important to consider vaccinations in lymphopenic patients and to use prophylactic antibiotics and antivirals. Venous thromboembolism prophylaxis is advised due to the increased thrombotic risk in these patients. Supportive agents like erythropoietin-stimulating agents and thrombopoietin receptor agonists (eltrombopag) may benefit VEXAS-MDS patients.[17] Note that the data on AHSCT in VEXAS is limited, and its efficacy remains inconclusive.

12.4 TUBULOINTERSTITIAL NEPHRITIS AND UVEITIS (TINU) SYNDROME

12.4.1 Introduction

Tubulointerstitial nephritis and uveitis (TINU) syndrome, first described in 1975 by Dobrin et al., is a disorder characterized by the concurrent presence of idiopathic acute tubulointerstitial nephritis and uveitis in the absence of other systemic diseases that could cause either condition.[19, 20] TINU is believed to be an immune-mediated process that can be triggered by certain drugs or infections, though most cases are idiopathic, lacking a clear precipitating factor.[20] Typically, TINU presents as bilateral, sudden-onset anterior uveitis, characterized by symptoms like redness, pain, and photophobia. However, recent literature suggests that TINU can also manifest with different subtypes of uveitis, indicating that the absence of anterior uveitis does not rule out the diagnosis.[20]

Tubulointerstitial nephritis (TIN) accounts for approximately 15% of all acute kidney injuries (AKI). Drug-induced TIN is the most common manifestation, with NSAIDs and antibiotics being the two most common etiologies. Histologically, TIN is marked by glomerular interstitial edema, inflammatory cell infiltration, and tubular damage. Diagnostic markers include urine sediment containing immune cells such as eosinophils and red blood cells, red cell casts, and proteinuria, often with high levels of albumin.[20]

12.4.2 Epidemiology

Historically, TINU syndrome was thought to develop predominantly in adolescent females, with a 3:1 female-to-male ratio and a median onset age of approximately 15 years.[19] However, the female predominance of TINU is largely being challenged, and it is thought to occur equally amongst male and female. Interestingly, males typically experience an earlier onset of the disease.[21] Mackensen et al. reported an incidence of TINU in about 1.7% of uveitis patients.[20] As more cases are studied, the female predominance seems to be less pronounced, and the disease has been observed in patients well into middle age.[21] TINU has been described across most ethnic groups, showing no specific racial or geographical preference. Notably, in Japan, it is the second-most-common cause of uveitis in children aged 10 to 15 years, following sarcoidosis. TINU accounts for approximately 32% of cases involving sudden-onset bilateral anterior uveitis in children and adolescents under 20 years of age.[21]

TINU syndrome has been associated with specific human leukocyte antigens (HLAs), including HLA-A2, HLA-A24, HLA-DQA101, HLA-DGB105, and most notably HLA-DRB101, which shows the strongest correlation.[21] While HLA-DRB101 exhibits a stronger correlation in individuals of European ancestry, no conclusive geographic, ethnic, or racial link has been established.

12.4.3 Etiology and Pathogenesis

The precise pathogenesis of TINU syndrome remains a subject of ongoing research and discussion. The prevailing theory posits that an environmental factor triggers an immune-mediated response in individuals with a specific genetic predisposition.[21] This process involves both cellular and humoral immunity. In the early stages of cellular immunity, HLA-class II receptors on immune cells present exogenous antigens to CD4+ T helper cells. Subsequently, this interaction stimulates a humoral response by B-lymphocytes, evidenced by the presence of autoantibodies against modified C-reactive protein (mCRP) in renal and ocular tissues. The possibility of a shared antigen between these tissues could account for the simultaneous renal and ocular involvement observed in TINU syndrome. Notably, elevated levels of anti-mCRP antibodies have been associated with the development of uveitis.[21]

12.4.3.1 Genetics and Environmental Factors

Mandeville et al. suggested a link between HLA-A2 and HLA-A24 in TINU patients, with these genotypes present in approximately 75% of cases in one Japanese case series. However, it's important to note that these two HLA genotypes are commonly found in the Japanese population, which may influence these findings.

In a separate case series, Levinson et al. reported associations of TINU with HLA-DQA1*01, HLA-DQB1*05, and HLA-DRB1*01, showing relative risks (RR) of 19.5, 16.3, and 25.5, respectively, and a lower RR of 8.5 with HLA-B14.

Although HLA-DRB1*01 is often cited as having the largest RR, other research indicates a much higher RR with a subtype of this HLA, specifically HLA-DRB1*0102, found in about 72% of TINU patients. Reddy et al. discovered that 14 out of 15 pediatric patients with unexplained panuveitis and TIN possessed the HLA haplotype HLA-DRB1*01 – HLA-DQB1*05. While other case studies and reports have identified links with various other HLA haplotypes, the associations with these haplotypes remain inconclusive.[20]

12.4.3.2 Medications as Risk Factors

The primary categories of medications implicated in the development of TINU syndrome include NSAIDs and antibiotics, as reported by Okafor. In the case series conducted by Mandeville et al., the use of antibiotics emerged as the most frequently reported risk factor, identified in 29 out of 122 patients. This was followed by NSAID use, noted in 22 out of 122 patients. However, there has not been a head-to-head analysis comparing different antibiotics or NSAIDs to determine specific associations with TINU syndrome.[20] It is also important to note that medications known to induce uveitis, such as cidofovir, rifabutin, sulfonamides, and bisphosphonates, have not been linked to TINU.

12.4.3.3 Infections as Risk Factors

Mandeville et al. identified infections, particularly respiratory infections, as a potential risk factor for the development of TINU syndrome. Several specific infectious agents have been suggested as possible contributors, including *Mycobacterium tuberculosis*, systemic toxoplasmosis, Epstein–Barr virus (EBV), and reactivation of varicella zoster. However, in cases of TINU associated with viral infections, the direct connection between the infectious agent and the syndrome is often less certain. This uncertainty is partly due to the high prevalence of IgG antibodies for EBV in the general population, making it difficult to establish a definitive link.[20] Amaro and colleagues also identified Chlamydia trachomatis infections as another infectious agent potentially associated with TINU.

12.4.3.4 Histopathology for TIN Diagnosis

On renal biopsy, glomeruli can show infiltration of mononuclear cells, largely composed of lymphocytes with few plasma cells and neutrophils.[22] Fibrosis involving approximately 80% of the interstitium is usually present with tubular edema, epithelial degeneration, and focal necrosis.[21] Immunofluorescent microscopy reveals IgG staining in the glomeruli with no complement components or other immunoglobulin subtype.[22]

12.4.4 Clinical Presentation

The onset of renal and intraocular inflammatory symptoms in TINU syndrome typically occurs at different times. On average, uveitis develops after TIN, typically with a delay of about 3 months, although this can extend to as long as 14 months. In approximately 20% of cases, ocular symptoms precede kidney disease. There are rare instances in which both renal and ocular manifestations present concurrently. Patients may experience prolonged nonspecific constitutional symptoms during the renal manifestation of the disease that are linked to a hypersensitivity reaction, including weight loss, malaise, fever, rash, arthralgia, and abdominal pain.[21] Additionally, a patient may experience symptoms of acute kidney injury, including decreased urine output and fluid retention. Urinalysis often reveals proteinuria and glucosuria.

12.4.4.1 Ocular Symptoms and Manifestations

The predominant ocular symptom in TINU syndrome is eye redness (hyperemia). Additional symptoms commonly include eye pain, blurred vision, and photophobia. Bilateral involvement occurs in approximately 92% of patients. Slit lamp examination typically reveals conjunctival injection and iridocyclitis. Generally, 1–2+ cell and flare are observed in the anterior chamber; a small case series in the *American Journal of Ophthalmology* noted that 3+ cell was seldom seen. In the same study, fine keratic precipitates were identified in 78% of patients, while posterior synechiae were present in about 33%. Posterior segment findings are not uncommon and include anterior vitreous cell, snowflake-like vitreous opacities, retinal exudates, and optic disc hyperemia, choroidal neovascular membranes, multifocal choroiditis, optic disc hyperemia, and edema[19, 23] (Figure 12.1). Recurrent or exacerbated uveitis is quite common in TINU syndrome. In cases of recurrent uveitis, more severe symptoms such as 3+ cell and posterior synechiae tend to be more frequent. Both fine and mutton-fat keratic precipitates, as well as hypopyon, are also more commonly observed. More severe posterior segment findings, including optic disc edema and hyperemia and retinal edema, are typically more pronounced during recurrent flares.[19] Most patients with TINU syndrome experience bilateral, non-granulomatous anterior uveitis.[21]

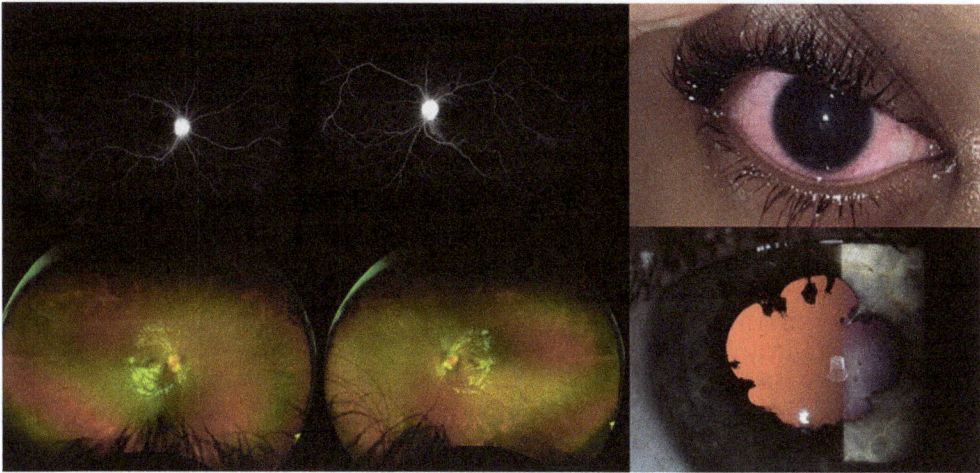

Figure 12.1 TINU anterior and posterior segment findings. Fluorescein angiography showing disc leakage (upper left) with accompanying fundus photography (lower left) illustrating optic disc edema in a patient with TINU. Slit lamp photos displaying fine keratic precipitates with injection (upper right) and posterior synechiae in a patient with TINU (lower right). (Acknowledgment to Dr. Sapna Gangaputra for photographs.)

12.4.5 Diagnosis

TINU syndrome is a diagnosis of exclusion, where other diseases that simultaneously cause uveitis and nephritis must be ruled out. It is typically diagnosed in the context of azotemia of unknown origin or a range of ophthalmic symptoms, such as visual impairment, eye pain, or eye redness. The diagnosis should be considered in young patients presenting with bilateral uveitis or tubulointerstitial nephritis. Historically, a renal biopsy is necessary for a confirmatory diagnosis of TIN. However, the patient must also present with the uveitis component for the diagnosis to be made.[21] In present day, the diagnosis can be confirmed with an elevated urine beta-2 microglobulin and creatinine with concomitant uveitis.[24]

Over 90% of TINU patients show increased urinary β-2 microglobulin, making it a proposed screening tool for clinicians.[21] Levels of N-acetylglucosaminidase may also be elevated. Typically, blood urea nitrogen (BUN) levels remain normal, while serum creatinine may be slightly elevated. Normocytic anemia, along with elevated ESR and CRP, is also observed in TINU. Microscopic urinalysis frequently indicates urinary eosinophils, pyuria, hematuria without infection, and white cell casts.[21] ANA, RF, angiotensin-converting enzyme and human T cell lymphotropic virus type I antibodies are generally normal. During uveitic flares, fluorescein angiography often reveals hyperfluorescence of the optic disc with leakage from the retinal microvasculature in the posterior pole.[19]

12.4.6 Treatment and Management

Long-term follow-up in TINU syndrome remains under-researched. However, treatments tend to yield generally favorable outcomes for both kidney and ocular health. It is important to note that the kidney and uveitis manifestations may follow independent courses and vary in severity. Treatment is not standardized. During active phases of both TIN and uveitis, ocular inflammation and renal function respond to corticosteroids. Nevertheless, managing ocular disease can be more challenging; uveitis may persist or relapse even after periods exceeding 10 years, whereas renal disease typically does not relapse.

12.4.6.1 Treatment of Uveitis

For most cases of anterior uveitis, topical corticosteroids and cycloplegic agents are the initial treatments. During the active phase, approximately 80% of anterior uveitis cases will require more intensive immunosuppression with systemic steroids. Recent case series suggest that systemic corticosteroids alone may not prevent recurrence – about 70% of patients need additional immune-modulating therapy (IMT).[19] Younger patients are more prone to develop chronic uveitis, which can last beyond 3 months. More than half of the individuals experience a recurrence of ocular inflammation after stopping corticosteroids, often with more severe symptoms.

Successful management of refractory cases, or those seeking to reduce corticosteroid use, has been reported with methotrexate (MTX), azathioprine (AZA), and mycophenolate mofetil (MMF). Current studies show no superiority of one IMT over another in terms of outcomes. IMT should be introduced in a stepwise manner, typically starting with a low dose of MTX once a week. AZA and MMF may be more beneficial for renal conditions. Sobolewska et al. reported in a retrospective case series that sustained IMT treatment, averaging between 13 and 40 months, with a median of 29.5 months, effectively managed ocular disease.[26] It is advised to aim for 12 to 24 months of disease quiescence before ceasing IMT. While IMT is generally effective in controlling TINU, biologics like adalimumab are seldom required. However, if patients experience adverse effects from IMT, particularly MTX, biologics may be considered. It is also important to note that TINU is a pediatric uveitide, so MMF should be considered as first-line treatment over MTX due to its safer side effect profile.

In a study by Goda et al. of 12 patients, systemic corticosteroids successfully managed initial episodes of uveitis and TIN, with dosages ranging from 20 mg to 60 mg of prednisone orally over a duration of 2 months for both adults and children.[19] Notably, about 45% of patients experienced a recurrence or worsening of their uveitis after weaning treatment with corticosteroids. Although the initial dose did not prevent recurrence, higher doses of prednisone above 40 mg orally have been associated with lower recurrence rates.

12.4.6.2 Renal Treatment

Immediate administration of systemic corticosteroids is crucial for TIN management. These steroids lessen interstitial inflammation and fibrosis, leading to quicker recovery from renal symptoms and increased glomerular filtration rate (GFR).[19] Although less common than uveitis flares, renal relapses can occur after discontinuing corticosteroids. One study indicated that chronic kidney disease was present in about 30% of patients despite treatment. The role of IMT in TIN treatment, particularly in TINU cases, is not well established. However, some practitioners have found that adding MMF to corticosteroid regimens can improve outcomes and help prevent nephritis.[19]

12.4.7 Prognosis and Screening

Currently, there is no established criterion for the monitoring and screening of patients with TINU syndrome. Nonetheless, beta-2 microglobulin (β2M) has been suggested as a marker for monitoring anterior uveal activity as well as regular ophthalmic exams checking for active inflammation. A prospective study demonstrated a strong correlation between urinary β2M levels and the presence of cells and flare in the anterior chamber.[21] It has been proposed that patients diagnosed with TINU syndrome undergo ophthalmologic screenings every 3 months, although no official follow-up interval has been formalized. Additionally, the annual monitoring of serum creatinine levels has been recommended for these patients.

12.4.7.1 Visual Outcomes

With appropriate treatment, visual outcomes tend to be positive. Research by Goda et al. indicated that the best-corrected visual acuity could decrease to 0.2 (equivalent to 20/200 on the Snellen chart) due to significant vitreous floaters. However, the final best-corrected visual acuity observed was 1.2, which is approximately 20/18 on the Snellen chart, indicating an excellent level of vision restoration.[19]

12.5 VOGT–KOYANAGI–HARADA (VKH) SYNDROME

12.5.1 Introduction

Vogt–Koyanagi–Harada (VKH) syndrome is a rare, progressive autoimmune disorder characterized by bilateral granulomatous panuveitis, accompanied by auditory, neurological, and integumentary manifestations.[26] Initially recognized by Alfred Vogt, a Swiss physician who reported the first case, the syndrome was later comprehensively delineated by Japanese researchers Yoshizo Koyanagi and Einosuke Harada.[26] Early ocular indicators of VKH include multifocal serous retinal detachments and choroidal thickening, which may advance to granulomatous anterior uveitis and progressive posterior segment depigmentation, termed 'sunset glow fundus.'[27]

12.5.2 Epidemiology

The prevalence of VKH syndrome exhibits marked geographic and ethnic variations, being notably more common in Asian, Latin American, Middle Eastern, and Native American populations. In the

United States, VKH is relatively rare, constituting approximately 3% to 4% of cases in tertiary uveitis care centers.[28] A Southern California case series of patients of VKH found a female majority (69%) and a significant representation of the Hispanic population (75%), with the mean age at onset being 33.4 years.[28] A case series of VKH in the Great Plains of Oklahoma by Reddy et al. found Native American ancestry is a significant risk factor.[29] Young patients, particularly those under 15 years of age, are more likely to experience severe complications such as glaucoma (50%), papillitis (53%), epiretinal membranes (16%), and retinal detachments (4%).[28]

12.5.3 Etiology and Pathogenesis

The environmental trigger for VKH is a matter of ongoing debate, with various infectious triggers associated with the syndrome in the literature. VKH shows a strong correlation with HLA DR4 and HLA DRB1*04:05.[30] Immunological and histopathological studies suggest that VKH is an autoimmune inflammatory condition mediated by CD4+ T cells that target melanocytes. These activated T cells induce an inflammatory cascade by producing cytokines including IL 17 and IL 23. Clinically, vitiligo and the characteristic sunset flow fundus represent a loss of melanocytes at the site of immune cell infiltration. Histopathology of chronic VKH shows a loss of choroidal melanocytes and the presence of both T and B lymphocytes in the choroid with a predominance of CD4+ lymphocytes.[28] Immunohistochemical analysis of patches of vitiligo in patients with VKH show the loss of skin melanocytes with the presence of melanin-laden macrophages and infiltration of mononuclear T lymphocytes with expression of HLA DR.[28] Rat models of VKH show thickening of the choroid due to lymphocyte and epithelioid cell infiltration surrounding melanocytes – suggesting they are the antigenic target. Kobayashi and colleagues demonstrated that VKH patients' T lymphocytes in serum will react to tyrosinase peptide within melanocytes, and these peptides were recognized by HLA DRB1*0405, suggesting tyrosinase peptide antigens as an autoantigen target in VKH.[28]

12.5.3.1 Viral Infections as Risk Factors for VKH Onset

Cross reactivity between tyrosinase peptide and a cytomegalovirus peptide (CMV-egH 290-302) has been demonstrated, leading to the hypothesis that VKH may develop due to molecular mimicry in patients with CMV. Epstein–Barr virus (EBV) has also been detected via PCR in the cerebrospinal fluid in patients with active VKH.[28] No definitive correlation with viral infection has been established in the development of VKH. However, a six-patient case series described coworkers, friends, and neighbors all diagnosed with VKH, suggesting an environmental factor.[28]

12.5.4 Clinical Presentation and Features

VKH typically manifests in four distinct phases: prodromal, acute uveitic, convalescent, and chronic recurrent. Identifying the unique clinical features of each phase is crucial for accurate diagnosis.[28]

12.5.4.1 Prodromal Phase

During the prodromal phase, patients often exhibit symptoms resembling a viral infection, lasting from a few days to several weeks. Symptoms are primarily systemic rather than ocular, including headaches, meningismus, fever, nausea, vertigo, orbital pain, and auditory disturbances. The presentation can vary significantly, with some patients showing multiple symptoms and others none until later stages.[28] If lumbar puncture occurs during this phase cerebrospinal fluid analysis (CSF) can demonstrate pleocytosis.

12.5.4.2 Acute Uveitic Phase

Progression from the prodromal phase leads to the acute uveitic phase, characterized by decreased visual acuity, bilateral granulomatous uveitis, serous retinal detachments (often multifocal), and choroidal thickening. If untreated, the initial posterior uveitis can extend to the vitreous and anterior chamber. However, the presence of anterior uveitis and vitritis is not essential for diagnosis. The anterior segment may exhibit a granulomatous reaction with mutton-fat keratic precipitates. Elevated intraocular pressure is responsive to steroids, especially in patients with shallow anterior chambers.[28]

12.5.4.3 Convalescent Phase

The convalescent phase usually begins weeks to months after the acute uveitic stage and often lasts several months. Patients may develop choroid depigmentation, vitiligo, poliosis (patches of white hair), and perilimbal depigmentation (Sugiura sign). Typically, choroid depigmentation occurs 2 to 3 months after the acute uveitic phase begins, leading to a distinct 'sunset glow fundus' appearance.

Table 12.8 Overview of VKH Diagnostic Criteria[28, 30, 31, 32]

Revised VKH Diagnostic Criteria

1. No history of penetrating ocular trauma or surgery
2. No clinical or laboratory evidence of other ocular disease entities
3. Bilateral ocular involvement; criterion [a] or [b] must be met depending on stage
   a. Early manifestations
      1. Diffuse choroiditis, subretinal fluid, bullous serous retinal detachment
      2. Focal areas of delays in choroidal perfusion, multiple areas of pinpoint leakage, large areas of placoid hyperfluorescence, pooling within subretinal fluid, optic nerve staining, and choroidal thickening without posterior scleritis diagnosed on ultrasound
   b. Late manifestations
      1. History suggestive of prior disease based on subsequent findings
      2. Ocular depigmentation: Sunset glow fundus or Sugiura sign
      3. Nummular chorioretinal depigmented scars, RPE clumping, recurrent or chronic anterior uveitis
      4. Neurological signs (past or present): Headache, meningismus, tinnitus, CSF pleocytosis
      5. Integumentary findings (not preceding uveitis): Vitiligo, poliosis, or alopecia

- *Complete VKH:* Criteria 1–5 present
- *Incomplete VKH:* Criteria 1–3 present and either criteria 4 or 5
- *Probable VKH:* Criteria 1–3 present

Source: Adapted from Holland et al. and O'Keefe et al. Table 1: Diagnostic Criterion of VKH and text.

This specific change in the fundus is highly indicative of VKH, with a positive predictive value of 94.5%.

The chronic recurrent phase typically starts 6 to 9 months after initial disease onset. This phase is characterized by a resurgence of granulomatous anterior uveitis, often showing resistance to systemic steroids. During this stage, patients can experience a range of complications, including retinal pigment epithelium (RPE) proliferation, subretinal fibrosis, subretinal neovascularization, posterior sub-capsular cataract, posterior synechiae, open-angle glaucoma, band keratopathy, and, in some cases, acute angle-closure glaucoma.[28] Repeated episodes of ocular inflammation in this phase lead to deterioration of the blood–aqueous barrier, resulting in more pronounced inflammation. The onset of the chronic recurrent phase may occur earlier, approximately 6.5 months post-initial presentation, in Hispanic patients compared to non-Hispanic patients.[28] Table 12.8 summarizes the findings in the four phases of VKH.

12.5.4.4 Systemic Manifestations

Neurological symptoms, including headache, meningismus, and cerebrospinal fluid pleocytosis, are more prevalent during the prodromal phase of VKH disease. Notably, headaches are reported in 82% of patients in this phase. Neurological complications including meningitis, focal cranial neuropathies, transverse myelitis, aphasia, and hemiparesis have been documented. Sensory hearing loss, particularly at higher frequencies (4, 6, and 8 kHz), occurs in 18% to 50% of patients, and tinnitus is present in 42% of patients.[28]

Integumentary findings, which typically manifest during the convalescent phase, include depigmentation of the choroid, eyebrows, eyelashes, hair, and skin, leading to poliosis and vitiligo. The rate of depigmentation varies based on race, but one study noted that skin changes occur in about 30% of patients with VKH. These symptoms usually develop after the onset of uveitis.[28]

12.5.5 Diagnosis

Given the lack of specific laboratory tests for VKH diagnosis and the overlap of its systemic and ocular manifestations with other diseases, standardized diagnostic criteria were established. The revised diagnostic criteria are included in Table 12.8 and establish the need to exclude other causes of ocular inflammation and the absence of penetrating ocular trauma or surgery (suggestive of sympathetic ophthalmia) in making the diagnosis of VKH. Subsequent validation by a 2005 retrospective case series showed that all 49 patients in the series were diagnosed with VKH by their final visit using these revised criteria, although initial diagnosis within the first 2 weeks was often missed. These criteria have demonstrated 100% specificity and have been validated in several case series.[28]

A recent multinational study highlighted that the presence of bilateral intraocular inflammation in the absence of ocular trauma or surgery with exudative retinal detachments has a 100% positive predictive value for VKH in the acute phase, indicating that this combination is highly indicative of VKH.[28]

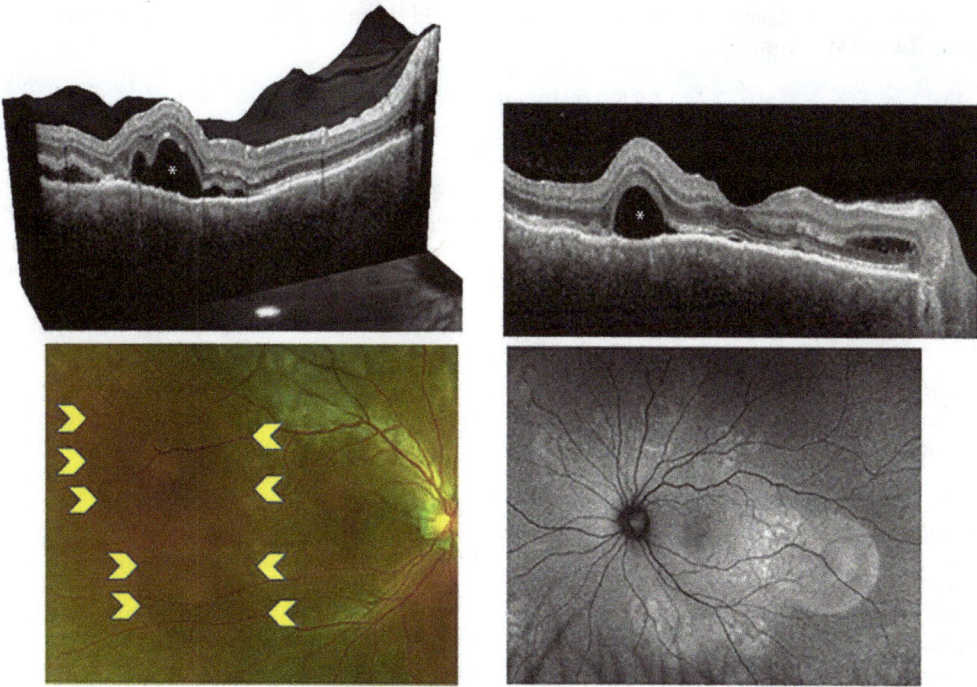

Figure 12.2 VKH posterior segment findings. Optical coherence tomography (OCT) showing multifocal exudative subretinal fluid (top photos, asterisks indicating subretinal fluid) in a VKH patient. Correlated fundus photograph (lower left) and fundusautofluorescence (lower right) showing corresponding areas of subretinal fluid (yellow arrows) in a VKH patient.

12.5.5.1 Ancillary Diagnostic Tools

In the United States, retinal fluorescein angiography is a common diagnostic procedure for VKH disease. Other valuable imaging techniques in VKH diagnosis include indocyanine green (ICG) angiography for detecting choroidal changes and ultrasonography for identifying choroidal thickening and exudative retinal detachments. Classic VKH findings on fluorescein angiography include hyperfluorescent spots and late leakage, with optic disc hyperfluorescence and disseminated spotted choroidal hyperfluorescence seen in the majority of patients. In the chronic uveitic stage, common findings are spotted hyperfluorescence, hypofluorescence, and optic disc hyperfluorescence. The convalescent stage is marked by spotted hyperfluorescence, hypofluorescence, and blockage of choroidal fluorescence due to retinal pigment epithelial migration. Early pinpoint peripapillary hyperfluorescence on FA in the hyperacute phase (< 14 days from symptom onset) may indicate a better prognosis, suggesting the need for more aggressive treatment in its absence. In contrast, retinal ICG angiography often indicates diffuse delayed choroidal perfusion, alongside segmental hyperfluorescence and hypofluorescence.[28]

Recent advancements in optical coherence tomography (OCT) and fundus autofluorescence photography have enhanced non-invasive imaging capabilities, offering detailed insights into the retina, retinal pigment epithelium (RPE), and choroid in VKH patients (Figure 12.2). For example, in the acute phase, enhanced-depth (ED)-OCT is particularly effective in assessing increased choroidal thickness and detecting subretinal fluid and exudative retinal detachments, with typical findings including subretinal fluid with septae and heightened choroidal thickness. This multifocal serous retinal detachment, visualized on OCT, is a characteristic finding in VKH.[28]

12.5.5.2 Differential Diagnosis of VKH

The differential diagnosis for VKH includes sympathetic ophthalmia, infectious uveitis, malignant masquerades (intraocular lymphoma, bilateral diffuse melanocytic hyperplasia, diffuse uveal lymphoid hyperplasia), and other inflammatory conditions including posterior scleritis, sarcoidosis, lupus choroidopathy, acute posterior multifocal placoid pigment epitheliopathy (APMPPE), and uveal effusion syndrome.[28]

12.5.6 Treatment and Management

Proposed by Silpa-Archa and colleagues in a large VKH review article summarizing the primary literature, the primary objectives in treating VKH disease are to (1) promptly suppress the acute intraocular inflammation using high-dose systemic corticosteroids and (2) gradually reduce the systemic steroid dosage while concurrently introducing IMT.[33] Despite efforts to establish early non-steroidal immunosuppressive drug therapy as the first-line treatment, systemic corticosteroids remain essential as the initial step in immunosuppression. This is because most IMTs take several weeks to exhibit therapeutic effects.[33]

12.5.6.1 Corticosteroids

Systemic corticosteroids can be administered either intravenously or orally. Hosoda et al. demonstrated a protocol starting with intravenous methylprednisolone, followed by a tapered oral prednisolone regimen while monitoring disease activity. Typical dosing varies from 1 to 2 mg/kg/day of prednisone orally. These findings were confirmed by Chee and colleagues, who observed that corticosteroids were effective for most patients presenting within 2 months of a uveitic attack. However, in cases of recurrent granulomatous anterior uveitis or chronic recurrent phase, both corticosteroids and IMT are necessary.[33] Early and high-dose corticosteroids are associated with quicker disease resolution and fewer complications and recurrences compared to later and lower doses. Oral prednisone alone as primary treatment can achieve a visual acuity of 20/50 or better in a subset of patients, as proven by Arevalo et al. in a 12-year prospective case series following VKH patients' visual outcomes from 1999 to 2011.[34] Arevalo and colleagues found that all patients remained on oral corticosteroids, with some patients needing pulse dosing of intravenous methylprednisolone. They found that 76% of patients also required concomitant IMT therapy to remain inactive. Other methods, like a series of sub-tenons triamcinolone acetonide injections (up to four), have shown 78% success in disease resolution, especially in patients presenting solely with ocular symptoms and no systemic signs.[33] Sustained-release steroidal implants, such as fluocinolone and dexamethasone, have shown benefits in some case series, but their role as primary treatment remains uncertain. Additionally, topical prednisolone 1% and cycloplegic agents are recommended for initial or chronic anterior chamber inflammation to alleviate pain and prevent synechiae. As inflammation decreases, topical steroids should be tapered. In chronic or refractory VKH cases, longer-term corticosteroid eye drops may prove beneficial.[33]

12.5.6.2 Conventional-Synthetic DMARDs/Immunomodulatory Therapy (IMT)

Disease-modifying agents are necessary for VKH patients with systemic manifestations, refractory or chronic uveitis requiring ongoing corticosteroids or those experiencing significant side effects from prolonged corticosteroid use.[33] While Parades et al. concluded better visual outcomes in patients promptly treated with a combination of IMT and corticosteroids compared to corticosteroids alone or delayed IMT introduction, other studies have not found significant differences between early versus late IMT in conjunction with systemic corticosteroids.[33, 35]

Considering VKH's pathogenesis as a T cell–mediated autoimmune response against melanocytes, cyclosporine A (CSA) and tacrolimus, calcineurin inhibitors targeting T cells, are effective treatment in VKH.[33] Azathioprine, mycophenolate, and methotrexate have also been shown as effective corticosteroid-sparing agents. Mycophenolate mofetil (2 grams daily) as first-line therapy combined with systemic corticosteroids significantly reduced the recurrence of uveitis and development of late complications in VKH and improved visual outcomes opposed to corticosteroid monotherapy or late initiated IMT.[33] A comparative study by Cuchacovich et al. found similar long-term outcomes in complications comparing treatment with a combination of prednisolone and azathioprine versus prednisone and cyclosporine, although the group receiving azathioprine needed higher average and cumulative doses of prednisone compared to the cyclosporine group.[36] Combination therapy with oral prednisolone, azathioprine, and cyclosporine demonstrated rapid and effective control of inflammation, along with favorable visual outcomes in particularly severe and persistent VKH cases. Methotrexate has proven effective and safe in VKH patients in both children and adults.[33]

Although less commonly used, alkylating agents such as cyclophosphamide and chlorambucil have been employed successfully in VKH treatment, albeit in a limited number of cases. The primary concerns with these agents are bone marrow suppression, a frequent side effect, and the risk of secondary malignancies, which have limited their use.

12.5.6.3 Biologics

Anti-TNF-alpha monoclonal antibodies, such as infliximab and adalimumab, have the most evidence for treatment of VKH. Infliximab has shown a 90% success rate in 12 refractory VKH cases that did not respond to systemic prednisolone and IMT, achieving rapid clinical remission within 1 to 2 months and maintaining disease-free remission for up to 24 months post-discontinuation. Adalimumab has also been effective, sustaining disease-free remission for up to 26 months.[33]

Rituximab, which targets B cells, has been effective in prolonging disease quiescence for up to 27 months following four doses over 18 months. The effectiveness of rituximab in VKH, a T cell-mediated disease, suggests a potential role for B lymphocytes in VKH and warrants further research to clarify and solidify rituximab's role in treating refractory VKH cases.[33]

12.5.7 Prognosis and Complications

The prognosis of VKH disease is closely linked to the timing of diagnosis and the chosen treatment approach. Patients who are diagnosed early tend to have better outcomes, often achieving visual acuity of 20/40 (Snellen) or better after treatment. These patients also tend to have a shorter treatment duration, averaging around 20 months, compared to those diagnosed during the chronic stages of the disease, who usually require treatment for about 36 months and are more prone to complications.[30]

12.6 SUMMARY

This chapter has provided an in-depth exploration of five rare autoimmune or autoinflammatory conditions that share overlapping multisystemic features yet remain distinct in their pathophysiology, clinical presentation, and treatment challenges: Cogan's syndrome, relapsing polychondritis, VEXAS syndrome, TINU syndrome, and Vogt–Koyanagi–Harada disease. Cogan's syndrome is an immune-mediated vasculitis primarily affecting ocular and auditory systems, marked by interstitial keratitis and neurosensory hearing loss, and often requires a combination of corticosteroids and immunosuppressive therapies. Relapsing polychondritis, on the other hand, is characterized by recurrent inflammation of cartilage and proteoglycan-rich tissues, including the ears, nose, and respiratory tract, leading to systemic manifestations. Treatment often involves corticosteroids and immunosuppressants, with biologics as a consideration for severe cases. VEXAS syndrome, recently identified, represents an intersection of autoinflammation and hematologic disorders, predominantly affecting older men and presenting with systemic inflammation and hematological abnormalities. Diagnosis relies on genetic testing, and while treatment options are evolving, hematopoietic stem cell transplantation remains the only curative approach. TINU syndrome combines tubulointerstitial nephritis and uveitis, often requiring systemic corticosteroids and long-term immunosuppressive management for recurrent uveitis. Lastly, VKH disease presents as a progressive autoimmune attack against melanocytes, affecting the eyes, skin, and auditory and neurological systems, with treatment primarily focused on high-dose corticosteroids and immunosuppressive therapy to control the inflammatory process and prevent chronic complications. Together, these entities underscore the complexity and diversity of autoimmune and autoinflammatory diseases that require a multidisciplinary approach for effective diagnosis, treatment, and management, highlighting the ongoing need for research to better understand and target these conditions at the molecular and clinical levels.

REFERENCES

1. D'Aguanno V, Ralli M, de Vincentiis M, et al. Optimal management of Cogan's syndrome: a multidisciplinary approach. *J Multidiscip Healthc.* 2017 Dec.;11:1–11. doi:10.2147/jmdh.s150940. Accessed 10 Dec. 2023.
2. Iliescu DA, Timaru CM, Batras M, et al. Cogan's syndrome. *Rom J Ophthalmol.* 2015 Jan.–Mar.;59(1):6–13. PMID:27373108; PMCID:PMC5729811.
3. Durtette C, Hachulla E, Resche-Rigon M, et al. Cogan syndrome: characteristics, outcome and treatment in a French nationwide retrospective study and literature review. *Autoimmun Rev.* 2017 Dec.;16(12):1219–1223. doi:10.1016/j.autrev.2017.10.005. Accessed 10 Dec. 2023.
4. Grasland, A. Typical and atypical Cogan's syndrome: 32 cases and review of the literature. *Rheumatology.* 2002 June 1;43(8):1007–1015. doi:10.1093/rheumatology/keh228. Accessed 10 Dec. 2023.
5. Kessel A, Vadasz Z, Toubi E. Cogan syndrome – pathogenesis, clinical variants and treatment approaches. *Autoimmun Rev.* 2014 Apr.;13(4–5):351–354. doi:10.1016/j.autrev.2014.01.002. Accessed 10 Dec. 2023.

6. Wang Y, Tang S, Shao C, et al. Cogan's syndrome is more than just keratitis: a case-based literature review. *BMC Ophthalmol*. 2023 May 12;23:212. www.ncbi.nlm.nih.gov/pmc/articles/PMC10176949/. doi:10.1186/s12886-023-02966-6. Accessed 29 Dec. 2023.

7. Espinoza GM, Wheeler J, Temprano KK, et al. Cogan's syndrome: clinical presentations and update on treatment. *Curr Allergy Asthma Rep*. 2020 Jun. 16;20(9):46. doi:10.1007/s11882-020-00945-1. PMID:32548646.

8. Fukuda K, Mizobuchi T, Nakajima I, et al. Ocular involvement in relapsing polychondritis. *J Clin Med*. 2021 Oct. 26;10(21):4970–4970. www.ncbi.nlm.nih.gov/pmc/articles/PMC8584789/. doi:10.3390/jcm10214970. Accessed 24 Jul. 2023.

9. Gallagher K, Al-Janabi A, Wang A. The ocular manifestations of relapsing polychondritis. *Int J Ophthalmol*. 2023 Mar. 1;43(8):2633–2641. doi:10.1007/s10792-023-02662-w. Accessed 11 Dec. 2023.

10. Rednic S, Damian L, Talarico R, et al. Relapsing polychondritis: state of the art on clinical practice guidelines. *RMD Open*. 2018 Oct. 18;4(Suppl 1):e000788. doi:10.1136/rmdopen-2018-000788. Accessed 11 Dec. 2023.

11. Sangle SR, Hughes CD, Barry L, et al. Relapsing polychondritis – a single centre study in the United Kingdom. *Autoimmun Rev*. 2023 Aug.;22(8):103352. doi:10.1016/j.autrev.2023.103352. Accessed 11 Dec. 2023.

12. Vitale A, Sota J, Rigante D, et al. Relapsing polychondritis: an update on pathogenesis, clinical features, diagnostic tools, and therapeutic perspectives. *Curr Rheumatol Rep*. 2015 Dec. 29;18(1). doi:10.1007/s11926-015-0549-5. Accessed 11 Dec. 2023.

13. Petitdemange A, Sztejkowski C, Damian L, et al. Treatment of relapsing polychondritis: a systematic review. *Clin Exp Rheumatol*. 2022 May 1;40((5)Suppl 134):81–85. www.pubmed.ncbi.nlm.nih.gov/35238756. doi:10.55563/clinexprheumatol/h9gq1o. Accessed 30 Dec. 2023.

14. Georgin-Lavialle S, Terrier B, Guedon AF, et al. Further characterization of clinical and laboratory features in VEXAS syndrome: large-scale analysis of a multicentre case series of 116 French patients. *Br J Dermatol*. 2021 Nov. 28;186(3):564–574. doi:10.1111/bjd.20805. Accessed 21 Dec. 2023.

15. Abumanhal M, Leibovitch I, Zisapel M, et al. Ocular and orbital manifestations in VEXAS syndrome. *Eye (London)*. 2024 Mar. 28. doi:10.1038/s41433-024-03014-3. Epub ahead of print. PMID:38548942.

16. Myint K, Patrao N, Vonica O, et al. Recurrent superior orbital fissure syndrome associated with VEXAS syndrome. *J Ophthalmic Inflamm Infect*. 2023 Sept. 7;13(1). doi:10.1186/s12348-023-00362-1. Accessed 21 Dec. 2023.

17. Al-Hakim A, Savic S. An update on VEXAS syndrome. *Expert Rev Clin Immunol*. 2022 Dec. 26;19(2):203–215. doi:10.1080/1744666x.2023.2157262. Accessed 21 Dec. 2023.

18. Grayson PC, Patel BA, Young NS. VEXAS syndrome. *Blood*. 2021 May 10. doi:10.1182/blood.2021011455. Accessed 21 Dec. 2023.

19. Goda C, Kotake S, Ichiishi A, et al. Clinical features in tubulointerstitial nephritis and uveitis (TINU) syndrome. *Am J Ophthalmol*. 2005 Oct.;140(4):637–641. doi:10.1016/j.ajo.2005.04.019. Accessed 23 Dec. 2023.

20. Okafor LO, Hewins P, Murray PI, et al. Tubulointerstitial nephritis and uveitis (TINU) syndrome: a systematic review of its epidemiology, demographics and risk factors. *Orphanet J Rare Dis*. 2017 Jul. 14;12(1). doi:10.1186/s13023-017-0677-2. Accessed 23 Dec. 2023.

21. Amaro D, Carreño E, Steeples LR, et al. Tubulointerstitial nephritis and uveitis (TINU) syndrome: a review. *Br J Ophthalmol*. 2019 Nov. 12;104(6):742–747. doi:10.1136/bjophthalmol-2019-314926. Accessed 23 Dec. 2023.

22. Matsumoto K, Fukunari K, Ikeda Y, et al. A report of an adult case of tubulointerstitial nephritis and uveitis (TINU) syndrome, with a review of 102 Japanese cases. *Am J Case Rep*. 2015 Feb. 28;16:119–123. doi:10.12659/AJCR.892788. PMID:25725230; PMCID:PMC4347719.

23. Koreishi AF, Zhou M, Goldstein DA. Tubulointerstitial nephritis and uveitis syndrome: characterization of clinical features. *Ocul Immunol Inflamm*. 2021 Nov. 17;29(7–8):1312–1317. doi:10.1080/09273948.2020.1736311. Epub 2020 May 28. PMID:32463299.

24. Hettinga YM, Scheerlinck LM, Lilien MR, et al. The value of measuring urinary beta2-microglobulin and serum creatinine for detecting tubulointerstitial nephritis and uveitis syndrome in young patients with uveitis. *JAMA Ophthalmol*. 2015;133(2):140–145.

25. Sobolewska B, Bayyoud T, Deuter C, et al. Long-term follow-up of patients with tubulointerstitial nephritis and uveitis (TINU) syndrome. *Ocul Immunol Inflamm*. 2018;26(4):601–607. doi:10.1080/09273948.2016.1247872. Epub 2016 Dec. 12. PMID:27937079.

26. Choo CH, Acharya NR, Shantha JG. Comprehensive and updated review on the diagnosis and treatment of Vogt-Koyanagi-Harada disease. *Ann Eye Sci.* 2023 June;8:4. doi:10.21037/aes-23-3. Accessed 28 Dec. 2023.

27. Bykhovskaya I, Thorne JE, Kempen JH, et al. Vogt-Koyanagi-Harada disease: clinical outcomes. *Am J Ophthalmol.* 2005 Oct.;140(4):674.e1–674.e6. doi:10.1016/j.ajo.2005.04.052. Accessed 28 Dec. 2023.

28. O'Keefe, GAD, Rao NA. Vogt-Koyanagi-Harada disease. *Surv Ophthalmol.* 2017 Jan.;62(1):1–25. doi:10.1016/j.survophthal.2016.05.002. Accessed 28 Dec. 2023.

29. Reddy AK, John FT, Justin GA, et al. Vogt-Koyanagi-Harada disease in a Native American population in Oklahoma. *Int. Ophthalmol.* 2021 Jan. 5;41(3):915–922. doi:10.1007/s10792-020-01647-3. Accessed 30 Jan. 2024.

30. Diallo K, Revuz S, Clavel-Refregiers G, et al. Vogt-Koyanagi-Harada disease : a retrospective and multicentric study of 41 patients. *BMC Ophthalmol.* 2020 Oct. 7;20(1). doi:10.1186/s12886-020-01656-x. Accessed 28 Dec. 2023.

31. Damico FM, Marin ML, Goldberg AC, et al. Revised diagnostic criteria for Vogt-Koyanagi-Harada disease : considerations on the different disease categories. *Am J Ophthalmol.* 2009 Feb.;147(2):339–345.e5. doi:10.1016/j.ajo.2008.08.034. Accessed 28 Dec. 2023.

32. Holland GN, Rao NA, Tabbara KF, et al. Revised diagnostic criteria for Vogt-Koyanagi-Harada disease : report of an international committee on nomenclature. *Am J Ophthalmol.* 2001 May;131(5):647–652. doi:10.1016/s0002-9394(01)00925-4. PMID:11336942.

33. Silpa-Archa S, Silpa-Archa N, Preble JM, et al. Vogt-Koyanagi-Harada syndrome : perspectives for immunogenetics, multimodal imaging, and therapeutic options. *Autoimmun Rev.* 2016 Aug.;15(8):809–819. doi:10.1016/j.autrev.2016.04.001. Accessed 28 Dec. 2023.

34. Arevalo JF, Lasave AF, Gupta V, et al. Clinical outcomes of patients with Vogt-Koyanagi-Harada disease over 12 years at a tertiary center. *Ocul Immunol Inflamm.* 2016 Oct.;24(5):521–529. doi: 10.3109/09273948.2015.1025984. Epub 2015 Sept. 23. PMID:26399962.

35. Paredes I, Ahmed M, Foster CS. Immunomodulatory therapy for Vogt-Koyanagi-Harada patients as first-line therapy. *Ocul Immunol Inflamm.* 2006 Apr;14(2):87–90. doi:10.1080/09273940500536766. PMID:16597537.

36. Cuchacovich M, Pacheco P, Díaz G, et al. Eficacia de la azatioprina en la enfermedad ocular inflamatoria no infecciosa resistente a tratamiento esteroidal sistémico [Role of azathioprine in steroid resistant non infectious ocular inflammatory diseases]. *Rev Med Chil.* 2007 Jun;135(6):702–707. Spanish. doi:10.4067/s0034-98872007000600003. Epub 2007 Aug. 22. PMID:17728895.

13 Ophthalmologic Disease in Systemic Sclerosis, Polymyositis and Dermatomyositis

Tina Brar, Noor Bazerbashi, Saitiel Sandoval Gonzalez, and Edmund Tsui

13.1 SYSTEMIC SCLEROSIS

13.1.1 Epidemiology and Classification

Systemic sclerosis (scleroderma, SSc) is a complex multisystem autoimmune connective-tissue disease classified by autoimmunity and vasculopathy with skin and internal organ fibrosis conventionally divided into two subgroups: limited cutaneous and diffuse cutaneous.[1] SSc has a high morbidity and mortality with a reduced quality of life. The reported prevalence and incidence of SSc in studies varies widely based on different geographic areas and times. Collective prevalence was noted to be 23 per 100,000 with the highest observed in the Indigenous people of Canada at 47 per 100,000.[2] The age at disease onset will vary according to ethnic background as well as gender. This disease is more prevalent in females versus males, about 4 to 1, commonly occurring in middle age between 45 and 64 years. There are several classification criteria used to define SSc cases, which include the 1980 ACR (American College of Rheumatology) criteria, 2001 LeRoy and Medsger criteria and the 2013 ACR & EULAR (European League Against Rheumatism) criteria. Although SSc is an uncommon disease, it remains an important one as it carries with it significant morbidity.[1]

13.1.2 Pathogenic Mechanisms/Markers

The pathogenesis of ocular involvement as well as other internal organs is poorly understood. The vasculopathy in SSc is portrayed by obliteration of microvasculature, which contributes to generalized tissue hypoxia. The etiology of systemic sclerosis remains unknown. Assorted environmental exposures, especially exposure to organic solvents and silica dust, have been noted to be associated with the development of systemic sclerosis.[3]

The majority of patients with SSc will test positive for antinuclear antibody on indirect immunofluorescence assay plus one of the three mutually exclusive antibodies, which include anticentromere, anti-topoisomerase I (also known as Scl-70) and anti-RNA polymerase III antibodies. These autoantibodies tend to be positive at the time of and sometimes even prior to symptom onset and very rarely switch during the disease course.[1]

13.1.3 Clinical Features

Typically, Raynaud phenomenon is the earliest symptom in patients with SSc and is seen in > 95% of these cases. Initial presentations may also include fatigue, arthralgia and myalgia. Organ systems affected most commonly in SSc include the skin and the pulmonary and gastrointestinal tracts. Gastrointestinal involvement is nearly universal in SSc patients and often shows up as the first non-Raynaud symptom. Skin changes present in three stages, with the initial being an inflammatory stage, which may occur for months. This edematous state is accompanied by puffiness of the hands and fingers with associated paronychia, sores and pruritis. An extended phase of progressive skin fibrosis occurs next, beginning distally and potentially progressing proximally, involving not only the upper extremities but also the chest/abdomen and face as well as lower extremities. In patients with diffuse SSc, the final stage is skin softening, commonly seen 2 years after skin disease onset, which may allow return to clinically normal skin. By late stages, patients will have atrophied skin, and although softer, it tends to be bound to underlying fibrotic tissue. A validated tool for SSc used for grading skin thickness in 17 body areas is the modified Rodnan skin score. Pulmonary disease is the main disease-related cause of mortality and commonly includes interstitial lung disease and/or pulmonary arterial hypertension. Renal disease is another important cause of morbidity and mortality in these patients. Scleroderma renal crisis occurs in ~5% of patients with SSc and is characterized by malignant hypertension and acute renal failure.[3]

13.1.4 Management/Treatment

Treatment of SSc remains a challenge, and it is vital to take a systematic approach to diagnosis and evaluation in each patient. Staging and classifying subsets of patients with varying organ involvement is particularly important because not all patients require the same level of therapeutic intervention at the same time.

DOI: 10.1201/9781003453710-13

13.1.5 Ocular Manifestations

SSc is a rare syndrome, with only a few case reports and series of ocular manifestations existing in the literature. While many of its dermatologic and systemic findings have been well documented, it is suspected that ocular involvement remains underreported. Some studies of small groups have discovered that up to 93% of patients have at least one ocular manifestation.[4] These range from mild findings such as eyelid stiffness to severe manifestations such as retinopathy.[5, 6]

13.1.5.1 Eyelids

Several eyelid manifestations have been documented in patients with SSc. Eyelid thickening and stiffness are perhaps some of the most common ocular findings of SSc, with some studies reporting between 77% and 93% prevalence among patients.[4, 6, 7] Eyelid thickening is thought to be due to over-production and accumulation of collagen and extracellular matrix proteins, resulting in fibrosis. This thickening may lead to stiffness, blepharophimosis (narrowed eye opening), and lagophthalmos (inability to fully close the eyelids) which in turn may result in poor tear film distribution and excessive tear loss.[5, 6] Prognosis for eyelid thickening is promising and can be managed surgically if eyelid malformation leads to visual impairment.

Eyelid telangiectasias can also commonly be found during routine examination and are present in 21% to 51% of patients with SSc.[5, 8] Ciliary madarosis is a type of alopecia that causes loss of the eyelashes and is seen more commonly in patients with the diffuse cutaneous subtype.[9]

13.1.5.2 Dry Eye Disease

Keratoconjunctivitis sicca, or dry eye disease (DED), is among the most common ocular manifestations of SSc. Studies have reported a prevalence of 37% to 79% of DED in patients with SSc.[10] The pathophysiology of DED in SSc appears to be multifactorial. Fibrosis of the tear ducts results in a reduced production of the aqueous layer of tears.[6] This lower production of tears is exacerbated by the eyelid malformations caused by SSc. As previously described, eyelid malformations are common in SSc and lead to excessive evaporation and poor distribution of the tear film. Surface dryness can lead to irritation and redness if not treated properly. If left uncontrolled, corneal scarring may occur and lead to vision impairment. Assessment for dry eye can be done by the Schirmer's test or by corneal fluorescein staining. Initial management of DED in patients with SSc includes the use of artificial tears to replace the aqueous tear layer and punctal plugs to reduce tear loss. The prognosis of DED is good with adequate intervention but may result in corneal scarring and a compromised epithelial layer if left untreated. Sjögren's syndrome has also been reported in association with SSc ranging from 14% to 23%.[8]

13.1.5.3 Conjunctiva

Conjunctival vascular congestion, neovascularization and telangiectasia are commonly observed in patients with SSc, likely because of the rich vascularization of this tissue. Fifty percent to 73% of study patients with SSc have been shown to have conjunctival vasodilation.[8] This spectrum of changes is thought to result from the progressive fibrotic process that affects the microvasculature, leading to alterations in vessel morphology and function. Subepithelial fibrosis of the conjunctiva may also lead to shallow fornices in up to 15% of patients.[7, 8]

13.1.5.4 Cornea

At this time, there are no clear corneal findings associated with SSc. Corneal thinning has been observed in some cases, suggesting potential structural alterations in the corneal tissue in SSc patients.[11] Other studies, however, have shown corneal thickening or a lack of statistically significant change in corneal thickness.[8] This highlights the need for further studies to clarify the impact of SSc on corneal health.

13.1.5.5 Iris

Between 8% and 13% of patients with SSc have been reported to have transillumination defects and vascular deformation of the iris.[6, 9] These findings are more common in people with lighter-colored irises. The pathophysiology behind these changes is likely a result of iris epithelial atrophy caused by SSc-associated vasculopathy. Management of transillumination defects is largely dependent on treating systemic disease.

13.1.5.6 Retina

Primary retinal manifestations in patients with SSc remain unclear. Some studies have found that up to 34% of patients with SSc have hard exudates, vascular tortuosity, microhemorrhage, and macular degeneration when compared to only 8% of control patients.[10, 12] These studies, however, did not properly control for hypertensive comorbidities, which are very common in patients with SSc. Because of this, it is difficult to attribute many of these findings to a primary SSc manifestation. Kök et al. recently demonstrated a decrease in retinal superficial and deep capillary plexus vessel density using optical coherence tomography angiography (OCTA) while controlling for hypertension and retinopathy.[13] This would suggest a primary retinal manifestation of SSc independent of hypertension. Further studies are nevertheless needed to completely assess the role of SSc in retinal pathology.

Comprehensive evaluation of retinal health in SSc patients remains crucial due to the role of hypertensive retinopathy. If not properly managed, patients may experience long-term reduction in visual acuity and an increased risk of retinal artery occlusions. Staging and regular monitoring of hypertensive retinopathy using the Modified Scheie Classification and fluorescein angiogram (FA) imaging are key to preventing vision loss in these patients. Medical management of patients' hypertension is the most important factor in preventing hypertensive retinopathy.

13.1.5.7 Choroid

Ocular manifestations involving the choroid in patients with SSc are largely characterized by a spectrum of vascular and structural changes. The dense vascularization of the choroid makes it highly susceptible to the effects of SSc-associated vasculopathy. Several studies utilizing FA and OCTA have demonstrated that up to 50% of patients with SSc have choroidal hypoperfusion (Figure 13.1).[6, 10, 13, 14] These findings have been made independent of the effects of hypertension, which is a common comorbidity of SSc patients due to renal disease. The pathophysiology of these findings is still unclear, but histopathological samples suggest that thickening of the precapillary basement membrane, obliteration of small-vessel lumen and swelling of endothelial cells may all play a role. Although rare among patients with SSc, severe choroidal hypoperfusion may lead to vision loss. Regular FA and OCTA imaging can help clinicians track and manage any reductions in choroidal perfusion.

13.1.5.8 Glaucoma

Glaucoma, a condition characterized by progressive optic nerve damage often associated with elevated intraocular pressure (IOP), has been noted as a significant ocular manifestation in patients with SSc. Studies have reported a higher prevalence of open-angle glaucoma among SSc patients (11% to 21%) compared to the general population, suggesting a potential predisposition to glaucoma in individuals with SSc.[6–8] The pathogenesis of glaucoma in SSc is complex and may involve both systemic factors related to the underlying disease process and iatrogenic effects of systemic therapy. While the exact mechanisms underlying the increased prevalence of glaucoma in SSc remain unclear, vascular abnormalities, including vasculopathy and ischemia associated with SSc, are implicated in the pathophysiology of glaucoma.[6] Because glaucoma can lead to irreversible vision loss, it is imperative to identify and treat early.

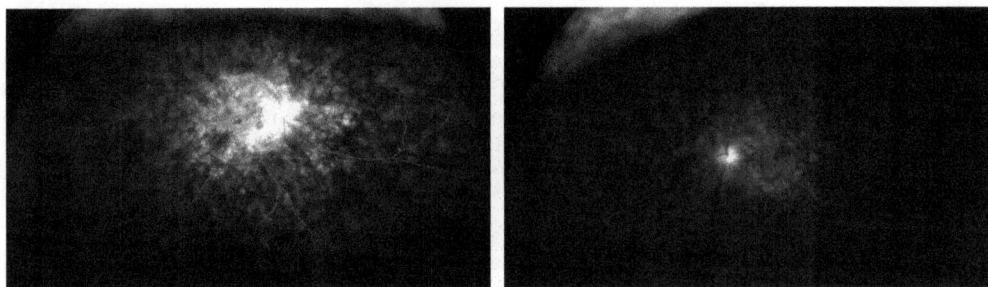

Figure 13.1 Fluorescein angiography of a patient with systemic sclerosis (SSc). Late-phase fluorescein angiograms of the right eye (left photo) and left eye (right photo) of a patient with systemic sclerosis showing widespread choroidal hypoperfusion and retinal vasculitis. (Image courtesy of Laura J. Kopplin, MD, PhD. Used with permission.)

13.2 SUMMARY

SSc is a rare autoimmune connective tissue disease characterized by skin and internal organ fibrosis. Ocular manifestations in SSc are varied, ranging from eyelid thickening and stiffness to severe complications including retinopathy. Common ocular findings include eyelid telangiectasias, ciliary madarosis, and dry eye disease (DED), with studies reporting a prevalence of DED in SSc patients ranging from 37% to 79%. While treatment of systemic disease is crucial for the best prognosis, early detection and management of ocular manifestations are necessary to prevent vision loss.

13.3 POLYMYOSITIS AND DERMATOMYOSITIS

13.3.1 Epidemiology and Classification Criteria

Recognition of the idiopathic inflammatory myopathies (IIM), like dermatomyositis (DM) and polymyositis (PM), has seen notable improvement, yet it remains a relatively rare autoimmune disease with an estimated incidence of 1.2 cases per 1,000,000 person-years.[15] Similar to many rheumatologic disorders, IIM exhibits a notable predilection for females, with approximately 70% of reported cases affecting women.[16] While both children and adults may suffer from this disease, it more commonly presents at a later age, with mean age of diagnosis at 57.2 years.[15] There were debates regarding the classification of IIM for years; our understanding of the distinct course of the disease subtypes improved after more autoantibodies were identified. ACR/EULAR IIM classification criteria were published in 2017 utilizing our improved understanding of this autoimmune disease.[17, 18]

13.3.2 Pathogenic Mechanism/Markers

Muscle biopsy is an indispensable tool in diagnosing myositis and has been instrumental in shaping our foundational understanding of its pathogenesis. Infiltration of CD4 and antigen-directed cytotoxic CD8+ cells is a known key driving factor of inflammation, but both the adaptive and the innate immune system play an interchangeable role in the disease's pathogenesis.[19] Histologic characterization of the location of the inflammatory infiltrates (i.e., perimysium versus endomysium) corresponds with different patterns of the disease. Subtypes of inflammatory myositis have several distinct features, and their etiology remains unclear. Identification of the associated autoantibody has helped with our understanding and prognostication of these disease subcategories. Some autoantibodies like Jo-1 and anti-TIF-1 gamma are found with cancer-associated dermatomyositis,[19] and treatment of underlying malignancy in these cases typically helps control the autoimmune process as well. Anti-SRP antibody and AntiMDA5 are associated with severe, rapidly progressive disease and with pulmonary involvement in the latter.[19]

13.3.3 Clinical Features

IIM is characterized by cellular infiltration of the skeletal muscles, resulting in the hallmark clinical feature of proximal muscle weakness.[19] This weakness is not confined to the skeletal muscles but rather may extend to encompass other muscles, including the pharyngeal and diaphragmatic muscles, leading to significant morbidity and mortality. Recent decades have witnessed an expanded understanding of IIM and revealed varied extra-muscular manifestations. These encompass potential links to malignancy and pulmonary, dermatologic and gastrointestinal involvement with certain subtypes of the disease.[20] Skin involvement, marked by features such as malar rash, Gottron papules, periorbital heliotrope rash, V-sign and shawl sign, stand out as pivotal characteristics of dermatomyositis and may precede or accompany the onset of muscular weakness. Ocular manifestations, on the other hand, are considered extremely rare when compared to other connective tissue diseases and might arise in up to 0.07% of the cases.[21]

13.3.4 Management/Treatment

Non-pharmacologic interventions like physical therapy and rehabilitation are used in combination with medications for management of patients with IIM. Immunosuppressive medications remain the cornerstone in the treatment of this disease, and it prevents progression of extra-muscular disease.

13.3.5 Ocular Manifestations

Due to the rarity of IIM, most of the available information regarding ocular involvement comes from case reports and small case studies. As previously mentioned, ocular pathology is suspected to occur in only 0.07% of cases of inflammatory myositis. It is also important to note that ocular manifestations in DM may differ from those of PM despite their many similarities.

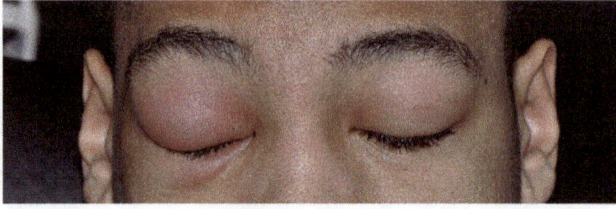

Figure 13.2 Heliotrope rash and periorbital edema in dermatomyositis. Blue-purple discoloration of the periorbital skin (heliotrope rash) with accompanying periorbital edema in a patient with dermatomyositis. (Image courtesy of Laura J. Kopplin, MD, PhD. Used with permission.)

13.3.5.1 Dermatomyositis
13.3.5.1.1 Eyelid

Perhaps the most common ocular manifestation of dermatomyositis is the heliotrope rash eruption, which occurs in 30% to 60% of patients with ocular features.[22] Heliotrope rash is characterized by blue-purple discoloration of the periorbital skin, often bilaterally, and may sometimes be accompanied by periorbital edema (Figure 13.2). The rash can be identified with careful examination of the face and is in itself benign. Periorbital edema may lead to eyelid ptosis and obstruction of vision if severe enough. Heliotrope rashes and associated edema often improve with the systemic steroid treatments used to treat overall dermatomyositis symptoms.[21, 22]

13.3.5.2 Extraocular Muscles

Ophthalmoplegia from extraocular muscle (EOM) involvement has been documented in some case reports. Although EOM involvement has often been seen as an exclusionary feature of dermatomyositis, the pathophysiology that affects other muscle groups can likely also occur here. Ophthalmoplegia can be assessed in patients with dermatomyositis by testing a patient's conjugate gaze abilities. A thorough history and clinical workup should be performed, since ophthalmoplegia in dermatomyositis patients may sometimes be associated with periorbital redness, edema, ptosis and pain that may mimic orbital cellulitis.[21] Lagophthalmos has also been documented in patients with EOM involvement.[21, 23] Full closure of the eyelid should be assessed in these patients. The size of the gap should be documented, and the clinician should look for the presence of Bell's phenomenon, which is the upward and lateral rotation of the eyeball during eyelid closure. EOM involvement has been successfully treated with the use of steroids and steroid-sparing immunosuppressive agents.[23]

13.3.5.3 Dry Eye Disease

Incomplete eyelid closure resulting from weakened EOM may lead to dry eye disease due to excessive tear evaporation. Recent studies, however, have shown a decrease in tear breakup time and Schirmer test measurements in patients with dermatomyositis with no eyelid abnormalities.[24] This would suggest an association between dry eye disease and dermatomyositis that is independent of excessive evaporation due to incomplete eyelid closure. The mechanism for this finding is, unfortunately, not yet fully understood since it is likely multifactorial. Assessment of eye dryness using fluorescein staining as well as Schimer testing should be performed in patients reporting dry eye symptoms. Prognosis of dry eye disease is good but may lead to excessive irritation and scarring of the corneal surface if left untreated. Lubricating artificial tears may be used as the initial treatment for dry eye disease in these patients.

13.3.5.4 Lens

Cataracts are common ocular manifestations in patients with DM, particularly following prolonged or high-dose steroid therapy, which is often a mainstay of treatment for these conditions.[25] In patients with DM and PM, cataracts typically present with symptoms such as progressive vision loss, night halos and glare, significantly affecting visual acuity and quality of life.[25] The cause is thought to be iatrogenic, since no primary association between dermatomyositis and cataracts has been made. Regular visual acuity and eye examination using slit lamp microscopy are necessary for detecting cataract formation in patients with DM. Management of cataracts in these patients may involve the use of steroid-sparing systemic agents and surgical extraction of the opacified lens.

13.3.5.5 *Retina*

Abnormalities in the retina are among the most common ocular manifestations of DM, preceded only by eyelid changes. A spectrum of posterior segment findings manifesting as cotton-wool spots, macular hemorrhages, edema and retinal nerve fiber layer infarctions can be found in patients with DM.[21] Of note, these findings are more common in children with juvenile dermatomyositis (JDM). This may be due to the fact that vasculitis is more common in JDM than in adult dermatomyositis.[26, 27] Patients with dermatomyositis-associated retinopathy are often asymptomatic and may present with vision loss as their first symptom.[21, 26, 27] Vision loss in these cases may be severe but is usually reversible if adequate treatment is started early. Severe retinopathy may also result in optic neuropathy as a late manifestation of the disease. Vision loss, relative afferent pupillary defect, and dyschromatopsia may be present in these patients. Fundus examination by an ophthalmologist should be performed in patients with dermatomyositis presenting with any of these symptoms to assess for retinopathy and optic neuropathy. Treatment with systemic steroids and other immunosuppressive agents may help reverse these changes in vision. If neovascularization of the retina has developed, argon-laser photocoagulation or intravitreal anti-VEGF injections may be indicated.

13.3.5.6 *Polymyositis*

Dry eye disease, cataracts, and posterior segment findings in PM are more rare but similar in presentation to those found in DM. Other ocular manifestations, including the heliotrope rash, are absent in PM. Despite this, some corneal abnormalities have been found in PM but not in DM.

13.3.5.6.1 *Cornea*

A recent study including patients with PM and DM demonstrated that corneal volume and thickness were reduced in patients with PM when compared to both patients with DM and healthy controls.[24] Thinner corneas may place patients at a greater risk of developing complications after refractive surgery and must thus be considered during presurgical evaluation.

13.4 SUMMARY

IIM, including PM and DM, are rare autoimmune diseases that primarily affect women. Myositis is characterized by proximal muscle weakness with some well-known extra-muscular findings. Ocular pathologies associated with IIM, however, are rare. These range from mild periorbital rashes to vision-threatening retinopathy. Treatment of the systemic disease remains the best way to manage ocular pathologies, but the existence of these pathologies highlights the importance of early ophthalmologic intervention in patients with ocular or vision-related symptoms.

REFERENCES

1. Volkmann ER, Andréasson K, Smith V. Systemic sclerosis. *Lancet*. 2023 Jan. 28;401(10373):304–318.
2. Calderon LM, Pope JE. Scleroderma epidemiology update. *Curr Opin Rheumatol*. 2021 Mar. 1;33(2):122–127.
3. Hochberg MC, Silman AJ, Smolen, JS, et al. *Rheumatology expert consult*, 6th edn. Mosby, 2014.
4. Waszczykowska A, Goś R, Waszczykowska E, et al. Prevalence of ocular manifestations in systemic sclerosis patients. *Arch Med Sci*. 2013 Dec. 30;9(6):1107–1113.
5. Kemeny-Beke A, Szodoray P. Ocular manifestations of rheumatic diseases. *Int Ophthalmol*. 2020 Feb.;40(2):503–510.
6. Kozikowska M, Luboń W, Kucharz EJ, et al. Ocular manifestations in patients with systemic sclerosis. *Reumatologia*. 2020;58(6):401–406.
7. Szucs G, Szekanecz Z, Aszalos Z, et al. A wide spectrum of ocular manifestations signify patients with systemic sclerosis. *Ocul Immunol Inflamm*. 2021 Jan. 2;29(1):81–89.
8. Gomes B de AF, Santhiago MR, Magalhães P, et al. Ocular findings in patients with systemic sclerosis. *Clinics (Sao Paulo)*. 2011;66(3):379–385.
9. West RH, Barnett AJ. Ocular involvement in scleroderma. *Br J Ophthalmol*. 1979 Dec.;63(12):845–847.
10. Tailor R, Gupta A, Herrick A, et al. Ocular manifestations of scleroderma. *Surv Ophthalmol*. 2009;54(2):292–304.
11. Nagy A, Rentka A, Nemeth G, et al. Corneal manifestations of systemic sclerosis. *Ocul Immunol Inflamm*. 2019;27(6):968–977.
12. Ushiyama O, Ushiyama K, Yamada T, et al. Retinal findings in systemic sclerosis: a comparison with nailfold capillaroscopic patterns. *Ann Rheum Dis*. 2003 Mar.;62(3):204–207.

13. Kök M, Ayan A, Fatih Küçük M, et al. Evaluation of the direct effects on retinal and choroidal microvascularity of systemic scleroderma. *Microvasc Res.* 2021 Jul.;136:104166.

14. Rommel F, Prangel D, Prasuhn M, et al. Correlation of retinal and choroidal microvascular impairment in systemic sclerosis. *Orphanet J Rare Dis.* 2021 Jan. 13;16(1):27.

15. Essouma M, Noubiap JJ, Singwe-Ngandeu M, et al. Epidemiology of idiopathic inflammatory myopathies in Africa: a contemporary systematic review. *J Clin Rheumatol.* 2022 Mar. 1;28(2):e552–e562.

16. Yang SH, Chang C, Lian ZX. Polymyositis and dermatomyositis – challenges in diagnosis and management. *J Transl Autoimmun.* 2019 Dec.;2:100018.

17. Leclair V, Lundberg IE. New myositis classification criteria – what we have learned since Bohan and Peter. *Curr Rheumatol Rep.* 2018 Apr 17;20(4):18.

18. Bottai M, Tjärnlund A, Santoni G, et al. EULAR/ACR classification criteria for adult and juvenile idiopathic inflammatory myopathies and their major subgroups: a methodology report. *RMD Open.* 2017;3(2):e000507.

19. Venalis P, Lundberg IE. Immune mechanisms in polymyositis and dermatomyositis and potential targets for therapy. *Rheumatology.* 2014 Mar. 1;53(3):397–405.

20. Findlay AR, Goyal NA, Mozaffar T. An overview of polymyositis and dermatomyositis. *Muscle Nerve.* 2015 May;51(5):638–656.

21. Ruiz-Lozano RE, Velazquez-Valenzuela F, Roman-Zamudio M, et al. Polymyositis and dermatomyositis: ocular manifestations and potential sight-threatening complications. *Rheumatol Int.* 2022 Jul. 21;42(7):1119–1131.

22. Al-Awqati MZ, Sokumbi O, Gold KG, et al. Periorbital masses in dermatomyositis. *Rheumatology (Oxford).* 2020 Dec. 1;59(12):e136–e137.

23. Roesler J, Jenkins D. Lagophthalmos as a presenting sign in dermatomyositis with muscle involvement limited to the ocular muscles. *JAAD Case Rep.* 2021 Apr;10:44–46.

24. Griger Z, Danko K, Bodoki L, et al. Corneal involvement of patients with polymyositis and dermatomyositis. *Ocul Immunol Inflamm.* 2020;28(1):58–66.

25. Santiago S, Enwereji N, Jiang C, et al. Ocular and eyelid involvement in collagen vascular diseases. Part II: dermatomyositis, scleroderma, and sarcoidosis. *Clin Dermatol.* 2024;42(1):9–16.

26. Yılmaz Tuğan B, Sönmez HE, Güngör M, et al. Preclinical ocular microvascular changes in juvenile dermatomyositis: a pilot optical coherence tomography angiography study. *Microvasc Res.* 2022 Sept.;143:104382.

27. Choi RY, Swan RJ, Hersh A, et al. Retinal manifestations of juvenile dermatomyositis: case report of bilateral diffuse chorioretinopathy with paracentral acute middle maculopathy and review of the literature. *Ocul Immunol Inflamm.* 2018;26(6):929–933.

14 Inflammatory Ocular Syndromes without Systemic Associations

Lorenzo E. Bosque and Meghan Berkenstock

14.1 SYMPATHETIC OPHTHALMIA

14.1.1 Epidemiology

Sympathetic ophthalmia (SO) is a rare, bilateral, granulomatous uveitis that typically occurs following a penetrating eye injury or intraocular surgery.[1–3] The exact incidence of SO is difficult to ascertain due to its rarity. According to the data from the Collaborative Ocular Melanoma Study (COMS), the incidence of SO is estimated to be 0.03% after ocular trauma and 0.01% after intraocular surgery.[1] Although the incidence has significantly declined over the years due to advancements in surgical techniques and the use of prophylactic corticosteroids, SO remains a significant cause of visual morbidity.[4–6]

14.1.2 Ocular Manifestations

The clinical manifestations of SO can affect all parts of the uveal tract and typically present between 2 weeks and even years post-injury.[1, 2, 5] Common symptoms include decreased vision, eye pain, redness, and photophobia.[1, 2] Key clinical signs include anterior chamber cells and vitreous cells or haze. Posterior segment involvement includes choroidal inflammation and exudative retinal detachments.[1–3, 5] Dalen-Fuchs nodules, which are clusters of epithelioid cells and lymphocytes between the retinal pigment epithelium (RPE) and Bruch's membrane, are a characteristic feature of SO.[1–3]

14.1.3 Key Pathogenic Mechanisms/Markers

The pathogenesis of SO is thought to be an autoimmune response triggered by exposure of hidden antigens from the injured eye to the immune system[3, 4] (see Chapter 1 for more detail). Several antigens have been implicated, including arrestin (S antigen), recoverin, and tyrosinase.[3] The autoimmune response is believed to be primarily against the uveal melanocytes.[3] Histopathological findings from enucleated eyes show a diffuse infiltration of the choroid with lymphocytes, plasma cells, and macrophages, as well as granulomas composed of epithelioid cells and multinucleated giant cells.[1–3]

14.1.4 Diagnostics Used for Ocular Manifestations

The diagnosis of SO is primarily clinical, based on the history of ocular trauma or surgery and the interval between the inciting event and the onset of uveitic clinical findings.[1–3] Imaging techniques such as fluorescein angiography (FA), indocyanine green angiography, and enhanced depth imaging optical coherence tomography (OCT) can be helpful in diagnosing and monitoring the disease.[3]

14.1.5 Natural History

SO is a chronic disease that can lead to severe visual impairment or blindness due to complications such as cataract, glaucoma, retinal scarring, and retinal detachment if left untreated.[1–3, 5] The disease's progression is unpredictable, with periods of exacerbation and remission.[3, 5]

14.1.6 Management and Treatment

The primary goal of treatment for SO is to suppress the inflammatory response to prevent or limit the damage to the ocular structures.[3–5] The mainstay of treatment for SO is systemic corticosteroids.[1–3, 5] Intravenous methylprednisolone pulse therapy can swiftly mitigate changes in the posterior segment during the acute stage. In patients who cannot tolerate corticosteroid side effects, cannot taper down to a dose of 7.5 mg or less per day, or who do not respond to them, other immunosuppressive agents are required.[3–5] Immunosuppressive drugs (IMT) include T cell inhibitors or antimetabolites, such as cyclosporine, azathioprine, methotrexate, and mycophenolate mofetil.[3–5] In refractory cases, biological agents including tumor necrosis factor-alpha inhibitors (infliximab, adalimumab) and interleukin-6 receptor inhibitors (tocilizumab) have also been shown to be effective.[3, 4] Surgical interventions may be required to manage complications such as cataract and glaucoma.[1–3, 5]

14.1.7 Prognosis

The prognosis for SO depends on several factors, including the severity of the disease at presentation, the response to treatment, and the presence of complications.[1–3, 5] In half of the cases, patients'

DOI: 10.1201/9781003453710-14

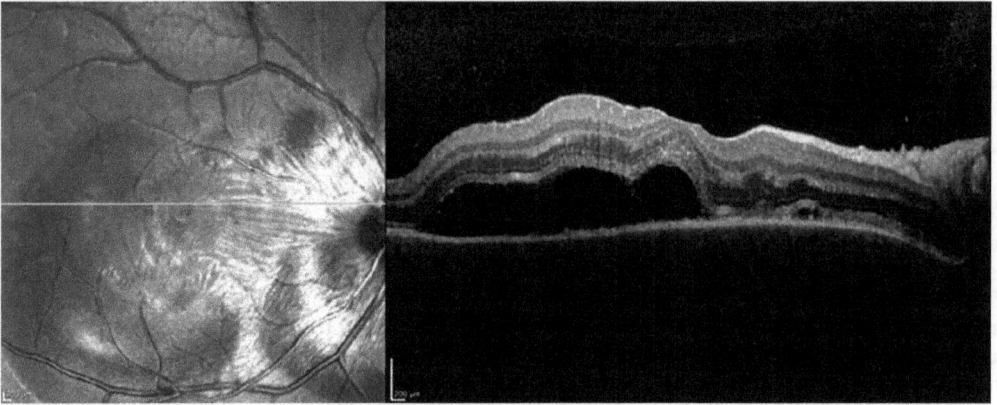

Figure 14.1 Sympathetic ophthalmia. Image of an OCT scan of the right eye showing subretinal fluid in a patient with sympathetic ophthalmia.

vision will deteriorate to 20/40 or worse, and 1 in 3 patients will become legally blind.[7] With early diagnosis and aggressive treatment, patients can maintain good visual acuity and avoid irreversible damage to the ocular structures leading to vision loss.[1-3,5]

14.1.8 National Guidelines

The Standardization of Uveitis Nomenclature (SUN) Working Group, comprised of an international consortium of uveitis specialists, has proposed classification criteria for SO.[5] These criteria were determined using a machine learning technique known as a classification and regression tree (CART) analysis, which allows for the identification of the best combination of features for diagnosing a disease.[5] The proposed classification criteria for SO are as follows:

1. *Mandatory criteria:* History of penetrating ocular injury or intraocular surgery in one eye, followed by the onset of uveitis in both eyes. Evidence of more than isolated anterior uveitis (either panuveitis with choroidal involvement or anterior chamber and vitreous inflammation).

2. *Common clinical features:* These include exudative retinal detachment, non-granulomatous anterior uveitis, and lack of keratic precipitates. The presence of any of these features increases the probability of SO.

3. *Exclusion criteria:* The presence of certain features suggestive of other types of uveitis (e.g., syphilis, Behçet's disease, Vogt–Koyanagi–Harada disease, sarcoidosis) can help to rule out SO.

These criteria were found to have a misclassification rate of 4% to 6.7% for SO, making them a useful tool for clinicians.[5] While these criteria provide guidance for the diagnosis of SO, it's important to note that the management and treatment of SO should be individualized based on the severity of the disease, the response to treatment, and the presence of complications.

14.2 BIRDSHOT CHORIORETINOPATHY

14.2.1 Epidemiology

Birdshot chorioretinopathy (BCR) is a rare but distinctive subtype of chronic posterior uveitis, with a genetic association to the HLA-A29 haplotype. Although the gene is present in around 7% of Caucasians, 80% to 98% of BCR patients are HLA-A29 positive.[7,8] The estimated prevalence of BCR is just 0.1–0.6/100,000[7,8] implying that these individuals face a relative risk, potentially as high as 224 times, of developing BCR.[9] Typically manifesting between the ages of 30 and 60, BCR shows a slight female predominance.[7] Although cases are reported globally, Caucasian populations with northern European ancestry have the highest prevalence.[7]

14.2.2 Ocular Manifestations

The hallmark of BCR is creamy, yellow-white lesions scattered across the retina with variable amounts of vitritis, vasculitis, and cystoid macular edema (CME). These lesions evolve slowly and

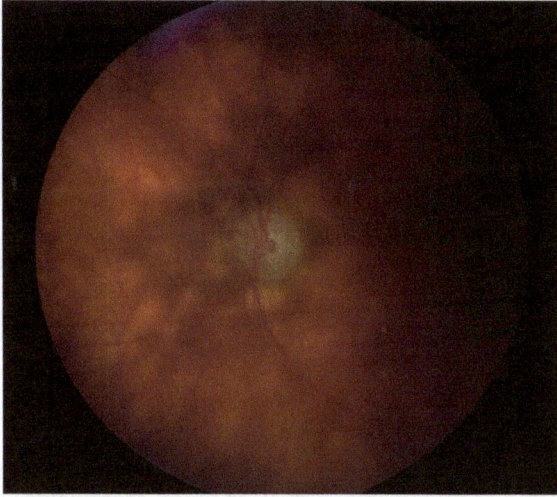

Figure 14.2 Birdshot chorioretinopathy. A color fundus image of a left eye showing the characteristic yellow, ovoid lesions surrounding the optic nerve in a patient with birdshot chorioretinopathy.

can lead to retinal degeneration.[10] Without treatment, disease progression and the development of complications, such as CME, can result in loss of visual acuity, emphasizing the significance of early detection and intervention.[7-9]

14.2.3 Key Pathogenic Mechanisms/Markers

The strong association with the HLA-A29 gene hints at an autoimmune origin; however, additional theories, such as molecular mimicry, have been posited, including an antigenic trigger leading to the development of BCR in those with a genetic predisposition.[7, 8]

14.2.4 Diagnostics Used for Ocular Manifestations

Birdshot lesions in fundoscopy, multiple white-creamy choroidal ovoid lesions, remain central to the diagnosis (Figure 14.2). Functional testing includes visual acuity assessments with 34% of patients maintaining 20/20 or better.[11] Visual field testing reveals common abnormalities such as peripheral constriction and central/paracentral scotoma, with about only one-third of patients displaying central field abnormalities.[11, 12]

Multimodal imaging includes FA, revealing retinal venular vasculitis and increased arteriovenous transit time.[13] Indocyanine green angiography (ICG-A) is crucial for identifying less apparent birdshot lesions.[14] Fundus autofluorescence (FAF) frequently shows peripapillary hypoautofluorescence (70% to 80% of cases) suggestive of retinal inflammation and damage. OCT, OCT-A, and enhanced depth imaging (EDI) OCT detect macular edema and, in late stages, choroidal thinning. Effective monitoring of the progression of BCR requires a multifaceted diagnostic approach, as the degenerative process can often be gradual and subtle, eluding detection through dilated fundus exams or single-modality assessments alone.

14.2.5 Natural History

In the progression of BCR, patients may encounter serious complications like cystoid macular edema, retinal vasculitis, and optic disc edema, which can lead to vision loss without treatment.[13] A notable aspect of BCR is the maintenance of central visual acuity until later stages of the disease. To mitigate these effects and preserve visual function, early diagnosis followed by immediate institution of local or systemic corticosteroids with concurrent use of IMT is required.

14.2.6 Management and Treatment

Recent data from a study of patients shows that corticosteroid-sparing success was achieved in 95.4% of patients treated with oral corticosteroids, typically within 12 months. Additionally, 76.5%

were able to discontinue corticosteroids successfully within a median time of 2.0 years. However, sustained drug-free remission was less common, achieved by about 25% of patients within 4 years of follow-up, with a relapse rate of 0.24 per person-year post-remission.[14] The treatment regimen often starts with systemic corticosteroids as initial or rescue therapy, transitioning to systemic IMT as a long-term solution. Early and adequately dosed immunosuppression can prevent the appearance of typical BCR lesions. Treatment options include antimetabolites (i.e., methotrexate and mycophenolate mofetil), calcineurin inhibitors (i.e., cyclosporine A), and biologics. Mycophenolate mofetil is increasingly popular due to its efficacy and tolerability, achieving control of intraocular inflammation in about 67% of patients.[15, 16] Intravitreal implants like fluocinolone acetonide and dexamethasone are effective for local management, especially for treatment of macular edema and vitreous haze.

14.2.7 National Guidelines

The SUN Working Group has established specific criteria or BCR. These criteria, crucial for accurate diagnosis, combine distinct ocular features and serological tests while also ruling out similar conditions. The classification criteria are as follows:[17]

1. The presence of characteristic bilateral multifocal choroiditis visible on ophthalmoscopy, showing multifocal cream-colored or yellow-orange, oval, or round choroidal lesions ("birdshot spots"), combined with absent to mild anterior chamber inflammation (no anterior chamber cells, keratic precipitates, or posterior synechiae), and absent to moderate vitritis.

2. Or a positive HLA-A29 test and either the presence of characteristic "birdshot" spots on ophthalmoscopy or characteristic findings on indocyanine green angiogram without the "birdshot" spots visible on ophthalmoscopy.

3. Exclusion criteria include a positive serologic test for syphilis, evidence of sarcoidosis, or intraocular lymphoma.

14.3 PARS PLANITIS

14.3.1 Epidemiology

Pars planitis is a chronic intermediate uveitis with a distinct phenotype of snowbanks and vitritis without an underlying infectious or systemic etiology.[18] Bilateral involvement is seen in approximately 86% of cases, and onset occurs mostly in the first and second decades of life.[19] The estimated incidence is 1.3 to 2.15 cases per 100,000 without a predisposition toward any particular gender or race, although some studies suggest variations based on ethnicity along with a genetic association with the HLA-DR2 and HLA-DR15 locus.[19, 20]

14.3.2 Ocular Manifestations

Patients with pars planitis might experience minimal symptoms but commonly describe floaters and blurry vision. Significant complications can arise, including epiretinal membrane formation, cataracts, cystoid macular edema, retinal vasculitis, retinal neovascularization, peripheral vitreous traction, and vitreous hemorrhage. Furthermore, sudden vision loss due to complications like retinal detachment or acute vitreous hemorrhage is a potential risk.[21]

14.3.3 Key Pathogenic Mechanisms/Markers

Immunopathogenesis plays a vital role in pars planitis. Elevated levels of surrogate markers of immune activation have been found in the serum of patients, including IL-8, soluble intracellular adhesion molecule 1, and increased expression of HLA-DR on peripheral CD4+ T cells. Moreover, activated Muller cells in the eye can express class II MHC molecules, presenting antigens to T cells and perpetuating inflammation.[22]

14.3.4 Diagnostics

By definition, pars planitis is idiopathic, and other causes of intermediate uveitis need to be excluded through serologic testing for syphilis, Lyme disease, and tuberculosis. Chest radiographs are also helpful in assessing for sarcoidosis. In the presence of neurologic symptoms, an MRI of the brain is warranted to assess for multiple sclerosis.[23]

With advancements in imaging technologies, tools such as fluorescein angiography have become invaluable in identifying vascular abnormalities, including leakage and areas of non-perfusion. OCT plays a pivotal role, helping clinicians detect macular edema and epiretinal membranes.

14.3.5 Natural History

Pars planitis presents with about 10% of patients experiencing self-limited disease, 59% having a prolonged course with exacerbations, and 31% showing chronic smoldering symptoms.[24] Approximately 70% of patients develop vision-threatening complications, such as macular edema, leading to visual loss.[18] Children often present with more severe symptoms and a poorer prognosis compared to adults, with early onset (before age 7) linked to increased complications and visual impairment.[25] The most common causes of severe visual loss are macular edema, cataract, and retinal detachment. An important consideration is the association of pars planitis with multiple sclerosis (MS). Due to its potential to cause blindness, especially in children, pars planitis requires early and aggressive treatment, including corticosteroids, IMT, anti-TNF-α agents, and surgical interventions for complications. Regular screening for symptoms of MS is also recommended for long-term management.

14.3.6 Management and Treatment

The treatment strategy consists of early and aggressive treatment with topical corticosteroids (difluprednate 0.05%), subtenon triamcinolone acetonide injections, intravitreal corticosteroid injections (triamcinolone acetonide, fluocinolone 0.18 mg implant, fluocinolone 0.59 mg insert, or dexamethasone 0.7 mg implant), or oral corticosteroids with or without concurrent use of immunosuppressive agents (antimetabolites, TNF-α inhibitors).[26-28] Retinal neovascularization along the snowbanks is treated with cryotherapy or laser photocoagulation.

14.4 STEROID-INDUCED OCULAR HYPERTENSION AND GLAUCOMA

14.4.1 Epidemiology

Corticosteroids, while effective in controlling ocular inflammation, can lead to the development of elevated intraocular pressure (IOP). A "steroid responder" (SR) refers to individuals whose IOP elevates by more than 5 to 10 mmHg from baseline after steroid use.[29] The susceptibility to such IOP elevation varies with approximately 30% to 40% of the general population exhibiting a mild IOP elevation of 6 to 15 mmHg, while about 5% are highly responsive (IOP elevations ≥ 16 mmHg).[30]

Risk factors include individuals with a family history of primary open-angle glaucoma (POAG) and those with POAG, and myopes tend to be more susceptible to rises exceeding 15 mmHg.[30] Additionally, patients who have undergone ocular surgery, particularly involving the anterior segment, may also exhibit enhanced steroid responsiveness. Such post-surgical patients can experience IOP elevations within hours to weeks of starting corticosteroid therapy.[31] Both the elderly and children are more prone to elevated IOP,[32-34] with older individuals having an odds ratio of up to 1.72 for developing steroid-induced glaucoma following the use of topical cortisone eye drops.[35]

14.4.2 Key Pathogenic Mechanisms/Markers

Several theories have been posited on the etiology of steroid-induced IOP elevation and glaucoma. Changes in the trabecular meshwork's extracellular matrix result in thickening of the trabecular beams through alterations of the cytoskeletal structure and elevated myocilin levels.[33] This leads to increased resistance, decreased aqueous outflow, and rising IOP. Additionally, corticosteroids inhibit trabecular meshwork cell phagocytosis, leading to cellular debris accumulation.[36, 37]

14.4.3 Diagnostics

Diagnosis relies on a detailed clinical history, including prolonged steroid eye drop use. Notably, renal transplant recipients also have an increased risk for SR.[38] Evaluation is based on examination of the anterior chamber and posterior segment, with careful attention to the IOP, visual field assessments, retinal nerve fiber OCT, and gonioscopy. Assessment of the IOP, or tonometry, is best evaluated using the Goldmann applanator (GAT).[39] However, in scenarios where GAT is challenging – children, uncooperative individuals, or the bedridden – alternatives such as the iCare tonometer or the Tonopen® are recommended.

14.4.4 Natural History

Steroid-induced glaucoma is a subtype of secondary open-angle glaucoma. Corticosteroid use can lead to elevated IOP within hours to years; the most common interval for IOP response is 4 to 6 weeks after initiation of therapy.[29] The degree of IOP elevation also varies, with some experiencing mild increases and others seeing significant spikes.[40] If left unchecked, chronic elevated IOP can lead to optic nerve damage and visual field defects.[41] Once the corticosteroid is reduced or discontinued, IOP often decreases, though not always to baseline levels. However, prolonged exposure can cause irreversible trabecular meshwork damage, making IOP control challenging even after cessation. Guidelines stress the importance of meticulous IOP monitoring in those on corticosteroids, especially those with known risk factors or a family predisposition. Immediate therapeutic interventions are recommended to prevent irreversible visual damage.[30]

14.4.5 Management and Treatment

The management of steroid-induced glaucoma requires a customized approach, primarily involving the reduction or cessation of the causative corticosteroid. However, discontinuing steroid treatment is not always viable, particularly in cases requiring ongoing management of chronic inflammation. In such scenarios, where it is medically appropriate, loteprednol can be considered.[41] Importantly, managing this condition necessitates a collaborative effort with the patient's comprehensive care team, including primary care physicians, rheumatologists, and otolaryngologists, to evaluate the possibility of using alternative steroid-sparing therapies in place of systemic or inhaled steroids. This includes transitions to IMT for long-term control of inflammation.

For immediate IOP reduction, topical anti-glaucoma medications (prostaglandin analogs, beta-blockers, carbonic anhydrase inhibitors, and alpha agonists) can be initiated.[36] Refractory cases, or those with significant optic nerve damage, might necessitate surgical interventions such as trabeculectomy, tube shunt placement, goniotomy, canaloplasty, or minimally invasive glaucoma surgeries (MIGS).[40, 42] Another alternative to the use of drops includes selective laser trabeculoplasty (SLT) in non-surgical candidates.[32] However, regular monitoring of IOP is crucial for patients on corticosteroid therapy. Patient education, emphasizing the importance of regular ophthalmic checkups, is vital for early detection and intervention.

REFERENCES

1. Parchand S et al. Sympathetic ophthalmia: A comprehensive update. *Indian J Ophthalmol.* 2022;70(6):1931–1944. doi:10.4103/ijo.IJO_2363_21.

2. Agarwal M, Radosavljevic A, Tyagi M, Pichi F, Al Dhanhani AA, Agarwal A, Cunningham Jr ET. Sympathetic ophthalmia – an overview. *Ocul Immunol Inflamm.* 2023;31(4):793–809. doi:10.1080/09273948.2022.2058554.

3. Fromal OV, Swaminathan V, Soares RR, Ho AC. Recent advances in diagnosis and management of sympathetic ophthalmia. *Curr Opin Ophthal.* 2021 Nov.;32(6):555–560. doi:10.1097/ICU.0000000000000803.

4. Paulbuddhe V, Addya S, Gurnani B, Singh D, Tripathy K, Chawla R. Sympathetic ophthalmia: Where do we currently stand on treatment strategies ? *Clin Ophthalmol.* 2021 Oct. 20;15:4201–4218. doi:10.2147/OPTH.S289688.

5. Standardization of Uveitis Nomenclature (SUN) Working Group. Classification criteria for sympathetic ophthalmia. *Am J Ophthal.* 2021;228:212–219. doi:10.1016/j.ajo.2021.03.048.

6. Chan CC, Roberge RG, Whitcup SM, Nussenblatt RB. Thirty two cases of sympathetic ophthalmia. A retrospective study at the National Eye Institute, Bethesda, MD from 1982 –1992. *Arch Ophthalmol.* 1995;113:597–601.

7. Minos E et al. Birdshot chorioretinopathy: Current knowledge and new concepts in pathophysiology, diagnosis, monitoring and treatment. *Orphanet J Rare Dis.* 2016 May 12;11(1):61. doi:10.1186/s13023-016-0429-8.

8. Vitale AT. Birdshot retinochoroidopathy. *J Ophthalmic Vis Res.* 2014;9(3):350–361. doi:10.4103/2008-322X.143376.

9. American Academy of Ophthalmology. Birdshot retinochoroidopathy. *Section 9: Intraocular inflammation and uveitis.* Singapore, 2011–2012:152–155.

10. Bousquet E, Duraffour P, Debillon L, Somisetty S, Monnet D, Brézin AP. Birdshot chorioretinopathy: A review. *J Clin Med.* 2022 Aug. 16;11(16):4772. doi:10.3390/jcm11164772.

11. Shah KH, Levinson RD, Yu F, Goldhardt R, Gordon LK, Gonzales CR, Heckenlively JR, Kappel PJ, Holland GN. Birdshot chorioretinopathy. *Surv Ophthalmol.* 2005;50:519–541. doi:10.1016/j.survophthal.2005.08.004.

12. Thorne JE, Jabs DA, Kedhar SR, Peters GB, Dunn JP. Loss of visual field among patients with birdshot chorioretinopathy. *Am J Ophthalmol.* 2008;145:23–28.e2. doi:10.1016/j.ajo.2007.08.039.

13. Papadia M, Herbort CP. New concepts in the appraisal and management of birdshot retinochoroiditis, a global perspective. *Int Ophthalmol.* 2015;35:287–301. doi:10.1007/s10792-015-0046-x.

14. Crowell EL, France R, Majmudar P, Jabs DA, Thorne JE. Treatment outcomes in birdshot chorioretinitis: Corticosteroid sparing, corticosteroid discontinuation, remission, and relapse. *Ophthalmol Retina*. 2022;6(7):620–627. doi:10.1016/j.oret.2022.03.003.

15. Doycheva D, Zierhut M, Blumenstock G, Stuebiger N, Deuter C. Longterm results of therapy with mycophenolate mofetil in chronic noninfectious uveitis. *Graefes Arch Clin Exp Ophthalmol*. 2011;249(8):1235–1243.

16. Goldberg NR, Lyu T, Moshier E, Godbold J, Jabs DA. Success with single-agent immunosuppression for multifocal choroidopathies. *Am J Ophthalmol*. 2014;158(6):1310–1317. doi:10.1016/j.ajo.2014.08.039.

17. Standardization of Uveitis Nomenclature (SUN) Working Group. Classification criteria for birdshot chorioretinitis. *Am J Ophthalmol*. 2021;228:65–71. doi:10.1016/j.ajo.2021.03.059.

18. Quinones K, Choi JY, Yilmaz T, Kafkala C, Letko E, Foster CS. Pars plana vitrectomy versus immunomodulatory therapy for intermediate uveitis: A prospective, randomized pilot study. *Ocul Immunol Inflamm*. 2010;18:411–417.

19. Ozdal PC, Berker N, Tugal-Tutkun I. Pars planitis: Epidemiology, clinical characteristics, management and visual prognosis. *J Ophthalmic Vis Res*. 2015;10(4):469–480. doi:10.4103/2008-322X.176897.

20. Tang WM, Pulido JS, Eckels DD, Han DP, Mieler WF, Pierce K. The association of HLA-DR15 and intermediate uveitis. *Am J Ophthalmol*. 1997;123(1):70–75. doi:10.1016/s0002-9394(14)70994-8.

21. Malinowski SM, Pulido JS, Folk JC. Long-term visual outcome and complications associated with pars planitis. *Ophthalmology*. 1993;100(6):818–824; discussion 825.

22. Przeździecka-Dołyk J et al. Immunopathogenic background of pars planitis. *J Ophthalmic Vis Res*. 2016;11(3):314–322.

23. Miserocchi E, Fogliato G, Modorati G, Bandello F. Review on the worldwide epidemiology of uveitis. *Eur J Ophthalmol*. 2013;23(5):705–717.

24. Smith RE, Godfrey WA, Kimura SJ. Chronic cyclitis. I. Course and visual prognosis. *Trans Am Acad Ophthalmol Otolaryngol*. 1973;77:OP760–OP768.

25. Guest S, Funkhouser E, Lightman S. Pars planitis: A comparison of childhood onset and adult onset disease. *Clin Experiment Ophthalmol*. 2001;29:81–84.

26. Deschenes J, Murray PI, Rao NA, Nussenblatt RB. International uveitis study group (IUSG): Clinical classification of uveitis. *Ocul Immunol Inflamm*. 2008;16(1):1–2. doi:10.1080/09273940801899822.

27. Babu BM, Rathinam SR. Intermediate uveitis. *Indian J Ophthalmol*. 2010;58(1):21–27. doi:10.4103/0301-4738.58469.

28. Foster CS, Vitale AT. *Diagnosis and treatment of uveitis*, 2nd edn. Jaypee Brothers.

29. Sheppard JD, Comstock TL, Cavet ME. Impact of the topical ophthalmic corticosteroid loteprednol etabonate on intraocular pressure. *Adv Ther*. 2016 Apr.;33(4):532–552.

30. Kersey JP, Broadway DC. Corticosteroid-induced glaucoma: A review of the literature. *Eye (Lond)*. 2006;20(4):407–416.

31. Korenfeld MS, Silverstein SM, Cooke DL, Vogel R, Crockett RS, Difluprednate Ophthalmic Emulsion 0.05% (Durezol) Study Group. Difluprednate ophthalmic emulsion 0.05% for postoperative inflammation and pain. *J Cataract Refract Surg*. 2009;35(1):26–34.

32. Rubin B, Taglienti A, Rothman RF, Marcus CH, Serle JB. The effect of selective laser trabeculoplasty on intraocular pressure in patients with intravitreal steroid-induced elevated intraocular pressure. *J Glaucoma*. 2008;17(4):287–292.

33. Cho WJ et al. Association of trabecular meshwork height with steroid-induced ocular hypertension. *Sci Rep*. 2023;13(1):9143.

34. Lam DSC et al. Ocular hypertensive and anti-inflammatory responses to different dosages of topical dexamethasone in children: A randomized trial. *Clin Experiment Ophthalmol*. 2005;33:252–258.

35. Garbe E, LeLorier J, Boivin JF, Suissa S. Risk of ocular hypertension or open-angle glaucoma in elderly patients on oral glucocorticoids. *Lancet*. 1997 Oct. 4;350(9083):979–982.

36. Razeghinejad MR, Katz LJ. Steroid-induced iatrogenic glaucoma. *Ophthalmic Res*. 2012;47(2):66–80.

37. Jones R 3rd, Rhee DJ. Corticosteroid-induced ocular hypertension and glaucoma: A brief review and update of the literature. *Curr Opin Ophthalmol*. 2006;17(2):163–167.

38. Ticho U, Durst A, Licht A, Berkowitz S. Steroid-induced glaucoma and cataract in renal transplant recipients. *Isr J Med Sci*. 1977;13(9):871–874.

39. Salvetat ML, Zeppieri M, Tosoni C, Brusini P. Medscape. Baseline factors predicting the risk of conversion from ocular hypertension to primary open-angle glaucoma during a 10-year follow-up. *Eye (Lond)*. 2016 Jun.;30(6):784–795.
40. Phulke S, Kaushik S, Kaur S, Pandav SS. Steroid-induced glaucoma: An avoidable irreversible blindness. *J Curr Glaucoma Pract*. 2017;11(2):67–72.
41. Comstock TL, Sheppard JD. Loteprednol etabonate for inflammatory conditions of the anterior segment of the eye: Twenty years of clinical experience with a retrometabolically designed corticosteroid. *Expert Opin Pharmacother*. 2018;19(4):337–353. doi:10.1080/14656566.2018.1439920.
42. Brusini P, Tosoni C, Zeppieri M. Canaloplasty in corticosteroid-induced glaucoma. Preliminary results. *J Clin Med*. 2018;7(2):31.

15 Considerations for Pediatric Rheumatologic Patients with Ophthalmic Disease

Rachel Guess, Maleewan Kitcharoensakkul, and Kara C. LaMattina

15.1 EPIDEMIOLOGY

While children only make up a small portion (5% to 10%) of uveitis assessed at tertiary referral centers, pediatric uveitis carries significant morbidity, resulting in blindness in up to 22% of patients, making it a particularly important entity.[1-4] The estimated annual incidence of childhood uveitis in North America and Europe is 4.3 to 6.9/100,000.[5] In the pediatric population, uveitis is more commonly classified as chronic rather than acute or recurrent, typically presents as bilateral disease, and is most frequently localized to the anterior segment of the eye.[1-3]

15.2 UNIQUE CHALLENGES FOR HISTORY AND EXAM

As has been well-described in the preceding chapters, uveitis can be a challenging entity in terms of both diagnosis and treatment. Uveitis management in the pediatric population adds another layer of complexity for a variety of reasons. The history-taking itself can be challenging: the insidious nature of many forms of pediatric uveitis often results in a lack of symptoms until late in the disease. Even if children are symptomatic, they may be too young to verbalize those symptoms. As children age, they may begin to engage in high-risk behaviors such as drug or alcohol consumption or sexual activity that they do not disclose for fear of judgment or punishment. An inaccurate history may result in an incomplete laboratory evaluation that misses a critical diagnosis.

Unfamiliarity with eye diseases in general, let alone uveitis, may also make it challenging for parents to seek out timely care. Symptoms like red eye can be attributed to more common entities like conjunctivitis. It is often the case to be treated with allergy or antibiotic drops for months before a slit lamp examination confirms the diagnosis of uveitis. This raises an additional challenge of caring for children: successful examination. Thorough slit lamp examination of the anterior and posterior segments along with indirect ophthalmoscopy are required to characterize uveitis and its associated complications. Children, particularly those who may be light sensitive secondary to their intraocular inflammation or those who have behavioral changes such as autism spectrum disorder, may be difficult to examine. Portable slit lamps are not an adequate substitute for fixed slit lamps, as there is often inadequate illumination to accurately characterize anterior chamber cell and flare. This makes examinations under anesthesia suboptimal for these evaluations unless a slit lamp can be utilized in the operating room, which poses its own challenge from an anesthesia perspective.

The same challenges faced in the examination of children can also make imaging studies difficult. Testing such as optical coherence tomography and fluorescein angiography can be critical in diagnosis and monitoring of both the disease (as in cases of retinal vasculitis) and the complications (such as macular edema or glaucoma). While adaptations such as the administration of fluorescein orally rather than intravenously can make testing more feasible in children, these studies still necessitate cooperation. If patients are too young to be able to cooperate, the tests may need to be performed under anesthesia. Unfortunately, even many tertiary hospitals may not be equipped to perform these studies in the operating room, which can necessitate referral to another center, adding the challenge of access and potential further delay of appropriate care.

Fortunately for our patients, new techniques for disease diagnosis and monitoring are being studied. In the future, it may be possible to use tear-based biomarkers to detect disease activity. It also may be possible to use common imaging machines with new programming to get accurate anterior chamber cell counts (reducing inter-rater variability) or degree of retinal vessel leakage, both of which could be utilized to assess disease activity and treatment response.

15.3 UNIQUE CONSIDERATIONS FOR THE DIFFERENTIAL DIAGNOSIS

In North America and most of the Western world, infectious etiologies are a rare cause of uveitis in children. As most forms of pediatric uveitis are chronic and noninfectious, with a high likelihood that immunosuppressive therapy will be needed in disease management, infectious uveitis should always be considered and ruled out with appropriate testing. The main causes of infectious pediatric uveitis are toxoplasmosis and toxocariasis, although it is also important to exclude tuberculosis and syphilis (which may be congenital or acquired, necessitating consideration of sexual activity or abuse). As in adult uveitis, a significant proportion of pediatric uveitis is idiopathic, though it is

DOI: 10.1201/9781003453710-15

important to recognize that diseases evolve over time. A systemic diagnosis may declare itself later in the disease course.

In addition to these considerations, it is also important to recognize that disease entities may be unique to or present differently in the pediatric population compared to the adult population. We will highlight some of those discrepancies in what follows, starting with the most common cause of noninfectious pediatric uveitis, juvenile idiopathic arthritis (JIA).[6] Up to 77% of uveitis in pediatrics is associated with JIA per one population-based study.[7]

15.3.1 Juvenile Idiopathic Arthritis

Juvenile idiopathic arthritis (JIA) is the most common pediatric rheumatologic disease and has several subtypes with varying risks of comorbid uveitis, with up to 20% of JIA patients developing uveitis. The subcategories of JIA (Table 15.1) are subject to change as new classification systems are proposed. However, uveitis remains the most common extra-articular manifestation of JIA. The risks of developing uveitis are tied to several key features of the disease. The prevalence of JIA-associated uveitis (JIA-U) is variable depending on JIA subtype (Table 15.2).

Table 15.1 Juvenile Idiopathic Arthritis (JIA) Subtypes with Their Frequency, Gender Predilection, and Typical Age of Onset[8]

Subtype	% of JIA	Gender Predilection	Age of Onset

Oligoarticular
  Extended
  Persistent
	50%	Females	2–4 years

Polyarticular
  RF positive
  RF negative
	
	< 5%
	15–20%
		Females	
			9–12 years
			1–3 years, 9–14 years

Systemic	10%	None	< 5 years
Psoriatic arthritis	3–10%	Early onset – Females Adolescents – Male	1–2 years, 8–12 years
Enthesitis-related arthritis	5–10%	Males	>10 years
*Undifferentiated	5–10%		

Abbreviations: RF: rheumatoid factor antibody.

Source: LaMattina KC, Goldstein DA. Pediatric uveitis. In: Nelson LB: *Color Atlas and Synopsis of Clinical Ophthalmology: Pediatric Ophthalmology*, Wills Eye Institute Series, Lippincott Williams & Wilkins, Philadelphia, 2019.

Table 15.2 Prevalence of Juvenile Idiopathic Arthritis–Associated Uveitis (JIA-U) Based on JIA Subtype[9]

Subtype	Uveitis Prevalence

Oligoarticular
  Extended
  Persistent
	30–50%

Polyarthritis
  RF positive
  RF negative
	
	Rare
	5–10%

Systemic	< 1%
Psoriatic arthritis	10–20%
Enthesitis-related	10–15%

Source: LaMattina KC, Goldstein DA. Pediatric uveitis. In: Nelson LB: *Color Atlas and Synopsis of Clinical Ophthalmology: Pediatric Ophthalmology*, Wills Eye Institute Series, Lippincott Williams & Wilkins, Philadelphia, 2019.

15.3.1.1 Pathogenesis

The pathogenesis of JIA-U is still not well understood. The increased risk of JIA-U with a positive ANA suggests there could be antibody-mediated inflammation. Patients with JIA, with and without uveitis, have increased antibody binding to the iris and retina compared to healthy controls.[10] Biopsies of eyes in JIA-U patients have shown T and B cell presence, with a CD4-positive T cell predominance, that are reactive to normal intraocular antigens.[10, 11] One theory is that regulatory T cell dysfunction leads to a loss of self-antigen tolerance and autoimmunity.[10] There is also consideration for activation of the innate immune system in JIA-U. However, questions remain due to lack of a robust mouse model.[12] No specific genetics are necessary to induce JIA-U, although several human leukocyte antigen (HLA) subtypes increase risk of the disease, including HLA-DR5 haplotype, HLA-DRB1*1104, and HLA-DPB1*0201. HLA-DRB1 with the presence of a serine or aspartate amino acid at the 11th position will also increase risk of JIA-U, with an odds ratio of 2.59, in females but not for males.[11] The presence of HLA-DR1 appears protective against JIA-U.[10] At present, it is not common to screen patients for these HLA subtypes, as more study is needed to understand their implications to the patient. However, this practice may change in the future.[11]

15.3.1.2 Screening

Most JIA patients are diagnosed with JIA prior to uveitis, although 3% to 7% of patients may have uveitis preceding arthritis. Therefore, it is important to screen for systemic diseases including JIA in pediatric patients presenting with uveitis.[13] Based on a longitudinal study of more than 1,000 JIA patients in Canada, the mean time from diagnosis of JIA to diagnosis of uveitis was 1.8 years (range from 4.2 months to 10 years), and at least 7% of patients developed uveitis during the mean follow-up period of 7 years.[14]

Acutely painful, red eyes can be manifestations of uveitis associated with certain types of JIA, including enthesitis-related arthritis and inflammatory bowel disease arthritis, particularly if they have HLA B27-positivity.[10] However, the classic presentation of JIA-U is chronic anterior uveitis, which is mostly asymptomatic. Therefore, scheduled screening is necessary to prevent ocular complications including visual loss, which has been described in 10% to 20% of JIA-U cases.[15] Based on the 2019 American College of Rheumatology (ACR) recommendation, the interval for eye screenings for patients with JIA is based on risk. The patients at a high risk of developing uveitis (oligoarthritis, rheumatoid factor negative polyarthritis, psoriatic arthritis, or ANA positive undifferentiated arthritis, younger than 7 years of age at JIA onset, and JIA duration of 4 years or less) should be screened every 3 months.[10] Patients at moderate risk of developing uveitis should be screened every 6 months, and low risk should be screened every 12 months. There are helpful tables for quick reference through the American College of Rheumatology and the American Academy of Ophthalmology. These are updated as guidelines evolve.

Although most patients with JIA-U have good visual outcomes, ocular complications have been reported in JIA and include posterior synechiae, cataract, band keratopathy, glaucoma, macular edema, and ultimately visual loss (Figure 15.1). The risk of ocular complications is associated with steroid use and type of uveitis (panuveitis portends a greater risk than that of anterior uveitis).[14] Early initiation of methotrexate (MTX) in patients at high uveitis risk may reduce the risks of new-onset uveitis in patients with biologic-naive JIA.[16]

15.3.2 Sarcoidosis

Sarcoidosis in the pediatric population can present vastly differently to that in adults (as described in Chapter 7). While older children, typically ages 8 to 15, tend to present with a clinical picture similar to the adult population, with pulmonary involvement affecting up to 90% of patients, younger children present with very different findings. Early-onset sarcoidosis typically presents before age 4 with a classic triad of rash, arthritis, and uveitis.[17] Children are also more likely to present with peripheral lymphadenopathy than adults (40% to 70% versus 4.8%).[18, 19] This finding can assist in diagnosis, as it may offer more accessible biopsy sites. While adults with ocular sarcoid are more commonly female, this gender predilection is less clear in the pediatric population.[20, 21] As with adults, ocular sarcoid may be asymptomatic in children, with a third of patients diagnosed with intraocular inflammation on routine screening.[22] While children and adults frequently have findings of anterior uveitis on exam, there may be more posterior segment findings in children than in adults (up to 85% in children versus 25% to 50% in adults).[22] Similar to adults, this posterior involvement typically manifests as multifocal choroiditis or retinal periphlebitis.[21]

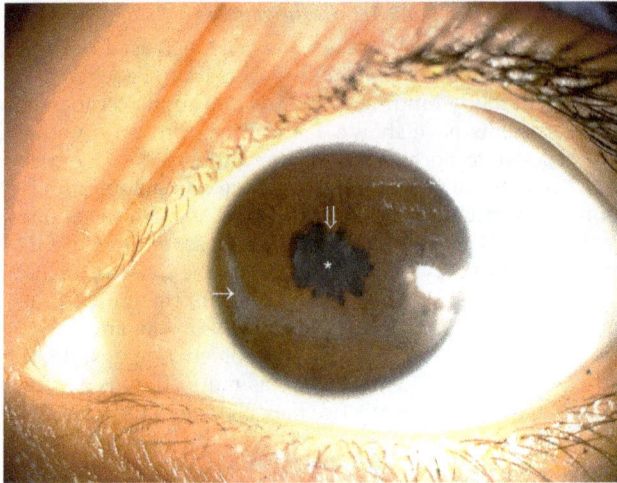

Figure 15.1 Band keratopathy (→), posterior synechiae (⇓), and a lenticular membrane (*) in a child with oligoarticular JIA.

When evaluating pediatric patients for sarcoidosis, laboratory studies such as angiotensin-converting enzyme (ACE) and lysozyme are less helpful than in adults.[23] This is a nonspecific marker, and many children have physiologically elevated levels of ACE,[24] which should be accounted for in assessing these levels. While screening with chest radiographs may be routine in both children and adults with uveitis, they are often normal in children with sarcoidosis. Chest CT is generally used with more caution in children and guided by clinical suspicion given the radiation exposure. Pulmonary function tests are another supportive (but non-diagnostic) test for children who are able to participate adequately.

15.3.3 Tubulointerstitial Nephritis and Uveitis

As reviewed in Chapter 12, our understanding of tubulointerstitial nephritis and uveitis (TINU) has evolved over the last decade. It was first described in a series in 1975, with two teenage girls who presented with bilateral anterior uveitis and eosinophilic interstitial nephritis.[25] In the following decades, TINU was typically classified as a bilateral anterior uveitis, which was more commonly seen in children.[26, 27] Recent studies, however, suggest that these findings may have been biased by a lack of suspicion and, therefore, testing in adults or patients who do not fit this classical clinical picture. Unfortunately, as the literature is still evolving, we do not yet have a clear picture on how the clinical presentation or prognosis for TINU may differ between children and adults. It remains an important entity to consider in any child with uveitis. If there is suspicion for TINU, a good screening tool is the urine beta-2 microglobulin test. See Chapter 12 for further details.

15.3.4 Pars Planitis

As described in Chapter 14, pars planitis describes idiopathic intermediate uveitis, which is typically characterized by vitreous snowballs and snowbanks (Figure 15.2). It typically demonstrates a bimodal distribution, affecting patients ages 5 to 15 years and 25 to 35 years.[28] While pars planitis in adulthood predominantly affects females (56% vs. 44%), in childhood, there is a male predisposition (61% vs. 39%). Paroli et al. found that children more often develop optic nerve edema than adults (15.5% vs. 9.2%) but are less likely than adults to develop ocular hypertension (7.5% vs. 15.6%).[29] Giles noted that children more commonly had aggressive anterior segment inflammation in pars planitis,[30] which would align with Paroli's finding of higher rates of band keratopathy in children than adults (3.5% vs. 0.3%, $p = 0.01$). Paroli also found that children with pars planitis are more likely to develop retinoschisis than their adult counterparts (5.8% vs. 1.7%, $p = 0.01$).[29]

As previously discussed, it is important to rule out multiple sclerosis (MS) in patients presenting with pars planitis through a thorough review of systems, with consideration of magnetic resonance imaging with suggestive symptoms. This is particularly important in cases utilizing immuno-modulatory therapy, as tumor necrosis factor inhibitors (TNFi) are contraindicated in patients with

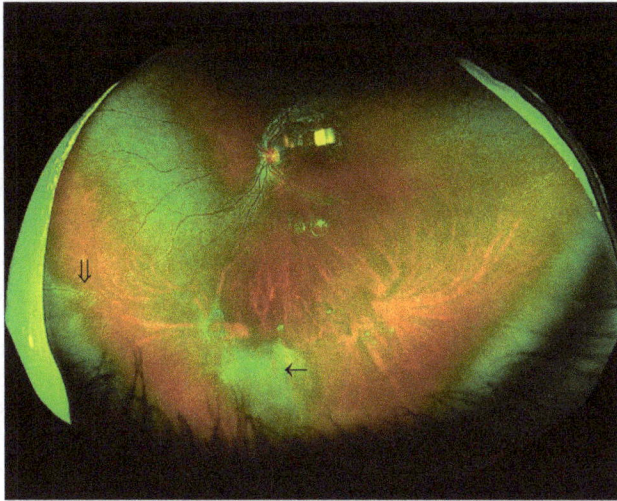

Figure 15.2 Inferior snowballs (←) and retinal vasculitis (⇊) in a patient with pars planitis. (Photo courtesy of Jennifer Jung, MD.)

demyelinating diseases. Fortunately, the rate of MS-associated pars planitis has been shown to be lower in the pediatric population than the adult population (2.4% vs. 6.7%).[29]

15.3.5 Vogt–Koyanagi–Harada Syndrome

As described in Chapter 12, Vogt–Koyanagi–Harada syndrome (VKH) is a multisystem disease that typically presents as a bilateral, chronic panuveitis characterized by exudative retinal detachments. While rare in children, it is more common in people of Southeast Asian descent and is the second most common cause of uveitis in Saudi Arabia.[31] Tabbara and colleagues found that children experience a more severe form of the disease than adults.[31] Children had worse visual outcomes: vision was 20/200 or worse in the better-seeing eye of 61% of children in their series (versus 26% in adults). Children were also more likely to develop complications of the disease and treatment, with more than 3 times the rates of glaucoma (46% compared with 14% in adults) and cataracts requiring surgery (61% compared with 17% in adults).[31] Improvement in our approach to pediatric uveitis, particularly with earlier implementation of newer steroid-sparing therapies, appears to have altered this course in a more recent Chinese study by Yang et al.[32] They found that fewer children had visual acuity less than or equal to 20/60 than adults between ages 16 and 65 (12.2% vs. 20.1%). Slightly fewer children developed glaucoma (24.2% vs. 26.0%) and required cataract surgery (14.9% vs. 22.0%) than adults in their series as well.[32]

15.3.6 Vasculitis

In pediatrics, there are several vasculitides that can cause ocular manifestations. Kawasaki disease (KD) is a medium-vessel vasculitis that presents in young children with rash, mucosal changes, lymphadenopathy, and fever longer than 5 days. Classically, children have bilateral non-exudative limbal-sparing conjunctivitis. Patients with KD could also have papillitis or uveitis (typically anterior). Kawasaki disease is treated with high-dose intravenous immunoglobulin and aspirin, with topical steroids as needed for uveitis. Consensus guidelines for treatment are available through the American Heart Association or the American College of Rheumatology.

Antineutrophilic cytoplasmic antibodies (ANCA)-associated vasculitis is a rare small-vessel vasculitis that classically affects the lungs and kidneys. Patients with ocular involvement, which is rare in children, typically present with episcleritis or scleritis.[33–35] Orbital pseudotumor is another rare manifestation of ANCA-associated vasculitis, but it is important to recognize because it can be sight threatening.[36]

Behçet's disease is a rare vasculitis of variable-vessel size that classically presents with severe oral and genital ulcers along with other manifestations such as CNS and/or GI involvement, arthritis, and rash. Patients with Behçet's frequently have ocular involvement, with up to 27% of children developing posterior uveitis and 18% developing anterior uveitis, which may be severe with hypopyon. Given the high rate of eye involvement, these patients should have routine eye examinations.[37]

Systemic lupus erythematosus (SLE) is one of the secondary vasculitic disorders. Patients with SLE can be found to have a vast array of eye manifestations that affect the skin, the orbit, the lacrimal system, the anterior or posterior segment of the eye, and the optic nerve. The most common ophthalmic involvement is keratoconjunctivitis sicca; other manifestations are rare in children and include episcleritis, uveitis, retinitis, cotton wool spots, retinal detachment, large-vessel occlusion, optic neuritis, and lupus choroidopathy.[38]

15.3.7 Inborn Errors of Immunity

Noninfectious uveitis and ocular inflammation are uncommon clinical manifestations of inborn errors of immunity (IEI), a heterozygous group of genetic disorders causing defects of the immune system.[39] It is important for clinicians to recognize these monogenic disorders because they could lead to targeted therapy based on mechanisms of disease and affect disease monitoring and prognosis. For example, haploinsufficiency of A20 and Blau syndrome are IEIs that have uveitis as their common manifestations. Blau syndrome shares several overlapping features with sarcoidosis, particularly the finding of noncaseating granulomas in affected tissues. However, Blau syndrome is a monogenic disorder due to gain-of-function in NOD2, commonly presenting before age 5 with a triad of granulomatous dermatitis, symmetrical polyarthritis, and recurrent uveitis. It is important to differentiate between the two conditions because Blau syndrome is more refractory to treatment with a higher risk for chronic morbidity and poor long-term outcomes.

For IEIs that can cause uveitis, the specific genetic defect and their main clinical features including uveitis are listed in Table 15.3.

Table 15.3 Monogenic Diseases Associated with Uveitis: Known Disease-Causing Genes at the Time of Publication and Common Extraocular Manifestations Are Included[39–44]

Disease	Gene Associated	Classic/Common Manifestations (Non-Exhaustive List)	Potential Ocular Manifestations
Cryoporin-Associated Periodic Fever Syndrome (CAPS)	NLRP3 NLRP12	▪ Fever ▪ Urticarial rash ▪ Arthritis/arthralgia ▪ Sensorineural hearing loss	▪ Conjunctivitis ▪ Episcleritis ▪ Uveitis ▪ Papilledema
Familial Mediterranean Fever (FMF)	MEFV	▪ Periodic noninfectious fever ▪ Arthritis/arthralgia ▪ Rash (erysipelas-like) ▪ Serositis	▪ Retinal vasculitis ▪ Uveitis ▪ Conjunctivitis ▪ Progressive thinning of the choroid
Tumor Necrosis Factor Receptor–Associated Periodic Fever Syndrome (TRAPS)	TNFRS1A	▪ Periodic noninfectious fever ▪ Painful migratory rash ▪ Myalgias/arthralgias ▪ Serositis	▪ Periorbital edema ▪ Uveitis ▪ Episcleritis
Blau Syndrome	NOD2	▪ Triad of: ▪ Arthritis ▪ Dermatitis ▪ Uveitis	▪ Granulomatous uveitis
Mevalonate Kinase Deficiency (MKD) including the spectrum of Hyper IgD syndrome (HIDS) to Mevalonate Aciduria (MA)	MVK	▪ Periodic noninfectious fever ▪ Abdominal pain ▪ Oral and genital ulcers ▪ Lymphadenopathy ▪ Hepatosplenomegaly ▪ Elevated IgD serum level	▪ Uveitis
NLRP1-Associated Autoinflammatory with Arthritis and Dyskeratosis (NAIAD)	NLRP1	▪ Fever ▪ Arthritis ▪ Immunodeficiency ▪ Vitamin A deficiency	▪ Uveitis ▪ Corneal dyskeratosis
Deficiency of Adenosine Deaminase 2 (DADA-2)	ADA2/CECR1	▪ Vasculopathy/Vasculitis ▪ Neurologic/Stroke ▪ Cytopenias ▪ Hypogammaglobulinemia	▪ Optic neuritis ▪ Optic atrophy ▪ Progressive thinning of the choroid

Table 15.3 (*Continued*)

Disease	Gene Associated	Classic/Common Manifestations (Non-Exhaustive List)	Potential Ocular Manifestations
Haploinsufficiency of A20 (A20)	*TNFAIP3/A20*	▪ Heterogenous ▪ Behçet's-like disease with oral and genital ulcers ▪ Gastrointestinal ulcers ▪ Fevers	▪ Uveitis
Autoinflammation and PLCg2 Antibody Deficiency (APLAID)	*PLCG2*	▪ Skin lesions ▪ Humoral immunodeficiency ▪ Enterocolitis ▪ Lung disease	▪ Uveitis ▪ Conjunctivitis ▪ Ocular ulcerations/erosions
Aicardi Goutieres	*TREX1* *RNASEH2A* *RNASEH2B* *RNASEH2C* *SAMHD* *ADAR1* *IFIH1* *LSM11* *RNU7–1* *ISG15*	▪ Encephalopathy early in life ▪ Intracranial calcifications ▪ Spasticity ▪ Developmental delays ▪ Epilepsy ▪ Chilblains ▪ Fever	▪ Glaucoma ▪ Optic neuritis ▪ Papillitis ▪ Cataracts
Chronic Atypical Neutrophilic Dermatosis with Lipodystrophy and Elevated Temperature (CANDLE)	*PSMB8* *PSMG2/PAC2* *PSMA3* *PSMB4* *PSMB9*	▪ Fever ▪ Chronic skin lesions with neutrophilic infiltrates ▪ Lipodystrophy	▪ Retinal vasculitis ▪ Uveitis
Autoimmune Polyendocrinopathy with Candidiasis and Ectodermal Dystrophy	*AIRE*	▪ Endocrinopathy ▪ Dental enamel hypoplasia ▪ Chronic mucocutaneous candidiasis	▪ Conjunctivitis ▪ Uveitis
Cytotoxic T Lymphocyte Antigen-4 (CTLA4) Haploinsufficiency	*CTLA4*	▪ Cytopenia ▪ Lymphoproliferation ▪ Hypogammaglobulinemia	▪ Uveitis
Lipopolysaccharide-Responsive and Beige-Like Anchor (LRBA) Deficiency	*LRBA*	▪ Infections ▪ Autoimmunity ▪ Hypogammaglobulinemia	▪ Uveitis
Common Variable Immunodeficiency (CVID)	Multiple associated genes	▪ Infections ▪ Bronchiectasis ▪ Hypogammaglobulinemia	▪ Uveitis
Chronic Granulomatous Disease	*CYBB, CYBA, NCF1, NCF3,* and *NCF4*	▪ Recurrent cutaneous and extracutaneous abscesses ▪ Colitis ▪ Recurrent bacterial pneumonias	▪ Chorioretinal lesions ▪ Corneal abnormalities ▪ Uveitis ▪ Optic nerve disease

15.4 UNIQUE CONSIDERATIONS FOR TREATMENT

In the realm of pediatric autoimmune eye disease, it is common for the ophthalmologist to partner with the rheumatologist for prescribing and administering systemic medications. The rheumatologist relies upon the ophthalmologist for regular updates on the state of the disease, indications for increasing therapy, and therapy response. The ophthalmologist may prefer for the rheumatologist to do the dosing and monitoring for treatment toxicity, evaluation of extraocular manifestations, and supervising of infusions of intravenous biologic agents based on their access to pediatric infusion centers. Most medications are dosed based on weight, and there may be alterations in dose to accommodate the accelerated drug metabolism seen in children. Tocilizumab is a prime example of this. Good communication between the rheumatologist and ophthalmologist is critical for effective and safe care. Communication tools have been developed to facilitate this in various institutions.

15.4.1 Corticosteroids

The American College of Rheumatology has developed consensus treatment guidelines for pediatric uveitis.[13] Topical corticosteroids are first-line therapy. Prednisolone acetate is the preferred first-line agent; loteprednol and fluorometholone offer insufficient potency to treat intraocular inflammation, and difluprednate carries a high risk of elevated intraocular pressure in children.[45] There may be a role for periocular or intraocular steroid injections in the management of pediatric uveitis, particularly in cases with vision-threatening complications such as cystoid macular edema or hypotony.[46] It is important to recognize that all of these treatment options are not generally meant as long-term solutions, given the risk of cataract or glaucoma. In severe or vision-threatening cases, oral or parenteral corticosteroids are commonly used.[13] In addition to carrying risks of side effects like weight gain as in adults, systemic steroids pose the unique risk to children of growth retardation. Because of this side effect profile, steroids are not meant to be used as a long-term treatment. Therefore, steroids in all forms are viewed as a bridge therapy in children until safer long-term treatment modalities can take effect.

15.4.2 Steroid-Sparing Chronic Therapies

Oral or subcutaneous (preferred) methotrexate is the most common initial steroid-sparing agent initiated.[13] In a large North American patient cohort, 85% of patients with JIA-U were treated with methotrexate,[47] although this is often not sufficient treatment.[48]

In severe cases, it is recommended to initiate biologic DMARD treatment early, with the preferred initial class being anti-TNF medications (specifically only ones that are monoclonal antibodies).[13] The most evidence supports adalimumab and infliximab with a paucity of data available for other anti-TNF medications.[13] Children with JIA-U often require increased frequency of dosing or above-standard dosing of anti-TNF medications. If they fail one anti-TNF, the recommendation is to trial a second anti-TNF medication and increase dosing as needed.

Other considerations for treatment in patients that have failed combination therapy of MTX with anti-TNF include replacing MTX with mycophenolate mofetil, cyclosporine, or leflunomide. Anti-TNF medication can be replaced with abatacept or tocilizumab.[13] There are limited case reports of using JAK inhibitors for treatment of adults with history of JIA-U. However, there is an ongoing trial evaluating the role of baricitinib for treatment of this patient population.[49]

15.4.3 Treatment Side Effects and Duration of Therapy

Pediatric patients may respond differently than adults to medications. For example, it is more common to see fatigue and nausea in children on methotrexate. This can be mitigated with subcutaneous administration, addition of folic acid daily, or dose reduction. Systemic steroids can impact growth, as mentioned, as well as the child's hormonal axis, mood, sleep, weight gain, self-image, bone health, and facial and body acne and slow their wound healing. Anti-TNF medications can induce psoriasis, which is typically a pustular psoriasis. Mycophenolate mofetil commonly causes gastrointestinal upset and diarrhea with onset, so it is common practice to start at a half dose for 1 to 2 weeks before ramping up to a full dose.

Another area of concern for pediatric patients is duration of therapy. Many children will require systemic immunosuppression for years if not life-long. Though there are multiple treatment options, in many cases, anti-drug antibody formation can threaten the effective list of medications for a patient.[50] The anti-TNF medication class is particularly susceptible to reduced efficacy and increased hypersensitivity reactions related to anti-drug antibodies.[51] Common practice is to continue DMARD therapy as tolerated while treating with anti-TNF medications to reduce the risk of forming anti-drug antibodies.[50] Another concern of long-term therapy is drug-related damage to the eye. This includes maculopathy or vortex keratopathy secondary to hydroxychloroquine toxicity (commonly used in SLE patients)[52] and formation of cataracts or glaucoma from extended steroid exposure (implant > topical > systemic).[53]

15.4.4 Environmental Factors and Impact on Treatment

Additionally, the treatment of children is complicated by their social environment. In those too young to self-manage medications, we rely on the family to reliably and effectively administer the medication. This includes remembering which type of eye drop to give at what frequency, remembering to shake the eye drops before giving them, remembering to keep the injectable medications in the refrigerator, and the ability to give an injectable medication at home. It is important for the prescribing office to provide teaching and training to the family on the necessary skills. Many children suffer from needle phobia and medication anxiety. This can be addressed over time with psychology, child life specialists, distraction techniques, and anesthetic options such as topical lidocaine gel. In extreme cases, it may be necessary to have the family go to the pediatrician's office for each injection to be done by a nurse or to switch to oral or infusion medications so that the onus is not on the family to inject the child. Additionally, children can participate better in their own care if they are given education at their level of understanding. Pediatric compliance improved and discontinuation of MTX was reduced for patients getting interactive education on their disease.[52] For adolescents, the impacts of drug use, sexual activity, and mental health should be considered and treatment tailored to reduce the individual's risk. Alcohol and tobacco products are to be avoided with methotrexate usage, and many medications are not considered safe for pregnancy. Not all adolescents feel comfortable with disclosing their social activities, and the treatment team should make regular confidential efforts to build trust and understanding to improve care.

15.4.5 Amblyopia Risk

A final consideration that is critical in discussing any eye disease in the pediatric population, including uveitis, is amblyopia. Particularly when considering a child with unilateral uveitis, one etiology for vision loss that must be evaluated early and treated appropriately is amblyopia.

15.5 SUMMARY

It is important to recognize that the approach to diagnosis and management of uveitis in children is different than that in adults. With incorporation of the discussed considerations, uveitis in children can be promptly and accurately diagnosed. Early implementation of steroid-sparing therapy is critical and will result in improved prognosis with fewer vision-threatening and systemic complications. Careful communication with families will help identify barriers to treatment and allow for individualized care that optimizes the child's ocular health. Partnership of ophthalmology and pediatric rheumatology for systemic treatment is common and often beneficial to the long-term outcome of the child.

REFERENCES

1. Paroli MP, Spinucci G, Liverani M, et al. Uveitis in childhood: an Italian clinical and epidemiological study. *Ocul Immunol Inflamm.* 2009 Jul.–Aug.;17(4):238–242. doi:10.1080/09273940802702561.
2. Curragh DS, O'Neill M, McAvoy CE, et al. Pediatric uveitis in a well-defined population: improved outcomes with immunosuppressive therapy. *Ocul Immunol Inflamm.* 2018;26(6):978–985. doi:10.1080/09273948.2017.1305420.
3. Smith JA, Mackensen F, Sen HN, et al. Epidemiology and course of disease in childhood uveitis. *Ophthalmology.* 2009 Aug.;116(8):1544–1551.e1. doi:10.1016/j.ophtha.2009.05.002.
4. Dajee KP, Rossen JL, Bratton ML, et al. A 10-year review of pediatric uveitis at a Hispanic-dominated tertiary pediatric ophthalmic clinic. *Clin Ophthalmol.* 2016 Aug. 22;10:1607–1612. doi:10.2147/OPTH.S96323.
5. Kump LI, Cervantes-Castañeda RA, Androudi SN, et al. Analysis of pediatric uveitis cases at a tertiary referral center. *Ophthalmology.* 2005 Jul.;112(7):1287–1292. doi:10.1016/j.ophtha.2005.01.044.
6. Maleki A, Anesi SD, Look-Why S, et al. Pediatric uveitis: a comprehensive review. *Surv Ophthalmol.* 2022 Mar.–Apr.;67(2):510–529. doi:10.1016/j.survophthal.2021.06.006.
7. Siiskonen M, Hirn I, Pesälä R, et al. Encouraging visual outcomes in children with idiopathic and JIA associated uveitis: a population-based study. *Pediatr Rheumatol Online J.* 2023 June 15;21(1):56. doi:10.1186/s12969-023-00841-8.
8. Stoll ML, Punaro M. Psoriatic juvenile idiopathic arthritis: a tale of two subgroups. *Curr Opin Rheumatol.* 2011 Sept.;23(5):437–443. doi:10.1097/BOR.0b013e328348b278.
9. LaMattina KC, Goldstein DA. Pediatric uveitis. In: Nelson LB, ed, *Color atlas and synopsis of clinical ophthalmology: Pediatric ophthalmology.* Wills Eye Institute Series. Lippincott Williams & Wilkins, 2019.
10. Clarke SL, Sen ES, Ramanan AV. Juvenile idiopathic arthritis-associated uveitis. *Pediatr Rheumatol Online J.* 2016 Apr. 27;14(1):27. doi:10.1186/s12969-016-0088-2.
11. Haasnoot AJW, Schilham MW, Kamphuis S, et al. Identification of an amino acid motif in HLA-DRβ1 that distinguishes uveitis in patients with juvenile idiopathic arthritis. *Arthritis Rheumatol.* 2018 Jul.;70(7):1155–1165. doi:10.1002/art.40484.

12. Sen ES, Dick AD, Ramanan AV. Uveitis associated with juvenile idiopathic arthritis. *Nat Rev Rheumatol.* 2015 Jun;11(6):338–348. doi:10.1038/nrrheum.2015.20.

13. Sen ES, Ramanan AV. Juvenile idiopathic arthritis-associated uveitis. *Clin Immunol.* 2020 Feb.;211:108322. doi:10.1016/j.clim.2019.108322.

14. Sabri K, Saurenmann RK, Silverman ED, et al. Course, complications, and outcome of juvenile arthritis-related uveitis. *J AAPOS.* 2008 Dec.;12(6):539–545. doi:10.1016/j.jaapos.2008.03.007.

15. Angeles-Han ST, Ringold S, Beukelman T, et al. 2019 American College of Rheumatology/ Arthritis Foundation Guideline for the screening, monitoring, and treatment of juvenile idiopathic arthritis-associated uveitis. *Arthritis Care Res (Hoboken).* 2019 June;71(6):703–716. doi:10.1002/acr.23871.

16. van Straalen JW, Akay G, Kouwenberg CV, et al. Methotrexate therapy associated with a reduced rate of new-onset uveitis in patients with biological-naïve juvenile idiopathic arthritis. *RMD Open.* 2023 Apr;9(2):e003010. doi:10.1136/rmdopen-2023-003010.

17. Gedalia A, Khan TA, Shetty AK, et al. Childhood sarcoidosis: Louisiana experience. *Clin Rheumatol.* 2016 Jul.;35(7):1879–1884. doi:10.1007/s10067-015-2870-9.

18. Hoffmann AL, Milman N, Byg KE. Childhood sarcoidosis in Denmark 1979–1994: incidence, clinical features and laboratory results at presentation in 48 children. *Acta Paediatr.* 2004 Jan.;93(1):30–36. https://onlinelibrary.wiley.com/doi/abs/10.1111/j.1651-2227.2004.tb00670.x?sid=nlm%3Apubmed. Accessed 17 Dec. 2023.

19. Melani AS, Bigliazzi C, Cimmino FA, et al. A comprehensive review of sarcoidosis treatment for pulmonologists. *Pulm Ther.* 2021 Dec.;7(2):325–344. doi:10.1007/s41030-021-00160-x.

20. Evans M, Sharma O, LaBree L, et al. Differences in clinical findings between Caucasians and African Americans with biopsy-proven sarcoidosis. *Ophthalmology.* 2007 Feb.;114(2):325–333. doi:10.1016/j.ophtha.2006.05.074.

21. Choi DE, Birnbaum AD, Oh F, et al. Pediatric uveitis secondary to probable, presumed, and biopsy-proven sarcoidosis. *J Pediatr Ophthalmol Strabismus.* 2011 May–June;48(3):157–162. doi:10.3928/01913913-20100518-01.

22. Obenauf CD, Shaw HE, Sydnor CF, et al. Sarcoidosis and its ophthalmic manifestations. *Am J Ophthalmol.* 1978 Nov.;86(5):648–655. doi:10.1016/0002-9394(78)90184-8.

23. Zheng SY, Du X, Dong JZ. Re-evaluating serum angiotensin-converting enzyme in sarcoidosis. *Front Immunol.* 2023 Oct. 5;14:950095. doi:10.3389/fimmu.2023.950095.

24. Bénéteau-Burnat B, Baudin B, Morgant G, et al. Serum angiotensin-converting enzyme in healthy and sarcoidotic children: comparison with the reference interval for adults. *Clin Chem.* 1990 Feb.;36(2):344–346. doi:10.1093/clinchem/36.2.344.

25. Dobrin RS, Vernier RL, Fish AL. Acute eosinophilic interstitial nephritis and renal failure with bone marrow-lymph node granulomas and anterior uveitis: a new syndrome. *Am J Med.* 1975 Sept.;59(3):325–333. doi:10.1016/0002-9343(75)90390-3.

26. Mackensen F, Smith JR, Rosenbaum JT. Enhanced recognition, treatment, and prognosis of tubulointerstitial nephritis and uveitis syndrome. *Ophthalmology.* 2007 May;114(5):995–999. doi:10.1016/j.ophtha.2007.01.002.

27. Okafor LO, Hewins P, Murray PI, et al. Tubulointerstitial nephritis and uveitis (TINU) syndrome: a systematic review of its epidemiology, demographics and risk factors. *Orphanet J Rare Dis.* 2017 Jul. 14;12(1):128. doi:10.1186/s13023-017-0677-2.

28. Kimura SJ, Hogan MJ. Chronic cyclitis. *Arch Ophthalmol.* 1964 Feb.;71:193–201. doi:10.1001/archopht.1964.00970010209011.

29. Paroli MP, Abicca I, Sapia A, et al. Intermediate uveitis: comparison between childhood-onset and adult-onset disease. *Eur J Ophthalmol.* 2014 Jan.–Feb.;24(1):94–100. doi:10.5301/ejo.5000336.

30. Giles CL. Pediatric intermediate uveitis. *J Pediatr Ophthalmol Strabismus.* 1989 May–June;26(3):136–139. doi:10.3928/0191-3913-19890501-10.

31. Tabbara KF, Chavis PS, Freeman WR. Vogt-Koyanagi-Harada syndrome in children compared to adults. *Acta Ophthalmol Scand.* 1998 Dec.;76(6):723–726. doi:10.1034/j.1600-0420.1998.760619.x.

32. Yang P, Liao W, Pu Y, et al. Vogt-Koyanagi-Harada disease in pediatric, adult and elderly: clinical characteristics and visual outcomes. *Graefes Arch Clin Exp Ophthalmol.* 2023 Sept.;261(9):2641–2650. doi:10.1007/s00417-023-06058-5.

33. Cabral DA, Canter DL, Muscal E, et al. Comparing presenting clinical features in 48 children with microscopic polyangiitis to 183 children who have granulomatosis with polyangiitis (Wegener's): an ARChiVe cohort study. *Arthritis Rheumatol.* 2016 Oct.;68(10):2514–2526. doi:10.1002/art.39729.

34. Tarsia M, Gaggiano C, Gessaroli E, et al. Pediatric scleritis: an update. *Ocul Immunol Inflamm.* 2023 Jan.;31(1):175–184. doi:10.1080/09273948.2021.2023582.
35. Junek ML, Zhao L, Garner S, et al. Ocular manifestations of ANCA-associated vasculitis. *Rheumatology (Oxford).* 2023 Jul. 5;62(7):2517–2524. doi:10.1093/rheumatology/keac663.
36. Durel CA, Hot A, Trefond L, et al. Orbital mass in ANCA-associated vasculitides: data on clinical, biological, radiological and histological presentation, therapeutic management, and outcome from 59 patients. *Rheumatology (Oxford).* 2019 Sept. 1;58(9):1565–1573. doi:10.1093/rheumatology/kez071.
37. Turk MA, Hayworth JL, Nevskaya T, et al. Ocular manifestations of Behçet's disease in children and adults: a systematic review and meta-analysis. *Clin Exp Rheumatol.* 2021 Sept.–Oct.;39((5) Suppl 132):94–101. doi:10.55563/clinexprheumatol/pt60bc.
38. Silpa-Archa S, Lee JJ, Foster CS. Ocular manifestations in systemic lupus erythematosus. *Br J Ophthalmol.* 2016 Jan.;100(1):135–141. doi:10.1136/bjophthalmol-2015-306629.
39. Maccora I, Marrani E, Mastrolia MV, et al. Ocular involvement in monogenic autoinflammatory disease. *Autoimmun Rev.* 2021 Nov.;20(11):102944. doi:10.1016/j.autrev.2021.102944.
40. Meyts I, Aksentijevich I. Deficiency of adenosine deaminase 2 (DADA2): updates on the phenotype, genetics, pathogenesis, and treatment. *J Clin Immunol.* 2018 Jul.;38(5):569–578. doi:10.1007/s10875-018-0525-8.
41. Chen Y, Ye Z, Chen L, et al. Association of clinical phenotypes in haploinsufficiency A20 (HA20) with disrupted domains of A20. *Front Immunol.* 2020 Sept. 23;11:574992. doi:10.3389/fimmu.2020.574992.
42. Liu A, Ying S. Aicardi-Goutières syndrome: a monogenic type I interferonopathy. *Scand J Immunol.* 2023 Oct.;98(4):e13314. doi:10.1111/sji.13314.
43. Volpi S, Picco P, Caorsi R, et al. Type I interferonopathies in pediatric rheumatology. *Pediatr Rheumatol Online J.* 2016 Jun 4;14(1):35. doi:10.1186/s12969-016-0094-4.
44. Marino A, Tirelli F, Giani T, et al. Periodic fever syndromes and the autoinflammatory diseases (AIDs). *J Transl Autoimmun.* 2019 Dec. 17;3:100031. doi:10.1016/j.jtauto.2019.100031.
45. Birnbaum AD, Jiang Y, Tessler HH, et al. Elevation of intraocular pressure in patients with uveitis treated with topical difluprednate. *Arch Ophthalmol.* 2011 May;129(5):667–668. doi:10.1001/archophthalmol.2011.82.
46. Taylor SR, Tomkins-Netzer O, Joshi L, et al. Dexamethasone implant in pediatric uveitis. *Ophthalmology.* 2012 Nov.;119(11):2412–2412.e2. doi:10.1016/j.ophtha.2012.07.025.
47. Tirelli F, Zannin ME, Vittadello F, et al. Methotrexate monotherapy in juvenile idiopathic arthritis associated uveitis: myth or reality? *Ocul Immunol Inflamm.* 2022 Oct.–Nov.;30(7–8):1763–1767. doi:10.1080/09273948.2021.1951303.
48. Henderson LA, Zurakowski D, Angeles-Han ST, et al. Medication use in juvenile uveitis patients enrolled in the Childhood Arthritis and Rheumatology Research Alliance Registry. *Pediatr Rheumatol Online J.* 2016;14(1):9. doi:10.1186/s12969-016-0069-5.
49. Maccora I, Land P, Miraldi Utz V, et al. Therapeutic potential of JAK inhibitors in juvenile idiopathic arthritis-associated uveitis. *Expert Rev Clin Immunol.* 2023 Jul.–Dec.;19(7):689–692. doi:10.1080/1744666X.2023.2207823.
50. Bots SJ, Parker CE, Brandse JF, et al. Anti-drug antibody formation against biologic agents in inflammatory bowel disease: a systematic review and meta-analysis. *BioDrugs.* 2021 Nov.;35(6):715–733. doi:10.1007/s40259-021-00507-5.
51. Petty RE, Laxer RM, Lindsley CB, et al. *Textbook of pediatric rheumatology,* 8th edn. Elsevier, 2020 [e-Book].
52. Dammacco R, Guerriero S, Alessio G, et al. Natural and iatrogenic ocular manifestations of rheumatoid arthritis: a systematic review. *Int Ophthalmol.* 2022 Feb.;42(2):689–711. doi:10.1007/s10792-021-02058-8.
53. Friedman DS, Holbrook JT, Ansari H, et al. Risk of elevated intraocular pressure and glaucoma in patients with uveitis: results of the multicenter uveitis steroid treatment trial. *Ophthalmology.* 2013 Aug.;120(8):1571–1579. doi:10.1016/j.ophtha.2013.01.025.

16 Ophthalmologic Side Effects of Rheumatologic Medications

Amy E. Pohodich, Justine Cheng, Akshay Thomas, and Christina Flaxel

16.1 INTRODUCTION

Rheumatic diseases are a group of disorders characterized by inflammation, typically affecting the joints, skin, and other connective tissues. These conditions encompass a wide range of autoimmune and inflammatory disorders, which are primarily managed with disease-modifying anti-rheumatic drugs and anti-inflammatory agents without an immunosuppressive effect. Though effective, several of these medications carry a risk of ocular side effects. This chapter highlights adverse ocular events associated with rheumatologic medications, offers insights into effective treatments and prognoses, and provides screening recommendations to enhance the care of these often-complex patients. It is crucial for healthcare providers, including rheumatologists and ophthalmologists, to be vigilant in monitoring patients for these potential ocular complications to enhance patient safety and optimize treatment outcomes.

16.2 DISCUSSION

16.2.1 General Considerations

Patients on immunomodulatory or immunosuppressive medications are at higher risk for opportunistic infections or reactivation of latent infections.[1] Prior to initiating biologic anti-rheumatic medications, providers should check for tuberculosis (TB), and, while not mandatory, current guidelines also recommend that patients be screened for TB prior to initiation of any corticosteroid, immunosuppressive, or disease-modifying drugs.[2] Similar to TB, other infectious diseases that can affect the eye in immunocompromised patients include cytomegalovirus (CMV), toxoplasmosis, herpes simplex virus (HSV), and varicella zoster virus (VZV). In many patients, ocular injury results from reactivation of latent infections in the setting of a weakened immune system rather than being a primary infection.[3–7] Ocular toxoplasmosis can present with floaters and blurry vision. In most immunocompetent patients with peripheral retinal involvement, no treatment is required, as disease is typically self-limited and resolves with formation of a chorioretinal scar at the site of infection.[8] With reactivation, new active lesions can be seen either adjacent to the old scar or at remote sites.[8] Given the presence of characteristic scarring, a dilated fundus exam at the time of immunosuppressive therapy initiation could help stratify risk for ocular toxoplasmosis. However, there are no formal recommendations for prophylactic treatment for inactive ocular toxoplasmosis.[8] CMV retinitis can also present with new onset blurred vision, flashes, and floaters, but nearly 50% of patients are asymptomatic.[3, 4, 7] Thus, it is important that immunocompromised patients receive annual eye exams even in the absence of ocular complaints, and consideration should be given to prophylactic antivirals for HSV in patients with known latent infection. Additionally, there should be a low threshold for referral to ophthalmology for patients with any vision changes on these medications.

16.2.2 Corticosteroids

While corticosteroids are strong immunosuppressants prescribed for a variety of systemic and ocular conditions, they have a long list of side effects.[9] In the eyes, they can cause ocular hypertension, cataract formation, delayed wound healing, and susceptibility to infections.[10–12] The latter two are seen elsewhere in the body, but in the eyes primarily manifest as reactivation of herpetic eye disease and persistent epithelial defects in patients with underlying neurotrophic corneal disease.[12, 13] The mechanism for ocular hypertension is thought secondary to remodeling of the trabecular meshwork, the drainage structure of the eye. Not all on corticosteroids will experience ocular hypertension – approximately a third will have a steroid response.[10] However, all patients who are on long-term corticosteroids will have cataract progression, most commonly a posterior subcapsular cataract, which forms as a result of glucocorticoid-protein adduct deposition in the lens.[11] It is important to note that these ocular effects become more pronounced as the route of administration gets closer to the eye. In other words, the effects of topical and periocular steroids are stronger than systemic steroids. Generally, we do not stop systemic corticosteroids unless there is a vision-threatening complication (e.g., uncontrolled intraocular pressure or acute retinal necrosis, a herpetic retinal infection). Most often, side effects of corticosteroids can be managed medically (e.g., topical anti-hypertensives, antiviral treatment, and prophylaxis) or surgically (cataract extraction).

DOI: 10.1201/9781003453710-16

16.2.3 Bisphosphonates

Bisphosphonates are prescribed to prevent bone resorption by preventing osteoclast function.[13] However, this class of medications is associated with a host of ocular side effects, ranging from mild conjunctivitis and acute anterior uveitis to more serious conditions like scleritis, optic neuritis, orbital inflammatory syndrome, and even idiopathic intracranial hypertension (IIH).[14, 15] The medication's propensity toward inducing ocular inflammation is thought to be from the activation of T cells and polarization of pro-inflammatory macrophages.[16] While the incidence for ocular inflammation is low (between 0.046% and 1.1%), and as a result, no formal ophthalmologic screening is indicated, those who have underlying rheumatologic conditions are at higher risk.[14, 17] Onset of symptoms is typically within 3 days of IV infusion but can be weeks after the start of oral administration. In some case reports, symptom onset can be months after initial challenge. The offending medication does not have to be stopped if the ocular symptoms can be managed with topical or systemic therapy. However, for severe adverse reactions, like IIH and severe panuveitis, the medication should be stopped promptly. For those who need to be on the medication, prophylactic corticosteroids and switching to a different agent are considerations, but there is no consensus amongst ophthalmologists about readministration of bisphosphonates.[18]

16.2.4 Non-Steroidal Anti-Inflammatory Drugs (NSAIDs)

Cases of tubulointerstitial nephritis and uveitis (TINU) syndrome have been attributed to the use of NSAIDs, with ibuprofen frequently reported.[19–21] Patients with acute interstitial nephritis often present with fever, weight loss, and fatigue, and the renal disease tends to precede ocular manifestations in most patients (65%).[19] Eye complaints vary from redness and pain to decreased vision, with specific symptoms dependent upon the location of intraocular involvement.[19, 20] The most common ophthalmic presentation is an acute bilateral anterior uveitis, but the wide spectrum of eye manifestations and variable timing between renal and ophthalmic involvement make diagnosis of this disease difficult.[19, 20] Definitive diagnosis does not necessarily require a renal biopsy, as a characteristic bilateral uveitis in the presence of elevated serum creatinine and urine beta-2 microglobulin are highly suggestive of TINU.[20] Given the temporal delay often seen between the kidney involvement and uveitis, patients with presumed NSAID-related tubulointerstitial nephritis should receive a baseline ophthalmologic exam at the time of diagnosis, with additional serial eye exams every 3 to 6 months for at least 1 year.[21] Treatment involves discontinuation of the offending drug, topical steroids for uveitis, and potentially systemic steroids for patients with severe or persistent renal or ocular disease.[19–21] Prognosis is generally good for both kidney and ocular function, but recurrences of uveitis are common.[19–21]

16.2.5 Tumor Necrosis Factor-Alpha (TNF-Alpha) Inhibitors

TNF-alpha inhibitors are used to treat a host of inflammatory conditions, including uveitis. However, these medications can infrequently cause a paradoxical inflammatory reaction. One of the most commonly reported ocular side effects is uveitis, with etanercept being the most frequently involved medication.[22] Etanercept, a soluble TNF receptor fusion protein, has also been implicated in rare cases of scleritis and ocular myositis.[23, 24] In addition to new-onset uveitis, adalimumab, a humanized monoclonal antibody against TNF-alpha, has been associated with recurrent immune corneal infiltrates after injections in one case report.[25] Infliximab is a mouse–human chimeric monoclonal antibody that has been associated with retinal vein thromboses and uveitis.[26–28] While optic neuritis has been reported with the use of TNF-alpha inhibitors, a safety analysis showed that rates of optic neuritis were not significantly different between patients receiving TNF-alpha inhibitors and patients on other disease-modifying therapies, suggesting no increased risk of optic neuritis with the use of TNF-alpha inhibitors.[29] Management of ocular adverse events depends on the type and severity of the presentation. It is important to rule out an infectious etiology for uveitis or scleritis. Some reports note an improvement in symptoms with discontinuation of the offending medication, and patients restarted on a TNF-alpha inhibitor after resolution of ocular inflammation should be monitored closely for recurrence.[22, 24]

16.2.6 Methotrexate

Methotrexate is a commonly prescribed disease-modifying antirheumatic drug (DMARD) that competitively inhibits dihydrofolate reductase, leading to disruption of DNA and RNA synthesis. Long-term use of methotrexate has also been associated with reduced serum folate levels.[30] Methotrexate has been linked to ocular surface disease, including burning, pruritis, and dry eye.[31]

Other rare side effects of methotrexate include macular dysfunction and optic neuropathy, and partial or complete recovery of vision has been reported with cessation of methotrexate therapy.[32-34] Methotrexate-induced optic neuropathy is thought to be related to folate deficiency, which can be an exacerbation of an underlying genetic disorder or through nutritional deficiency.[32] Given the potential reversible nature of vision loss, methotrexate should be discontinued immediately in patients reporting decreased vision, scotomas, or reduced color vision, with referral to ophthalmology for further workup before considering resumption. Additionally, patients receiving methotrexate should routinely use folate supplementation to limit methotrexate adverse effects.[30]

16.2.7 Hydroxychloroquine

Hydroxychloroquine (HCQ) has a well-documented side effect of retinal toxicity.[35] It is thought that HCQ binds melanin in the retinal pigment epithelium (RPE), which prevents macular cone function as well as inhibits lysosome activity within the RPE, causing accumulation of photoreceptor byproducts.[35-37] Late-stage HCQ toxicity is classically seen as a bulls-eye maculopathy on fundus exam. This is a descriptive term of pigmentary changes in a bulls-eye pattern, which correlates to outer retinal atrophy.[37] Patients will typically complain of central scotomas well before the pigmentary changes on exam. As such, it is important for all who will be started on the medication to have a baseline eye exam and to have periodic screenings. The American Academy of Ophthalmology has outlined screening protocols for patients on HCQ. Baseline exams are to assess for any underlying retinal conditions such as macular degeneration or other hereditary macular disease that would compromise retinal function or complicate retinal toxicity recognition. In patients without major risk factors for retinal toxicity and doses less than 5 mg/kg/day, yearly screening with automated visual fields to assess for scotomas, and an optical coherence tomography (OCT), an imaging modality of the macula, to assess for anatomic abnormalities should begin after 5 years of therapy (Figure 16.1). The retinal toxicity is dose dependent, and generally, toxicity will not manifest until

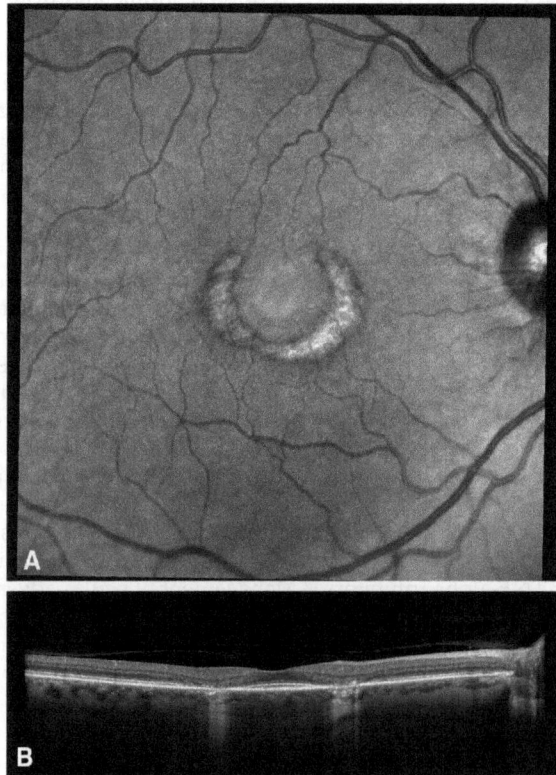

Figure 16.1 Hydroxychloroquine toxicity. (A) En face optical coherence tomography (OCT) image from a patient with hydroxychloroquine toxicity demonstrating the macular "bulls-eye" pattern. (B) OCT through bulls-eye shown in (A) that highlights the loss of the ellipsoid zone perifoveally, with sparing of the ellipsoid zone subfoveally.

Table 16.1 Noninfectious Ocular Side Effects of Common Rheumatologic Medications

Drug Name	Drug Class	Ocular Side Effects
Prednisone	Glucocorticoid	Steroid-induced ocular hypertension or glaucoma, cataracts, delayed wound healing, susceptibility to infections
Zoledronate (IV) Pamidronate (IV) Alendronate (oral) Risedronate (oral) Ibandronate (IV or oral)	Bisphosphonate	Conjunctivitis, scleritis, uveitis, optic neuritis, orbital inflammation, idiopathic intracranial hypertension
Ibuprofen	NSAID	TINU
Etanercept	TNF-α antagonist	Uveitis, scleritis, ocular myositis
Adalimumab	TNF-α antagonist	Uveitis, corneal infiltrates
Infliximab	TNF-α antagonist	Uveitis, retinal vein thrombosis
Methotrexate	Antimetabolite	Dry eye, macular dysfunction, optic neuropathy
Hydroxychloroquine	Antimalarial	Retinal toxicity

Abbreviations: NSAID: non-steroidal anti-inflammatory drug; TINU: tubulointerstitial nephritis and uveitis; TNF-α: tumor necrosis factor-alpha.

cumulative dose of HCQ is greater than 1 kilogram.[38, 39] However, those on daily doses greater than 5 mg/kg/day are also at risk. With treatment above the 5 mg/kg/day recommended dose, the risk of developing retinopathy in 20 years is 20%. Because retinal toxicity is not reversible, HCQ must be stopped if there are signs of early photoreceptor dysfunction. Importantly, even after discontinuation of the medication, photoreceptor damage can worsen for years to come.[39, 40]

16.3 SUMMARY

Many rheumatologic medications carry the risk of ocular side effects. It is crucial for healthcare providers, especially rheumatologists and ophthalmologists, to recognize the potential ocular complications associated with these medications. Patients prescribed rheumatologic medications should be informed about the possibility of ocular side effects and advised to report any visual disturbances or ocular complaints promptly. Establishing a collaborative relationship between rheumatologists and ophthalmologists is essential to ensure timely referrals and comprehensive eye examinations for patients on these medications. Early detection and management of ocular side effects are paramount in optimizing patient care and minimizing the risk of vision-related complications.

REFERENCES

1. Winthrop KL, Novosad SA, Baddley JW, et al. Opportunistic infections and biologic therapies in immune-mediated inflammatory diseases: consensus recommendations for infection reporting during clinical trials and postmarketing surveillance. *Ann Rheum Dis*. 2015;74(12):2107–2116.
2. Fragoulis GE, Nikiphorou E, Dey M, et al. 2022 EULAR recommendations for screening and prophylaxis of chronic and opportunistic infections in adults with autoimmune inflammatory rheumatic diseases. *Ann Rheum Dis*. 2023;82(6):742–753.
3. Downes KM, Tarasewicz D, Weisberg LJ, et al. Good syndrome and other causes of cytomegalovirus retinitis in HIV-negative patients-case report and comprehensive review of the literature. *J Ophthalmic Inflamm Infect*. 2016;6(1):3.
4. Munro M, Yadavalli T, Fonteh C, et al. Cytomegalovirus retinitis in HIV and non-HIV individuals. *Microorganisms*. 2019;8(1).
5. Puga M, Carpio D, Sampil M, et al. Ocular toxoplasmosis reactivation in a patient with inflammatory bowel disease under treatment with azathioprine. *J Clin Gastroenterol*. 2016;50(7):610.
6. Roux C, Breuil V, Albert C, et al. Ophthalmic herpes zoster infection in patients with rheumatoid arthritis who were treated with tocilizumab. *J Rheumatol*. 2011;38(2):399.
7. Rothova A, Hajjaj A, de Hoog J, et al. Uveitis causes according to immune status of patients. *Acta Ophthalmol*. 2019;97(1):53–59.
8. Kim SJ, Scott IU, Brown GC, et al. Interventions for toxoplasma retinochoroiditis: a report by the American academy of ophthalmology. *Ophthalmology*. 2013;120(2):371–378.
9. Schäcke H, Döcke WD, Asadullah K. Mechanisms involved in the side effects of glucocorticoids. *Pharmacol Ther*. 2002;96(1):23–43.

10. Roberti G, Oddone F, Agnifili L, et al. Steroid-induced glaucoma: epidemiology, pathophysiology, and clinical management. *Surv Ophthalmol.* 2020;65(4):458–472.
11. James ER. The etiology of steroid cataract. *J Ocul Pharmacol Ther.* 2007;23(5):403–420.
12. Gulkilik G, Demirci G, Ozdamar AM, et al. A case of herpetic keratitis after intravitreal triamcinolone injection. *Cornea.* 2007;26(8):1000–1001.
13. Ryu JS, Ko JH, Kim MK, et al. Prednisolone induces apoptosis in corneal epithelial cells through the intrinsic pathway. *Sci Rep.* 2017;7:4135.
14. Drake MT, Clarke BL, Khosla S. Bisphosphonates: mechanism of action and role in clinical practice. *Mayo Clinic Proc.* 2008;83(9):1032.
15. Chartrand NA, Lau CK, Parsons MT, et al. Ocular side effects of bisphosphonates: a review of literature. *J Ocul Pharmacol Ther.* 2023;39(1):3–16. doi:10.1089/jop.2022.0094.
16. Umunakwe OC, Herren D, Kim SJ, et al. Diffuse ocular and orbital inflammation after zoledronate infusion-case report and review of the literature. *Digit J Ophthalmol.* 2017;23(4):18–21.
17. Etminan M, Forooghian F, Maberley D. Inflammatory ocular adverse events with the use of oral bisphosphonates: a retrospective cohort study. *CMAJ* 2012;184(8):e431–e434.
18. Banal F, Briot K, Ayoub G, et al. Unilateral anterior uveitis complicating zoledronic acid therapy in prostate cancer. *J Rheumatol.* 2008;35(12):2458–2459.
19. Mandeville JT, Levinson RD, Holland GN. The tubulointerstitial nephritis and uveitis syndrome. *Surv Ophthalmol.* 2001;46(3):195–208.
20. Okafor LO, Hewins P, Murray PI, et al. Tubulointerstitial nephritis and uveitis (TINU) syndrome: a systematic review of its epidemiology, demographics and risk factors. *Orphanet J Rare Dis.* 2017;12(1):128.
21. Li C, Su T, Chu R, Li X, et al. Tubulointerstitial nephritis with uveitis in Chinese adults. *Clin J Am Soc Nephrol.* 2014;9(1):21–28.
22. Nicolela Susanna F, Pavesio C. A review of ocular adverse events of biological anti-TNF drugs. *J Ophthalmic Inflamm Infect.* 2020;10(1):11.
23. Caramaschi P, Biasi D, Carletto A, et al. Orbital myositis in a rheumatoid arthritis patient during etanercept treatment. *Clin Exp Rheumatol.* 2003;21(1):136–137.
24. Gaujoux-Viala C, Giampietro C, Gaujoux T, et al. Scleritis: a paradoxical effect of etanercept? Etanercept-associated inflammatory eye disease. *J Rheumatol.* 2012;39(2):233–239.
25. Matet A, Daruich A, Beydoun T, et al. Systemic adalimumab induces peripheral corneal infiltrates: a case report. *BMC Ophthalmol.* 2015;15:57.
26. Puli SR, Benage DD. Retinal vein thrombosis after infliximab (Remicade) treatment for Crohn's disease. *Am J Gastroenterol.* 2003;98(4):939–940.
27. Veerappan SG, Kennedy M, O'Morain CA, et al. Retinal vein thrombosis following infliximab treatment for severe left-sided ulcerative colitis. *Eur J Gastroenterol Hepatol.* 2008;20(6): 588–589.
28. Vergou T, Moustou AE, Maniateas A, et al. Central retinal vein occlusion following infliximab treatment for plaque-type psoriasis. *Int J Dermatol.* 2010;49(10):1215–1217.
29. Winthrop KL, Chen L, Fraunfelder FW, et al. Initiation of anti-TNF therapy and the risk of optic neuritis: from the safety assessment of biologic ThERapy (SABER) study. *Am J Ophthalmol.* 2013;155(1):183–189.e1.
30. Whittle SL, Hughes RA. Folate supplementation and methotrexate treatment in rheumatoid arthritis: a review. *Rheumatology (Oxford).* 2004;43(3):267–271.
31. Doroshow JH, Locker GY, Gaasterland DE, et al. Ocular irritation from high-dose methotrexate therapy: pharmacokinetics of drug in the tear film. *Cancer.* 1981;48(10):2158–2162.
32. Clare G, Colley S, Kennett R, et al. Reversible optic neuropathy associated with low-dose methotrexate therapy. *J Neuroophthalmol.* 2005;25(2):109–112.
33. Ponjavic V, Gränse L, Stigmar EB, et al. Reduced full-field electroretinogram (ERG) in a patient treated with methotrexate. *Acta Ophthalmol Scand.* 2004;82(1):96–99.
34. Sbeity ZH, Baydoun L, Schmidt S, et al. Visual field changes in methotrexate therapy: case report and review of the literature. *J Med Liban.* 2006;54(3):164–167.
35. Marmor MF, Kellner U, Lai TY, et al. Recommendations on screening for chloroquine and hydroxychloroquine retinopathy (2016 revision). *Ophthalmology.* 2016;123(6):1386–1394.
36. Browning DJ, Lee C. Somatotype, the risk of hydroxychloroquine retinopathy, and safe daily dosing guidelines. *Clin Ophthalmol.* 2018;12:811–818.
37. Melles RB, Marmor MF. The risk of toxic retinopathy in patients on long-term hydroxychloroquine therapy. *JAMA Ophthalmol.* 2014;132(12):1453–1460.

38. Kim JW, Kim YY, Lee H, et al. Risk of retinal toxicity in long-term users of hydroxychloroquine. *J Rheumatol*. 2017;44(11):1674–1679.
39. Marmor MF, Hu J. Effect of disease stage on progression of hydroxychloroquine retinopathy. *JAMA Ophthalmol*. 2014;132(9):1105–1112.
40. Yusuf I, Sharma S, Luqmani R, et al. Hydroxychloroquine retinopathy. *Eye* 2017;31:828–845.

17 Immunosuppressive Therapies for Inflammatory Ocular Disease

Sean T. Berkowitz and Sapna Gangaputra

Uveitis and other forms of ocular inflammation can require varying degrees of treatment to avoid potentially devastating and irreversible inflammatory sequela. Self-limited ocular inflammatory diseases may not require chronic treatment, while severe, recurrent, or chronic noninfectious ocular inflammation frequently requires escalation from topical, regional, and oral corticosteroids to corticosteroid-sparing agents: antimetabolites, T cell inhibitors, cytotoxic agents, and biologics including monoclonal antibodies.[1] The indications and rationale for immunomodulatory therapy (IMT) for ocular inflammation are complex and, if ophthalmologists are not comfortable, often managed in collaboration with rheumatology colleagues. Regardless, an understanding of indications and principles is critical for all clinicians managing ocular inflammation.

Most treatment paradigms utilize a stepladder approach: non-steroidal anti-inflammatory drugs when appropriate (scleritis, limited role in uveitis treatment), local and systemic corticosteroids, conventional immunomodulators, biologic agents, and cytotoxic agents in refractory cases. Surgical interventions (e.g., pars plana vitrectomy) are beyond the scope of the current text and are often reserved for extreme or recalcitrant cases.

The goal of treatment is "corticosteroid-free" remission using the least potent therapeutic with the best adverse event profile and, ultimately, "treatment-free" long-term quiescence.[2]

Corticosteroids are typically first-line management for many forms of uveitis and in many cases of scleral, corneal, and orbital inflammatory disease. Topical corticosteroids (prednisolone acetate 1%, difluprednate 0.05%) are very effective for anterior uveitis. Poor response, macular edema (ME), or intermediate, posterior, or panuveitis require periocular, intravitreal, or systemic corticosteroids to rapidly control ocular inflammation. The PeriOcular vs. INTravitreal (POINT) corticosteroids for uveitic macular edema trial found intravitreal approaches were superior for uveitic macular edema, though with increased rates of intraocular pressure elevation.[3] In terms of systemic approaches, typical corticosteroid regimens include prednisone doses of 1 mg/kg/day up to 60 mg/day tapered by 5 to 10 mg per week or intravenous methylprednisolone 1 gram pulse per day for 3 consecutive days followed by prednisone taper.[4] If there is no response or worsening after 2 to 4 weeks of high-dose oral steroids or flares occur at prednisone levels more than 10 mg per day, transition to steroid-sparing immunomodulatory therapy should be considered, typically with oral corticosteroid taper starting around 4 to 8 weeks after initiation.[4] While corticosteroid-free quiescence is the goal, clinical studies typically consider "corticosteroid-sparing" success as control of inflammation (inactive or trace inflammation) with less than 10 mg per day of oral prednisone or equivalent.

Disease location, severity, and etiology should be well defined for appropriate treatment escalation. There is evidence that certain disease states are considered an indication for early initiation of IMT. Behçet's has a well-established poor visual and overall prognosis despite corticosteroids,[5] classically managed with early chlorambucil,[6] cyclosporine,[7] azathioprine,[8] or more recently with anti-tumor necrosis factor (TNF) agents.[7] Birdshot chorioretinopathy is a chronic disease, frequently refractory to corticosteroids and needing early transition to IMT.[9] Diseases with high chronicity and poor visual prognosis such as multifocal choroiditis with panuveitis[10] or Vogt–Koyanagi–Harada (VKH)[11] may respond well to corticosteroid therapy, but IMT should be considered to avoid long-term side effects. Similarly, serpiginous choroidopathy classically demonstrates rapid progression and recurrence,[12] making IMT a reasonable consideration. In the pediatric population, juvenile idiopathic arthritis–associated uveitis (JIA) is associated with devastating inflammatory sequelae, and immunosuppression is well supported.[13] In addition to NIU, scleritis describes severe inflammation of the sclera, which is frequently associated with systemic rheumatologic disease including necrotizing vasculitis, which requires IMT. Likewise, mucous membrane pemphigoid can have devastating ocular consequences and requires escalation to IMT. In broad terms, more posterior disease with lasting visual impairment risk and development of ocular comorbidities (intraocular pressure rise due to steroid response, visual impairment due to uveitic macular edema, cataract progression from chronic corticosteroid use in a younger patient) will benefit from transition to IMT.

Evidence for the use of steroid-sparing immunomodulatory agents in the treatment of ocular inflammatory conditions comes from both randomized clinical trials and cohort studies. The Multicenter Uveitis Steroid Treatment (MUST) trial found local and systemic management to be efficacious for NIU;[14] however, local treatments or implants have variable pharmacokinetic and

DOI: 10.1201/9781003453710-17

pharmacodynamic properties, leading to risks of flare between treatments or for patients lost to follow-up and higher risk of cataract and glaucoma. Seven-year data from MUST showed systemic therapy had better visual acuity than intravitreal fluocinolone acetonide, likely due to the complexity of repeat dosing.[15] The Systemic Immunosuppressive Therapy for Eye Disease (SITE) cohort study was a landmark study composed of decades of tertiary uveitis referral clinical records, which established the safety (cancer incidence and cancer-associated mortality rate) and efficacy of many IMT commonly used for uveitides.[16] The evidence for use of various immunomodulatory therapeutic classes in ocular inflammatory conditions is reviewed later.

17.1 CONVENTIONAL IMMUNOSUPPRESSIVE AGENTS

17.1.1 Antimetabolites

Methotrexate (MTX) is a folate analog and inhibitor of dihydrofolate reductase. Dosage typically starts around 10 to 15 mg once weekly (up to maximum dose of 25 mg) either oral or subcutaneous to avoid gastrointestinal upset. Concurrent folate at 1 to 2 mg per day is recommended to prevent folate deficiency and help with nausea. Adverse side effects include stomatitis, hepatotoxicity, cytopenia, interstitial pneumonia, and GI disturbance. There is extensive history of MTX use in childhood rheumatic disease,[17] making MTX a mainstay for JIA-associated uveitis. Within the SITE cohort at 12 months, 66% of patients achieved sustained control with 58.4% corticosteroid sparing.[18] While effective for JIA, case series suggest long-term maintenance therapy is needed to prevent relapse.[19] Onset is expected after at least 6 to 8 weeks. Monitoring is described in Table 17.1.[2]

Mycophenolate mofetil (MMF) is a selective inhibitor of inosine monophosphate preventing guanosine synthesis. Oral dosage typically starts at 1 gram twice daily, with caution in those with GI comorbidities. Adverse effects noted in transplant trials include GI disturbance, cytopenia, potential malignancy, and opportunistic infection.[20] In the SITE cohort at 1 year, MMF achieved sustained control in 73% of a patients and corticosteroid sparing in 55%,[21] and in a separate cohort with higher dosage, corticosteroid sparing was achieved in 95% of posterior uveitis patients.[22] Onset is expected around 3 months. Monitoring is described in Table 17.1.[2]

In the First-Line Antimetabolite as Steroid-Sparing Treatment (FAST) uveitis trial, MMF did not result in superior control of inflammation when compared to MTX. Specifically, treatment success was achieved in 74.4% and 33.3% of posterior or panuveitis and intermediate uveitis patients managed with MTX, respectively, compared to 55.3% and 63.6% of posterior or panuveitis and intermediate uveitis patients managed with MMF.[23] MTX and MMF performed similarly with regard to uveitis macular edema, with frequent persistent UME at 12 months in each group of the FAST cohort.[24] Presentation-specific factors such as the presence of retinal vasculitis may be risk factors for failing both MMF and MTX.[25]

Azathioprine (AZA), a purine nucleoside analog, suppresses DNA replication and RNA transcription, which decreases the numbers and reactivity of T and B lymphocytes. AZA is typically dosed orally at 1 to 3 mg per kg per day, with dose adjustment in those with low thiopurine methyltransferase (TPMT) activity.[26] Severe side effects include bone marrow suppression (worsened by concomitant allopurinol), possible increased risk of malignant disease, and hepatotoxicity. It has been used for uveitis since the 1960s,[27, 28] and there is RCT trial evidence for efficacy for ocular and systemic manifestations of Behçet's.[8] In the SITE cohort, 62% achieved inactivity of inflammation with 47% achieving corticosteroid sparing at one year.[29] Onset is expected between 8 weeks and 3 months. Monitoring is described in Table 17.1.[2]

Leflunomide (LEF) is a non-biologic immunomodulatory medication that inhibits mitochondrial synthesis and cell cycle progression, reducing proliferation of lymphocytes. Dosage is typically 10 to 20 mg daily. Adverse effects include transaminitis, hypertension, gastrointestinal discomfort, pancytopenia, and interstitial lung disease. Early animal studies suggested higher potency of LEF compared to cyclosporin for S-antigen-induced autoimmune uveitis.[30] Human evidence primarily is case series level.[31] LEF showed worse control of JIA uveitis when compared to MTX,[32] though may be considered in patients intolerant to MTX.[33] Monitoring is described in Table 17.1.

17.1.2 T Cell Inhibitors

Cyclosporine A (CSA) is a natural peptide that inhibits immunocompetent T lymphocyte signaling and replication. Absorption is variable, and dosage typically ranges from 2 to 5 mg per kg per day divided equally twice daily. Higher doses are associated with nephrotoxicity, and it can also cause hypertension, hepatotoxicity, gingival hyperplasia, tremor, paresthesia, myalgias, electrolyte changes, and hirsutism. Randomized control trial evidence from the 1990s for severe uveitis showed

Table 17.1 Monitoring Immunosuppressive Therapies

Medication	Major Side Effects	Baseline Evaluations	Surveillance
Methotrexate (MTX)	Stomatitis, myelosuppression, GI distress, hepatotoxicity	Infectious testing, CBC & Diff, CMP (LFTs, BUN/Cr)	CBC & Diff, CMP every month for first 3 months, then q 3 months
Myocphenolate mofetil (MMF)	GI distress, infection, neutropenia	Infectious testing, CBC & Diff, CMP (LFTs, BUN/Cr)	CBC & Diff, CMP every month for first 3 months, then q 3 months
Azathioprine (AZA)	Myelosuppression, GI distress, hepatitis, pancreatitis, infection	Infectious testing, CBC & Diff, CMP (LFTs, BUN/Cr) TMPT Activity	CBC & Diff, CMP every month for first 3 months, then q 3 months
Leflunomide (LEF)	Diarrhea, neurologic side effects	Infectious testing, CBC & Diff, CMP (LFTs, BUN/Cr), BP	Monthly LFT for 6 months then every other month
Cyclosporine A (CSA)	Nephrotoxicity, hyperuricemia, hypercholesterolemia, hypertension, diabetes, neurotoxicity, gum hyperplasia	Infectious testing, CBC & Diff, CMP (LFTs, BUN/Cr) Cr clearance, fasting lipid profile, BP	CBC & Diff, CMP (LFTs, BUN/Cr), CSA trough level, BP, fasting lipid, Cr clearance 1–3 months
Tacrolimus	Nephrotoxicity, hypertension, diabetes, neurotoxicity, malignancy	Infectious testing, CBC & Diff, CMP (LFTs, BUN/Cr) Cr clearance, fasting lipid profile, BP	CBC & Diff, CMP (LFTs, BUN/Cr), trough level, BP, fasting lipid, Cr clearance 1–3 months
Chlorambucil	Myelosuppression, bone marrow aplasia, sterility, infections, malignancy	Infectious testing, CBC & Diff, CMP (LFTs, BUN/Cr)	CBC & Diff, CMP every 3 months
Cyclophosphamide	Hemorrhagic cystitis, myelosuppression, alopecia, infections, sterility, malignancy	Infectious testing, CBC & Diff, CMP (LFTs, BUN/Cr), UA	CBC & Diff, CMP (LFTs, BUN/Cr), UA every 4–8 weeks
Adalimumab	Sepsis, injection site infections, anaphylaxis, demyelination, drug-induced lupus, TB reactivation	Infectious testing, CBC & Diff, LFTs, TB testing, MRI if at risk	CBC & Diff, LFTs, every 3 months; annual TB testing and hepatitis B in at risk patients
Infliximab	TB reactivation, opportunistic infection, malignancy	Infectious testing, CBC & Diff, LFTs, ANA, TB testing	CBC & Diff, LFTs monthly; annual TB testing and hepatitis B in at risk patients
Tocilizumab	Infection, GI perforation, leucopenia	Infectious testing, CBC & Diff, LFTs, lipid profile, TB testing	CBC & Diff, LFT, lipid profile monthly

Abbreviations: CBC with Diff: complete blood count with differential, LFTs: liver function testing, BUN/Cr: serum blood urine nitrogen and creatine, UA: urinalysis, CMP: complete metabolic profile, BP: blood pressure.

* Some providers may prefer full chemistries in a CMP vs. just LFTs and BUN/Cr.

modest therapeutic efficacy relative to corticosteroids,[34] including in a pediatric population.[35] In the more recent SITE cohort, cyclosporine achieved sustained control in 51.9% of patients and corticosteroid sparing in 36.1% at 12 months, the lowest success rates of other single agents in the SITE cohort.[36] Onset is expected between 8 and 12 weeks. Monitoring is described in Table 17.1.[2]

Tacrolimus is an antibiotic produced by Streptomyces that inhibits T lymphocytes, which can be either intravenous or oral administration. Typical uveitis dosage may start with around 0.05 mg/kg/day. Case series in the 1990s showed reasonable evidence for efficacy in controlling intraocular inflammation.[37–39] Like cyclosporine, adverse events include nephrotoxicity, neurologic symptoms, hyperglycemia, hypertension, and paresthesia. Tacrolimus was infrequently prescribed in the SITE cohort, with a small study suggesting 85% probability of achieving corticosteroid sparing after 14 months of treatment.[40] Similar to cyclosporine, onset is expected between 8 and 12 weeks. Monitoring is described in Table 17.1.[2]

17.1.3 Cytotoxic Agents

Chlorambucil is an alkylating agent with a slow onset of activity. Early evidence suggests efficacy in Behçet's[41, 42] and induction of remission for sympathetic ophthalmia.[6] Dosage can range from 0.1 to 0.2 mg per kg per day to a short-term high-dose regimen of 2 mg daily for 1 week with escalation by 2 mg per day each week until inflammation is resolved or toxicity limits escalation. It has been shown to be effective for chronic NIU refractory to corticosteroid therapy;[28] however, there are numerous side effects such as sterility,[43] bone marrow suppression, opportunistic infections, and teratogenicity. There are significant concerns with alkylating agents for malignancy, and chlorambucil has been shown to increase the risk of malignancy.[44] Given these risks, usage is typically reserved for severe intractable disease in which short-term high-dose strategies are used to induce remission.[45] Onset is expected around 2 weeks. Monitoring is described in Table 17.1.[2]

Cyclophosphamide is an alkylating agent typically used for chemotherapy that has been used for uveitis since the 1950s.[46] Oral dosage typically starts around 1 to 2 mg per kg per day, and intravenous dosing is based on body surface area. More common and serious adverse side effects include hemorrhagic cystitis, myelosuppression, and gastrointestinal intolerance. Cyclophosphamide has classically been used for granulomatosis with polyangiitis and other rheumatologic conditions with ocular sequela, with limited evidence from small case series for uveitides.[47] However, there was stronger evidence in the SITE cohort, and at 12 months, 76% of patients achieved sustained control, with corticosteroid sparing in 61.2%.[48] For MMP, 91% of patients achieved drug-free remission at 2 years,[49] with similar results for serpiginous choroiditis.[50] Onset is expected around 2 weeks. Monitoring is described in Table 17.1.[2]

Alkylating agents such as chlorambucil and cyclophosphamide are typically used to induce remission, with a goal of short duration of therapy, ideally less than 24 months. While justifiable for severe disease such as necrotizing scleritis from systemic vasculitides, classically, there is concern for increased malignancy with these agents.[51] In 1995, the Systemic Immunosuppressive Therapy for Eye Disease (SITE) trial found no statistically significant increased risk of malignancy for immunomodulatory therapy (IMT) compared to systemic corticosteroids for ocular inflammatory disease.[52] Recent long-term follow-up corroborates prior evidence that antimetabolites and TNF inhibitors are not clearly associated with increased cancer mortality in the uveitis patient population.[53]

17.2 BIOLOGIC AGENTS

17.2.1 Tumor Necrosis Factor (TNF) Inhibitors

Adalimumab is a humanized monoclonal antibody to TNF-alpha. It is typically delivered via subcutaneous injection of 40 mg every 2 weeks. Adverse reactions include susceptibility to infections (mycobacterial, bacterial, viral, and fungal), rash, drug-induced lupus, thrombosis, demyelinating disease, congestive heart failure, transaminitis, and malignancy. An expert panel in 2014 recommended adalimumab as first-line therapy for Behçet's and second-line for JIA or other severe uveitidies.[54] Adalimumab was approved for NIU based on safety and efficacy data from two RCTs,[55, 56] with an extension study cohort showing reasonable safety data and increase in quiescence from 34% at entry to 85% by week 150.[57] In a JIA cohort on MTX, adjuvant adalimumab was associated with more effective inflammation control but higher adverse events.[58] Onset is expected around 1 to 2 weeks. Monitoring is described in Table 17.1.[2]

Infliximab is a chimeric monoclonal antibody to TNF-alpha. Dosage is typically via intravenous infusion of 5 to 20 mg per kg for three monthly infusions followed by maintenance every 2 months. In addition to infectious risk and common TNF-alpha risks mentioned already, there is a risk for development of anti-infliximab antibodies and subsequent infusion reaction.[59] Small case series for birdshot chorioretinopathy showed 88.9% of patients on infliximab achieved inflammation control at 1 year.[60] An expert panel in 2014 recommended infliximab as first-line therapy for Behçet's and second-line for JIA or other severe uveitidies.[54] Case series evidence showed 75% of patients with recalcitrant uveitis achieved remission off all corticosteroids[61] across a wide variety of NIU etiologies.[61] Infliximab has successfully treated pediatric NIU recalcitrant to adalimumab therapy.[62] Onset is expected around 1 to 2 weeks. Monitoring is described in Table 17.1.[2]

Anti-drug antibodies (ADA) can develop between 2 weeks and several years after initiation in roughly 12.7% of patients on TNFi (25.3% for infliximab, 14.1% for adalimumab), with reduction in odds of ADA formation by 74% when used with concomitant low-dose antimetabolite.[63] In the NIU population, adalimumab antibodies were found in 35.7% of patients (with no anti-infliximab antibodies attributed to small sample size); however, concomitant use of IMT was associated with lower rates of ADA formation and thus increased TNFi concentrations.[64] Immunogenicity is one factor related to monoclonal antibody clearance,[65] and more frequent weekly dosing of monoclonal antibodies is believed to lead to less ADA formation.[64] Pharmacokinetics may explain why increasing adalimumab dosage to weekly has been shown effective for refractory uveitis,[66] though it may not completely address refractory macular edema.[67] There is no standard drug level for therapeutic monitoring for NIU, though monitoring may be beneficial to support dosage or agent selection.[68] Fortunately, these biologics are believed to be interchangeable with limited case series evidence for NIU.[69, 70]

Infliximab and adalimumab are the most well-studied biologics, with more limited evidence for golimumab[71] and certolizumab.[72] Etanercept is thought less efficacious for intraocular inflammation than the other anti-TNF agents.[73]

17.3 INTERLEUKIN-6 INHIBITORS

Tocilizumab is a humanized monoclonal antibody that inhibits IL-6. Dosage is typically in the range of 4 to 8 mg/kg as a monthly infusion or 162 mg subcutaneously every 1 to 2 weeks, with similar risks to anti-TNF alpha inhibitors.[2] Tocilizumab (TCZ) has shown promising efficacy in a variety of uveitides in small case series as well as in 6-month outcomes from an RCT for NIU,[74] and some believe the effects are best captured through composite endpoint outcomes.[75] TCZ failed to reach the primary endpoint for JIA in the phase 2 APTITUDE trial,[76] but more frequent weekly subcutaneous dosing has been reported to be more successful in recalcitrant JIA in smaller case series.[77] Similarly, there is small case series support for TCZ for noninfectious retinal vasculitis,[78] Behçet's disease,[79] refractory pars planitis,[80] and MS-associated uveitis.[81] In a French multicenter study of uveitic ME refractory to steroids, tocilizumab showed promising improvement in complete response of uveitic ME compared to infliximab and adalimumab.[82] Onset can be as early as 1 to 2 months. Monitoring is described in Table 17.1.[2]

Sarilumab is a human anti-IL-6 receptor antibody that targets the alpha subunit to block IL-6 signaling cascade. Sarilumab is dosed as 200 mg subcutaneously every 2 weeks. Sarilumab has shown promising phase 2 RCT results from the SATURN trial for NIU and uveitic macular edema;[83] however, there is less data on the use of sarilumab in uveitis than tocilizumab. Like TCZ, sarilumab is believed to be efficacious for recalcitrant macular edema. IL-6 is believed to induce the production of vascular endothelial growth factor (VEGF), which is a well-established mediator of macular edema through retinal vascular leakage.[84] There are case reports of efficacy in rare cases such as recalcitrant CME in non-paraneoplastic autoimmune retinopathy.[85]

17.4 OTHER BIOLOGICS

Gevokizumab (anti-IL-1β)[86] appears ineffective for intraocular inflammation; however, there are myriad targets under active investigation. In addition to anti-TNF-alpha, there are several biologics which have been used to treat uveitis: anakinra (anti-IL-1R), canakinumab (anti-IL-1beta), daclizumab (anti-IL2 receptor/CD25), secukinumab (anti-IL-17A), ustekinumab (anti-IL-12/23), rituximab (anti-CD20), abatacept (T cell costimulator modulator), interferon alpha-2a/alpha-2b/beta, tofacitinib (Janus kinase inhibitor), and baricitinib (Janus kinase inhibitor).[87]

Anakinra and canakinumab have shown efficacy in Behçet's,[88, 89] HLA-B27 and MS-related uveitis,[90] and JIA.[91] Daclizumab showed some efficacy in reduction of other immunosuppressive agents in chronic NIU.[92] In a phase 2 RCT, secukinumab was well tolerated and effective when delivered by IV but not subcutaneous routes.[93] Ustekinumab has been reported successful in case series of psoriasis-associated uveitis,[94] with forthcoming phase 2 clinical trials.[95] Rituximab has shown mixed results across various uveitides,[96] including an RCT for Behçet's,[97] case series reports including JIA,[98] and pediatric VKH.[99] There have been mixed results for efficacy of abatacept for JIA.[100–102] Interferon-alpha-2 showed promising efficacy for Behçet's[103, 104] and uveitic macular edema,[105–107] with additional evidence for the less immunogenic interferon-alpha-2b.[108] There is mixed evidence for interferon beta.[109, 110] Limited case series data suggest efficacy of JAK inhibitors for JIA,[111, 112] which is under active clinical trial investigation with an open-label Bayesian trial for baricitinib.[113] A phase 3 randomized control trial of brepocitinib in intermediate, posterior, and panuveitis is also being conducted.

17.5 SUMMARY

In general, SITE and associated recent studies have provided some comparative efficacy data; however, there is a lack of large-cohort, robust comparative efficacy studies comparing biologics and other immunosuppressive agents for noninfectious uveitis. There is an emerging role for intravitreal immunosuppressive medication for inflammatory conditions, malignancy, and aberrant cellular proliferation (proliferative vitreoretinopathy, PVR) that is beyond the scope of the current text and under active investigation.[114] With the emergence of myriad biologics, the therapeutic landscape is shifting, and there is a potential for new robust treatment approaches to upend the classic step-wise approach. In the interim, conventional principles, early diagnosis, and aggressive control of inflammation can help prevent morbidity and mortality of treatable ocular inflammation. Close collaboration between ophthalmologists, subspecialty uveitis experts, and expert rheumatologists will facilitate optimal care for our patients.

REFERENCES

1. Jabs DA. Immunosuppression for the uveitides. *Ophthalmology*. 2018;125(2):193–202.
2. Foster CS, Kothari S, Anesi SD, et al. The Ocular Immunology and Uveitis Foundation preferred practice patterns of uveitis management. *Surv Ophthalmol*. 2016;61(1):1–17.
3. Thorne JE, Sugar EA, Holbrook JT, et al. Periocular triamcinolone vs. intravitreal triamcinolone vs. intravitreal dexamethasone implant for the treatment of uveitic macular edema: the PeriOcular vs. INTravitreal corticosteroids for uveitic macular edema (POINT) Trial. *Ophthalmology*. 2019;126(2):283–295.
4. Jabs DA, Rosenbaum JT, Foster CS, et al. Guidelines for the use of immunosuppressive drugs in patients with ocular inflammatory disorders: recommendations of an expert panel. *Am J Ophthalmol*. 2000;130(4):492–513.
5. Kitaichi N, Miyazaki A, Iwata D, et al. Ocular features of Behçet's disease: an international collaborative study. *Br J Ophthalmol*. 2007;91(12):1579–1582.
6. Tessler HH, Jennings T. High-dose short-term chlorambucil for intractable sympathetic ophthalmia and Behçet's disease. *Br J Ophthalmol*. 1990;74(6):353–357.
7. Masuda K, Nakajima A, Urayama A, et al. Double-masked trial of cyclosporin versus colchicine and long-term open study of cyclosporin in Behçet's disease. *Lancet*. 1989;1(8647):1093–1096.
8. Yazici H, Pazarli H, Barnes CG, et al. A controlled trial of azathioprine in Behçet's syndrome. *N Engl J Med*. 1990;322(5):281–285.
9. Vitale AT, Rodriguez A, Foster CS. Low-dose cyclosporine therapy in the treatment of birdshot retinochoroidopathy. *Ophthalmology*. 1994;101(5):822–831.
10. Dreyer RF, Gass DJ. Multifocal choroiditis and panuveitis: a syndrome that mimics ocular histoplasmosis. *Arch Ophthalmol*. 1984;102(12):1776–1784.
11. Bykhovskaya I, Thorne JE, Kempen JH, et al. Vogt-Koyanagi-Harada disease: clinical outcomes. *Am J Ophthalmol*. 2005;140(4):674–678.
12. Weiss H, Annesley WH, Jr., Shields JA, et al. The clinical course of serpiginous choroidopathy. *Am J Ophthalmol*. 1979;87(2):133–142.
13. Gregory AC, II, Kempen JH, Daniel E, et al. Risk factors for loss of visual acuity among patients with uveitis associated with juvenile idiopathic arthritis: the systemic immunosuppressive therapy for eye diseases study. *Ophthalmology*. 2013;120(1):186–192.
14. Multicenter Uveitis Steroid Treatment Trial Research Group, Kempen JH, Altaweel MM, et al. Randomized comparison of systemic anti-inflammatory therapy versus fluocinolone acetonide implant for intermediate, posterior, and panuveitis: the multicenter uveitis steroid treatment trial. *Ophthalmology*. 2011;118(10):1916–1926.
15. Writing Committee for the Multicenter Uveitis Steroid Treatment T, Follow-Up Study Research Group, Kempen JH, et al. Association between long-lasting intravitreous fluocinolone acetonide implant vs systemic anti-inflammatory therapy and visual acuity at 7 years among patients with intermediate, posterior, or panuveitis. *JAMA*. 2017;317(19):1993–2005.
16. Kempen JH, Daniel E, Dunn JP, et al. Overall and cancer related mortality among patients with ocular inflammation treated with immunosuppressive drugs: retrospective cohort study. *BMJ*. 2009;339:b2480.
17. Wallace CA. The use of methotrexate in childhood rheumatic diseases. *Arthritis Rheum*. 1998;41(3):381–391.
18. Gangaputra S, Newcomb CW, Liesegang TL, et al. Methotrexate for ocular inflammatory diseases. *Ophthalmology*. 2009;116(11):2188–2198.e2181.
19. Kalinina Ayuso V, van de Winkel EL, Rothova A, et al. Relapse rate of uveitis post-methotrexate treatment in juvenile idiopathic arthritis. *Am J Ophthalmol*. 2011;151(2):217–222.
20. Kilmartin DJ, Forrester JV, Dick AD. Rescue therapy with mycophenolate mofetil in refractory uveitis. *Lancet*. 1998;352(9121):35–36.
21. Daniel E, Thorne JE, Newcomb CW, et al. Mycophenolate mofetil for ocular inflammation. *Am J Ophthalmol*. 2010;149(3):423–432.e421–422.

22. Goldberg NR, Lyu T, Moshier E, et al. Success with single-agent immunosuppression for multifocal choroidopathies. *Am J Ophthalmol*. 2014;158(6):1310–1317.

23. Rathinam SR, Gonzales JA, Thundikandy R, et al. Effect of corticosteroid-sparing treatment with mycophenolate mofetil vs methotrexate on inflammation in patients with uveitis: a randomized clinical trial. *JAMA*. 2019;322(10):936–945.

24. Tsui E, Rathinam SR, Gonzales JA, et al. Outcomes of uveitic macular edema in the first-line antimetabolites as steroid-sparing treatment uveitis trial. *Ophthalmology*. 2022;129(6): 661–667.

25. Reddy AK, Miller DC, Sura AA, et al. Risk of failing both methotrexate and mycophenolate mofetil from the first-line antimetabolites as steroid-sparing treatment (FAST) uveitis trial. *J Ophthalmic Inflamm Infect*. 2023;13(1):29.

26. Dean L. Azathioprine therapy and TPMT and NUDT15 genotype. In: Pratt VM, Scott SA, Pirmohamed M, et al., eds, *Medical genetics summaries*. Bethesda, MD: National Center for Biotechnical Information, 2012.

27. Newell FW, Krill AE. Treatment of uveitis with azathioprine (Imuran). *Trans Ophthalmol Soc UK (1962)*. 1967;87:499–511.

28. Andrasch RH, Pirofsky B, Burns RP. Immunosuppressive therapy for severe chronic uveitis. *Arch Ophthalmol*. 1978;96(2):247–251.

29. Pasadhika S, Kempen JH, Newcomb CW, et al. Azathioprine for ocular inflammatory diseases. *Am J Ophthalmol*. 2009;148(4):500–509.e502.

30. Robertson SM, Lang LS. Leflunomide: inhibition of S-antigen induced autoimmune uveitis in Lewis rats. *Agents Actions*. 1994;42(3–4):167–172.

31. Steigerwalt RD, Jr., Bacci S, Valesini G. Severe uveitis successfully treated with leflunomide. *Retin Cases Brief Rep*. 2007;1(1):54–55.

32. Bichler J, Benseler SM, Krumrey-Langkammerer M, et al. Leflunomide is associated with a higher flare rate compared to methotrexate in the treatment of chronic uveitis in juvenile idiopathic arthritis. *Scand J Rheumatol*. 2015;44(4):280–283.

33. Garg N, Cohen E, Tsui E, et al. The effect of leflunomide as adjunctive therapy with a TNF inhibitor in pediatric patients with uveitis. *J Pediatr Ophthalmol Strabismus*. 2022:1–4.

34. Nussenblatt RB, Palestine AG, Chan CC, et al. Randomized, double-masked study of cyclosporine compared to prednisolone in the treatment of endogenous uveitis. *Am J Ophthalmol*. 1991;112(2):138–146.

35. Walton RC, Nussenblatt RB, Whitcup SM. Cyclosporine therapy for severe sight-threatening uveitis in children and adolescents. *Ophthalmology*. 1998;105(11):2028–2034.

36. Kacmaz RO, Kempen JH, Newcomb C, et al. Cyclosporine for ocular inflammatory diseases. *Ophthalmology*. 2010;117(3):576–584.

37. Mochizuki M, Masuda K, Sakane T, et al. A clinical trial of FK506 in refractory uveitis. *Am J Ophthalmol*. 1993;115(6):763–769.

38. Ishioka M, Ohno S, Nakamura S, et al. FK506 treatment of noninfectious uveitis. *Am J Ophthalmol*. 1994;118(6):723–729.

39. Kilmartin DJ, Forrester JV, Dick AD. Tacrolimus (FK506) in failed cyclosporin A therapy in endogenous posterior uveitis. *Ocul Immunol Inflamm*. 1998;6(2):101–109.

40. Hogan AC, McAvoy CE, Dick AD, et al. Long-term efficacy and tolerance of tacrolimus for the treatment of uveitis. *Ophthalmology*. 2007;114(5):1000–1006.

41. Mamo JG, Azzam SA. Treatment of Behçet's disease with chlorambucil. *Arch Ophthalmol*. 1970;84(4):446–450.

42. Abdalla MI, el-D Bahoat N. Long-lasting remission of Behçet's disease after chlorambucil therapy. *Br J Ophthalmol*. 1973;57(9):706–711.

43. Tabbara KF. Chlorambucil in Behçet's disease: a reappraisal. *Ophthalmology*. 1983;90(8):906–908.

44. Berk PD, Goldberg JD, Silverstein MN, et al. Increased incidence of acute leukemia in polycythemia vera associated with chlorambucil therapy. *N Engl J Med*. 1981;304(8):441–447.

45. Goldstein DA, Fontanilla FA, Kaul S, et al. Long-term follow-up of patients treated with short-term high-dose chlorambucil for sight-threatening ocular inflammation. *Ophthalmology*. 2002;109(2):370–377.

46. Roda Perez E. Nitrogen mustard therapy of uveitis of unknown etiology. *Rev Clin Esp*. 1952;44(3):173–180.

47. Rosenbaum JT. Treatment of severe refractory uveitis with intravenous cyclophosphamide. *J Rheumatol*. 1994;21(1):123–125.

48. Pujari SS, Kempen JH, Newcomb CW, et al. Cyclophosphamide for ocular inflammatory diseases. *Ophthalmology*. 2010;117(2):356–365.

49. Thorne JE, Woreta FA, Jabs DA, et al. Treatment of ocular mucous membrane pemphigoid with immunosuppressive drug therapy. *Ophthalmology*. 2008;115(12):2146–2152.e2141.

50. Akpek EK, Jabs DA, Tessler HH, et al. Successful treatment of serpiginous choroiditis with alkylating agents. *Ophthalmology*. 2002;109(8):1506–1513.

51. Kempen JH, Gangaputra S, Daniel E, et al. Long-term risk of malignancy among patients treated with immunosuppressive agents for ocular inflammation: a critical assessment of the evidence. *Am J Ophthalmol*. 2008;146(6):802–812.e801.

52. Lane L, Tamesis R, Rodriguez A, et al. Systemic immunosuppressive therapy and the occurrence of malignancy in patients with ocular inflammatory disease. *Ophthalmology*. 1995;102(10):1530–1535.

53. Kempen JH, Newcomb CW, Washington TL, et al. Use of immunosuppression and the risk of subsequent overall or cancer mortality. *Ophthalmology*. 2023;130(12):1258–1268.

54. Levy-Clarke G, Jabs DA, Read RW, Rosenbaum JT, Vitale A, Van Gelder RN. Expert panel recommendations for the use of anti-tumor necrosis factor biologic agents in patients with ocular inflammatory disorders. *Ophthalmology*. 2014;121(3):785–796.e783.

55. Jaffe GJ, Dick AD, Brezin AP, et al. Adalimumab in patients with active noninfectious uveitis. *N Engl J Med*. 2016;375(10):932–943.

56. Nguyen QD, Merrill PT, Jaffe GJ, et al. Adalimumab for prevention of uveitic flare in patients with inactive non-infectious uveitis controlled by corticosteroids (VISUAL II): a multicentre, double-masked, randomised, placebo-controlled phase 3 trial. *Lancet*. 2016;388(10050):1183–1192.

57. Suhler EB, Jaffe GJ, Fortin E, et al. Long-term safety and efficacy of adalimumab in patients with noninfectious intermediate uveitis, posterior uveitis, or panuveitis. *Ophthalmology*. 2021;128(6):899–909.

58. Ramanan AV, Dick AD, Jones AP, et al. Adalimumab plus methotrexate for uveitis in juvenile idiopathic arthritis. *N Engl J Med*. 2017;376(17):1637–1646.

59. Baert F, Noman M, Vermeire S, et al. Influence of immunogenicity on the long-term efficacy of infliximab in Crohn's disease. *N Engl J Med*. 2003;348(7):601–608.

60. Artornsombudh P, Gevorgyan O, Payal A, et al. Infliximab treatment of patients with birdshot retinochoroidopathy. *Ophthalmology*. 2013;120(3):588–592.

61. Kruh JN, Yang P, Suelves AM, Foster CS. Infliximab for the treatment of refractory noninfectious uveitis: a study of 88 patients with long-term follow-up. *Ophthalmology*. 2014;121(1):358–364.

62. Ashkenazy N, Saboo US, Abraham A, et al. Successful treatment with infliximab after adalimumab failure in pediatric noninfectious uveitis. *J AAPOS*. 2019;23(3):e151–e155.

63. Thomas SS, Borazan N, Barroso N, et al. Comparative immunogenicity of TNF inhibitors: impact on clinical efficacy and tolerability in the management of autoimmune diseases. A systematic review and meta-analysis. *BioDrugs*. 2015;29(4):241–258.

64. Bellur S, McHarg M, Kongwattananon W, et al. Antidrug antibodies to tumor necrosis factor alpha inhibitors in patients with noninfectious uveitis. *JAMA Ophthalmol*. 2023;141(2):150–156.

65. Ordas I, Mould DR, Feagan BG, et al. Anti-TNF monoclonal antibodies in inflammatory bowel disease: pharmacokinetics-based dosing paradigms. *Clin Pharmacol Ther*. 2012;91(4):635–646.

66. Roberts JE, Nigrovic PA, Lo MS, Chang MH. Weekly adalimumab, an effective alternative for refractory uveitis in children. *J Clin Rheumatol*. 2022;28(1):e301–e304.

67. Liberman P, Berkenstock MK, Burkholder BM, et al. Escalation to weekly adalimumab for the treatment of ocular inflammation. *Ocul Immunol Inflamm*. 2021;29(7–8):1564–1568.

68. Sejournet L, Kerever S, Mathis T, et al. Therapeutic drug monitoring guides the management of patients with chronic non-infectious uveitis treated with adalimumab: a retrospective study. *Br J Ophthalmol*. 2022;106(10):1380–1386.

69. Dhingra N, Morgan J, Dick AD. Switching biologic agents for uveitis. *Eye (London)*. 2009;23(9):1868–1870.

70. Simonini G, Katie D, Cimaz R, et al. Does switching anti-TNFalpha biologic agents represent an effective option in childhood chronic uveitis: the evidence from a systematic review and meta-analysis approach. *Semin Arthritis Rheum*. 2014;44(1):39–46.

71. Cordero-Coma M, Salom D, Diaz-Llopis M, et al. Golimumab for uveitis. *Ophthalmology*. 2011;118(9):1892, e1893–e1894.

72. Tosi GM, Sota J, Vitale A, et al. Efficacy and safety of certolizumab pegol and golimumab in the treatment of non-infectious uveitis. *Clin Exp Rheumatol*. 2019;37(4):680–683.

73. Wendling D, Joshi A, Reilly P, et al. Comparing the risk of developing uveitis in patients initiating anti-tumor necrosis factor therapy for ankylosing spondylitis: an analysis of a large US claims database. *Curr Med Res Opin.* 2014;30(12):2515–2521.

74. Sepah YJ, Sadiq MA, Chu DS, et al. Primary (month-6) outcomes of the STOP-uveitis study: evaluating the safety, tolerability, and efficacy of tocilizumab in patients with noninfectious uveitis. *Am J Ophthalmol.* 2017;183:71–80.

75. Hassan M, Sadiq MA, Ormaechea MS, et al. Utilisation of composite endpoint outcome to assess efficacy of tocilizumab for non-infectious uveitis in the STOP-uveitis study. *Br J Ophthalmol.* 2023;107(8):1197–1201.

76. Ramanan AV, Dick AD, Guly C, et al. Tocilizumab in patients with anti-TNF refractory juvenile idiopathic arthritis-associated uveitis (APTITUDE): a multicentre, single-arm, phase 2 trial. *Lancet Rheumatol.* 2020;2(3):e135–e141.

77. Marino A, Marelli L, Nucci P, Caporali R, Miserocchi E. Subcutaneous tocilizumab in juvenile idiopathic arthritis associated uveitis. *Ocul Immunol Inflamm.* 2023;31(10):1997–2000.

78. Karaca I, Uludag G, Matsumiya W, et al. Six-month outcomes of infliximab and tocilizumab therapy in non-infectious retinal vasculitis. *Eye (Lond).* 2023;37(11):2197–2203.

79. Khitri MY, Bartoli A, Maalouf G, et al. Tocilizumab in Behçet disease: a multicenter study of 30 patients. *J Rheumatol.* 2023;50(7):916–923.

80. Kongrat L, Maleki A, Rujkorakarn P, et al. Outcomes of intravenous tocilizumab treatment for refractory pars planitis. *Ocul Immunol Inflamm.* 2024:1–6.

81. Gil W, Lagrib H, Olagne L, et al. Multiple sclerosis-associated uveitis: a case report of refractory bilateral chronic granulomatous panuveitis successfully treated with tocilizumab. *Ocul Immunol Inflamm.* 2024:1–4.

82. Leclercq M, Andrillon A, Maalouf G, et al. Anti-tumor necrosis factor alpha versus tocilizumab in the treatment of refractory uveitic macular edema: a multicenter study from the French uveitis network. *Ophthalmology.* 2022;129(5):520–529.

83. Heissigerova J, Callanan D, de Smet MD, et al. Efficacy and safety of sarilumab for the treatment of posterior segment noninfectious uveitis (SARIL-NIU): the phase 2 SATURN study. *Ophthalmology.* 2019;126(3):428–437.

84. Yang JY, Goldberg D, Sobrin L. Interleukin-6 and macular edema: a review of outcomes with inhibition. *Int J Mol Sci.* 2023;24(5).

85. Grewal DS, Jaffe GJ, Keenan RT. Sarilumab for recalcitrant cystoid macular edema in non-paraneoplastic autoimmune retinopathy. *Retin Cases Brief Rep.* 2021;15(5):504–508.

86. Tugal-Tutkun I, Pavesio C, De Cordoue A, et al. Use of gevokizumab in patients with Behçet's disease uveitis: an international, randomized, double-masked, placebo-controlled study and open-label extension study. *Ocul Immunol Inflamm.* 2018;26(7):1023–1033.

87. Ferreira LB, Smith AJ, Smith JR. Biologic drugs for the treatment of noninfectious uveitis. *Asia Pac J Ophthalmol (Phila).* 2021;10(1):63–73.

88. Fabiani C, Vitale A, Emmi G, et al. Interleukin (IL)-1 inhibition with anakinra and canakinumab in Behçet's disease-related uveitis: a multicenter retrospective observational study. *Clin Rheumatol.* 2017;36(1):191–197.

89. Fabiani C, Vitale A, Rigante D, et al. The presence of uveitis is associated with a sustained response to the interleukin (IL)-1 inhibitors anakinra and canakinumab in Behçet's disease. *Ocul Immunol Inflamm.* 2020;28(2):298–304.

90. Lopalco G, Schiraldi S, Venerito V, et al. Effectiveness and safety profile of anakinra in a HLA-B27 positive patient with multiple sclerosis-associated uveitis. *Mult Scler Relat Disord.* 2020;42:102152.

91. Brambilla A, Caputo R, Cimaz R, et al. Canakinumab for childhood sight-threatening refractory uveitis: a case series. *J Rheumatol.* 2016;43(7):1445–1447.

92. Wroblewski K, Sen HN, Yeh S, et al. Long-term daclizumab therapy for the treatment of non-infectious ocular inflammatory disease. *Can J Ophthalmol.* 2011;46(4):322–328.

93. Letko E, Yeh S, Foster CS, et al. Efficacy and safety of intravenous secukinumab in noninfectious uveitis requiring steroid-sparing immunosuppressive therapy. *Ophthalmology.* 2015;122(5):939–948.

94. Mugheddu C, Atzori L, Del Piano M, et al. Successful ustekinumab treatment of noninfectious uveitis and concomitant severe psoriatic arthritis and plaque psoriasis. *Dermatol Ther.* 2017;30(5).

95. Pepple KL, Lin P. Targeting interleukin-23 in the treatment of noninfectious uveitis. *Ophthalmology.* 2018;125(12):1977–1983.
96. Lasave AF, You C, Ma L, et al. Long-term outcomes of rituximab therapy in patients with noninfectious posterior uveitis refractory to conventional immunosuppressive therapy. *Retina.* 2018;38(2):395–402.
97. Davatchi F, Shams H, Rezaipoor M, et al. Rituximab in intractable ocular lesions of Behçet's disease; randomized single-blind control study (pilot study). *Int J Rheum Dis.* 2010;13(3):246–252.
98. Miserocchi E, Modorati G, Berchicci L, et al. Long-term treatment with rituximab in severe juvenile idiopathic arthritis-associated uveitis. *Br J Ophthalmol.* 2016;100(6):782–786.
99. Umran RMR, Shukur ZYH. Rituximab for sight-threatening refractory pediatric Vogt-Koyanagi-Harada disease. *Mod Rheumatol.* 2018;28(1):197–199.
100. Birolo C, Zannin ME, Arsenyeva S, et al. Comparable efficacy of abatacept used as first-line or second-line biological agent for severe juvenile idiopathic arthritis-related uveitis. *J Rheumatol.* 2016;43(11):2068–2073.
101. Tappeiner C, Miserocchi E, Bodaghi B, et al. Abatacept in the treatment of severe, long-standing, and refractory uveitis associated with juvenile idiopathic arthritis. *J Rheumatol.* 2015;42(4):706–711.
102. Zulian F, Balzarin M, Falcini F, et al. Abatacept for severe anti-tumor necrosis factor alpha refractory juvenile idiopathic arthritis-related uveitis. *Arthritis Care Res (Hoboken).* 2010;62(6):821–825.
103. Sobaci G, Erdem U, Durukan AH, et al. Safety and effectiveness of interferon alpha-2a in treatment of patients with Behçet's uveitis refractory to conventional treatments. *Ophthalmology.* 2010;117(7):1430–1435.
104. Kotter I, Zierhut M, Eckstein AK, et al. Human recombinant interferon alfa-2a for the treatment of Behçet's disease with sight threatening posterior or panuveitis. *Br J Ophthalmol.* 2003;87(4):423–431.
105. De Simone L, Sangiovanni A, Aldigeri R, et al. Interferon alpha-2a treatment for post-uveitic refractory macular edema. *Ocul Immunol Inflamm.* 2020;28(2):322–328.
106. Fardeau C, Simon A, Rodde B, et al. Interferon-alpha2a and systemic corticosteroid in monotherapy in chronic uveitis: results of the randomized controlled BIRDFERON study. *Am J Ophthalmol.* 2017;177:182–194.
107. Stiefel HC, Kopplin LJ, Albini T, et al. Treatment of refractory cystoid macular edema with pegylated interferon alfa-2A: a retrospective chart review. *Ocul Immunol Inflamm.* 2021;29(3):566–571.
108. Celiker H, Kazokoglu H, Direskeneli H. Long-term efficacy of pegylated interferon alpha-2b in Behçet's uveitis: a small case series. *Ocul Immunol Inflamm.* 2019;27(1):15–22.
109. Mackensen F, Jakob E, Springer C, et al. Interferon versus methotrexate in intermediate uveitis with macular edema: results of a randomized controlled clinical trial. *Am J Ophthalmol.* 2013;156(3):478–486.e471.
110. Jouve L, Benrabah R, Heron E, et al. Multiple sclerosis-related uveitis: does MS treatment affect uveitis course? *Ocul Immunol Inflamm.* 2017;25(3):302–307.
111. Miserocchi E, Giuffre C, Cornalba M, et al. JAK inhibitors in refractory juvenile idiopathic arthritis-associated uveitis. *Clin Rheumatol.* 2020;39(3):847–851.
112. Bauermann P, Heiligenhaus A, Heinz C. Effect of Janus Kinase inhibitor treatment on anterior uveitis and associated macular edema in an adult patient with juvenile idiopathic arthritis. *Ocul Immunol Inflamm.* 2019;27(8):1232–1234.
113. Ramanan AV, Guly CM, Keller SY, et al. Clinical effectiveness and safety of baricitinib for the treatment of juvenile idiopathic arthritis-associated uveitis or chronic anterior antinuclear antibody-positive uveitis: study protocol for an open-label, adalimumab active-controlled phase 3 clinical trial (JUVE-BRIGHT). *Trials.* 2021;22(1):689.
114. Multicenter Uveitis Steroid Treatment Trial Research Group WC, Acharya NR, Vitale AT, et al. Intravitreal therapy for uveitic macular edema-ranibizumab versus methotrexate versus the dexamethasone implant: the MERIT trial results. *Ophthalmology.* 2023;130(9):914–923.

Index

Note: Page numbers in *italics* indicate a figure and page numbers in **bold** indicate a table on the corresponding page.

For Product Safety Concerns and Information please contact our EU
representative GPSR@taylorandfrancis.com
Taylor & Francis Verlag GmbH, Kaufingerstraße 24, 80331 München, Germany

9 781032 592312